SPACE PHYSIOLOGY AND MEDICINE

Editor

ARNAULD E. NICOGOSSIAN, M.D.
Director, Life Sciences Division
National Aeronautics and Space Administration (NASA)
Washington, D.C.

Associate Editors

Carolyn Leach Huntoon, Ph.D.
Director, Space and Life Sciences Directorate,
NASA, Johnson Space Center, Houston, Texas

Sam L. Pool, M.D.
Chief, Medical Sciences Division, NASA,
Johnson Space Center, Houston, Texas

SPACE PHYSIOLOGY AND MEDICINE

second edition

 LEA & FEBIGER, Philadelphia • London 1989

Lea & Febiger
600 Washington Square
Philadelphia, PA   19106-4198
U.S.A.
(215) 922-1330

Lea & Febiger (UK) Ltd.
145a Croydon Road
Beckenham, Kent BR3 3RB
U.K.

Library of Congress Cataloging-in-Publication Data

Space physiology and medicine/editor, Arnauld E. Nicogossian;
   associate editors, Carolyn Leach Huntoon, Sam L. Pool.—2nd ed.
      p.   cm.
   Rev. ed. of: Space physiology and medicine/Arnauld E.
Nicogossian and James F. Parker, Jr. 1982.
   Includes bibliographies and index.
   ISBN 0-8121-1162-1
   1. Space flight—Physiological aspects.   2. Space medicine.
I. Nicogossian, Arnauld E.   II. Huntoon, Carolyn Leach.   III. Pool,
Sam L.
   [DNLM: 1. Extraterrestrial Environment.   2. Space Flight.   WD 750
S7325]
RC1150.S63 1989
616.9'80214—dc19
DNLM/DLC
for Library of Congress

88-13855
CIP

Printed in the United States of America
Print number: 3 2 1

Dedication

To our families,
who provided encouragement and support
during the preparation of this textbook.

Foreword

Over the past three decades the quest for knowledge concerning space flight—and its impact on human physiology—has sparked new and exciting discoveries in a spectrum of medical disciplines. These advances have enhanced our understanding of the nature and extent of human capabilities and physiological responses in the unique environment of microgravity, and have enabled us to proceed wisely toward planning near-term manned missions and bolder, long-range missions envisioned for the future.

The second edition of *Space Physiology and Medicine* chronicles the ongoing work of scientists attempting to describe and understand the responses of man and his life processes in the space environment. These changes are largely adaptive in nature; many are benign, others present specific biomedical challenges for physicians attending returning crewmembers. Throughout the brief history of manned space flight, investigative biomedical research and its attendant development activities have helped in the formulation of engineering and medical criteria for enhancing the safety and health of space crewmembers. Complementary efforts have been directed toward maintaining relative comfort and hygiene in the closed spacecraft environment and toward providing the basic necessities for living and working on what many consider the new frontier.

We must remember, however, that the search for answers that will enable more sophisticated missions of longer durations has just begun. The knowledge we gain through contemporary biomedical and biological investigations in space will guide the course of the bolder space missions we will undertake in the 21st century and beyond.

Frederick C. Robbins, M.D.
University Professor Emeritus
Dean Emeritus, School of Medicine
Case Western Reserve University
Cleveland, Ohio

Preface

Significant new knowledge has been acquired since the first edition of *Space Physiology and Medicine* appeared in September 1982. In preparing the second edition, it became obvious that all the findings could not be incorporated in the present volume. Some of the data were too preliminary to be published and would have resulted in speculations rather than in a presentation of definitive knowledge. The discipline of space medicine is still in its infancy, and more experimentation is required before a comprehensive picture of how living systems adapt to the space environment over prolonged periods of time can be established. Space remains a novel and only partially explored environment. Thus, the contributors to this book have made a significant effort to provide the reader with a global view of the biological issues and, at the same time, an in-depth review of the practical aspects of space medicine.

Some areas, such as radiation, performance, neurophysiology, nutrition, and human capabilities, have been significantly upgraded. Other chapters have been updated with new information obtained from the United States Space Shuttle short-duration missions and the U.S.S.R. long-duration orbital missions. The last six years have been a testimony of many firsts for the space program. A new group of individuals, payload specialists, have joined professional astronaut pilots and mission specialists to work in space. Man's endurance in space has approached a year, at least for two individuals. More women have flown in space than in the preceding 20 years. And space exploration has become a true international endeavor, with gradually more spacefaring nations entering the arena of manned space flight.

It is our hope that this manual will serve as a general reference text for the reader and stimulate further inquiry into the field of space medicine. We plan to revise this manual on a periodic basis to keep pace with the new knowledge, especially in the area of space and gravitational biology, as it becomes available.

The authors wish to express their special gratitude to Lea & Febiger for helping with the publication of this manual, and for the special assistance provided by Mr. Ronald Teeter in compiling and preparing the manuscripts.

Arnauld E. Nicogossian, M.D.

Acknowledgements

The editors gratefully acknowledge the generous assistance provided by the following:

NASA Headquarters Graphics Department, which provided numerous illustrations.

Pamela Ewart and **Natalie Karakulko,** KRUG International, Houston, Texas, for their efforts in word processing during the initial stages of this book.

Victoria Garshnek, George Washington University, and **Ron Teeter,** Lockheed, Washington, D.C., for their help and dedication during the preparation of the second edition of **Space Physiology and Medicine.**

Jon Lomberg, who provided the cover art for this book.

We are particularly indebted to **Kenneth Bussy,** Executive Editor, Lea & Febiger Publishing Company, for his valued counsel and guidance.

Contributors

NANCY G. ALDRICH
Section Manager
KRUG International
Houston, Texas

JAMES H. BREDT, Ph.D.
Manager, Biological Systems Research
National Aeronautics and Space Administration
Washington, D.C.

JERI W. BROWN
Section Head, Crew Interface Analysis
Man Systems Division
National Aeronautics and Space Administration
Johnson Space Center
Houston, Texas

MICHAEL W. BUNGO, M.D.
Director, Space Biomedical Research Institute
National Aeronautics and Space Administration
Johnson Space Center
Houston, Texas
Clinical Assistant Professor
University of Texas Health Sciences Center
Houston, Texas
University of Texas Medical Branch
Galveston, Texas

NITZA M. CINTRON, Ph.D.
Chief, Biomedical Laboratories Branch
National Aeronautics and Space Administration
Johnson Space Center
Houston, Texas

MARTIN E. COLEMAN, Ph.D.
Toxicologist, Biomedical Laboratories Branch
National Aeronautics and Space Administration
Johnson Space Center
Houston, Texas

JEFFREY R. DAVIS, M.D.
Chief, Medical Operations Branch
National Aeronautics and Space Administration
Johnson Space Center
Houston, Texas

LAWRENCE F. DIETLEIN, M.D., Ph.D
Assistant Director for Life Sciences
Johnson Space Center
Houston, Texas
   U.S. Public Health Service
Medical Director (Retired)

MICHAEL B. DUKE, Ph.D.
Chief, Solar System Exploration Division
National Aeronautics and Space Administration
Johnson Space Center
Houston, Texas

VICTORIA GARSHNEK, Ph.D.
Senior Research Scientist
Science Communication Studies
Division of Continuing Education
George Washington University
Washington, D.C.

JERRY L. HOMICK, Ph.D.
Deputy Chief, Medical Sciences Division
National Aeronautics and Space Administration
Johnson Space Center
Houston, Texas

DAVID J. HORRIGAN, JR.
Head, Environmental Physiology
Space Biomedical Research Institute
Johnson Space Center
Houston, Texas

CAROLYN LEACH HUNTOON, Ph.D.
Director, Space and Life Sciences Directorate
National Aeronautics and Space Administration
Johnson Space Center
Houston, Texas
Associate Professor (Adjunct)
University of Texas Health Sciences Center
Houston, Texas

PHILIP C. JOHNSON, JR., M.D.
Chief Scientist, Medical Sciences Division
National Aeronautics and Space Administration
Johnson Space Center
Houston, Texas

ADRIAN LeBLANC, Ph.D.
Senior Research Scientist
KRUG International
Houston, Texas

PERCIVAL D. McCORMACK, M.D., Ph.D.
Manager, Operational Medicine Program
National Aeronautics and Space Administration
Washington, D.C.
Lecturer, Department of Physiology and
Biophysics
Georgetown Medical School
Washington, D.C.

EDWARD C. MOSELEY, Ph.D.
Technical Assistant, Medical Sciences Division
National Aeronautics and Space Administration
Johnson Space Center
Houston, Texas

D. STUART NACHTWEY, Ph.D.
Chief Scientist, Medical Sciences Space Station
Office
Johnson Space Center
Houston, Texas

ARNAULD E. NICOGOSSIAN, M.D.
Director, Life Sciences Division
National Aeronautics and Space Administration
Washington, D.C.
Assistant Professor, Department of Biometrics
and Preventive Medicine
Uniformed Services University of Health Sciences
Washington, D.C.

DONALD E. PARKER, Ph.D.
Universities Space Research Association
Houston, Texas

JAMES F. PARKER, JR., Ph.D.
President
Biotechnology, Inc.
Annandale, Virginia

SAM L. POOL, M.D.
Chief, Medical Sciences Division
National Aeronautics and Space Administration
Johnson Space Center
Houston, Texas

PAUL C. RAMBAUT, Sc.D.
Deputy Director, Division of Extramural Activities
National Cancer Institute
National Institutes of Health
Bethesda, Maryland

MILLARD F. RESCHKE, Ph.D.
Senior Vestibular Scientist, Space Biomedical
Research Institute
National Aeronautics and Space Administration
Johnson Space Center
Houston, Texas

FREDERICK C. ROBBINS, M.D.
University Professor Emeritus
Dean Emeritus, School of Medicine
Case Western Reserve University
Cleveland, Ohio

RICHARD L. SAUER, Ph.D.
Senior Aerospace Engineer, Biomedical
    Laboratories Branch
National Aeronautics and Space Administration
Johnson Space Center
Houston, Texas

VICTOR S. SCHNEIDER, M.D.
U.S. Public Health Service
National Institutes of Health
National Aeronautics and Space Administration
Director, Bone and Mineral Laboratory
Johnson Space Center
Houston, Texas
Associate Professor of Medicine
University of Texas Health Sciences Center
Houston, Texas

JAMES M. VANDERPLOEG, M.D.
Managing Physician, Kelsey-Seybold Clear Lake
Houston, Texas

JAMES M. WALIGORA, Ph.D.
Deputy Director, Space Biomedical Research
    Institute
National Aeronautics and Space Administration
Johnson Space Center
Houston, Texas

Contents

section **IV**

PHYSIOLOGICAL ADAPTATION TO SPACE FLIGHT

section **V**

HEALTH MAINTENANCE OF SPACE CREWMEMBERS

section **VI**

MEDICAL PROBLEMS OF SPACE FLIGHT

MANNED SPACE FLIGHT

section I

1 Historical Perspectives

ARNAULD E. NICOGOSSIAN
VICTORIA GARSHNEK

The late nineteenth century marked the invention of the first relatively crude vehicle for powered flight; in 1989, the unmanned Voyager spacecraft will rendezvous with the planet Neptune, to eventually leave the solar system. Clearly, the evolution of space flight has been rapid and progressive: six planets—and a number of their satellites—have been remotely studied, Apollo astronauts have worked on the lunar surface, and the scientific community and lay public have expressed enthusiasm for the prospects of a lunar base and a manned mission to Mars.

The need to sustain life and productive human function in space flight has presented an array of unique challenges in the fields of medicine and physiology. Concurrent advances in space flight capabilities and mission sophistication have spurred numerous technological breakthroughs in the biomedical sciences. The symbiotic relationship between the space sciences and medical sciences will continue to further space exploration and benefit terrestrial medicine.

THE SUPPORT OF MAN IN SPACE

The foundations for space medicine can be traced back many years to early programs in the fields of occupational and aviation medicine. However, it was not until World War II, and the development of the V-2 rocket, that serious consideration was given to the possibility of manned space flight and, in turn, the need for specialized space medicine. Major General H.G. Armstrong foresaw this need and, in 1948, at the USAF School of Aviation Medicine, organized a panel meeting on the topic of "Aeromedical Problems of Space Travel" (von Beckh, 1979). Presentations were made by (then Colonel) Armstrong, Professor Hubertus Strughold (later to be regarded as the "father of space medicine"), and the astrophysicist, Dr. Heinz Haber. From an historical perspective, this meeting may be regarded as the beginning point of a new and specialized practice within the field of medicine. Space medicine later emerged as an accepted and growing specialty within the broad domain of occupational medicine.

Subsequently, there was a rapid growth of interest on the parts of biomedical scientists in programs which might lead to manned space flight. By 1950, the United States had launched two primates into space on board V-2 rockets. While neither animal survived, useful information was obtained concerning the hazards of space flight for mammalian life forms. These early flights demonstrated the need for reliable life support systems, and began to define the parameters for protection against the rigors and stresses of weightlessness and reentry into gravity.

Scientists soon recognized the need for an organization to coordinate and exchange information concerning space medicine research. In 1950, during the 21st Annual Meeting of the Aeromedical Association, the Space Medicine Branch was formed. The committee which petitioned the Association for admission consisted of Drs. A.C. Ivy, J.P. Marbarger, R.J. Benford, P.A. Campbell, and A. Graybiel. In 1951, the petition was accepted, and space medicine was accorded formal recognition within the broader medical community.

The Schools of Aviation Medicine of both the Navy and the Air Force, as well as a number of laboratories in the armed services, soon undertook projects dealing with man in space. Topics such as life support, acceleration tolerance, and reactions to confinement—all of which had been studied in the aviation context—were investigated as a function of the environmental parameters it was believed man would face when he traveled into space. These early investigations generated a considerable knowledge base, which would prove quite useful in later space medicine activities.

Many early practitioners of space medicine were trained in the aviation medicine programs of the Navy and the Air Force. Beginning in the 1950s, these two organizations expanded their curricula to include additional topics of specific interest to space medicine. The new directions were reflected by new organizational designations. The Air Force facility became the School of Aerospace Medicine, while the Navy school became the Naval Aerospace Medical Institute. The schools of public health of Johns Hopkins, Harvard, and Ohio State Universities, which cooperated with the military facilities in providing required residency training, also reflected the changing orientation in their curricula.

Interest in the possibility of orbital space flight continued to grow in both the United States and the Soviet Union during the mid-1950's. On 4 October 1957, the Soviet Union successfully launched the Sputnik 1 satellite into Earth orbit. Public interest in U.S. space efforts surged after the flight of Sputnik 1, and the two nations became engaged in a "space race" which allowed little time for leisurely planning and development. The sense of urgency that permeated American space planning after 1957 had considerable implications for space medicine.

As the possibility of manned space flight drew closer to realization, biomedical scientists became more interested in the biological and medical aspects of human exposure to the space environment. Within this group, however, there was some controversy over the ability of the human organism to sustain useful function in space and, especially, to withstand the stresses of launch and reentry. The National Academy of Sciences—National Research Council Committee on Bioastronautics, meeting in 1958, identified a number of potential problems for astronauts, including such effects on human physiology as anorexia, nausea, inability to swallow, disorientation, and other effects which would be of real consequence for the conduct of manned space flight. A more comprehensive listing of these issues is provided in Table 1-1 (Dietlein, 1977). Some of these predictions were later confirmed; others were not.

The hectic pace of space activities during the late 1950's left little time for a step-by-step program to develop a medical basis for manned space flight. Issues of life support, safety, and health had to be addressed on an a priori basis, building principally on the tenets of established science of aviation medicine. The first space suits, for example, were a direct outgrowth of the Navy full-pressure suit used on high altitude aircraft. The rapid pace also meant that new knowledge was generated more from mission results than from research conducted in laboratories and ground-based simulations: the realities of space missions dictated progress in space medicine.

The following sections consider the manned space programs conducted by the United States and the Soviet Union and review key biomedical problems and findings. A summary presented at the end of this chapter lists all manned space missions and extravehicular activities conducted by these two nations to date.

THE AMERICAN PROGRAM

PROJECT MERCURY

The National Aeronautics and Space Administration (NASA), formed in 1958, was charged by the President of the United States with a twofold mission in manned space flight. The mission was given high national priority, second only to national defense. NASA was, at the earliest feasible time, to launch a man into space, provide him with an environment in which he could perform effectively, and recover him safely. These goals were soon realized on Project Mercury. At the same time, NASA, with the support of leading life scientists, was to develop a capability for extended manned space flight (Lovelace, 1965).

The mission given to NASA was accomplished with remarkable success (Figure 1-1). The original goal of orbiting a man in

---

TABLE 1-1

PREDICTED EFFECTS OF WEIGHTLESSNESS

Anorexia	Demineralization of bones
Nausea	Renal calculi
Disorientation	Motion sickness
Sleepiness	Pulmonary atelectasis
Sleeplessness	Tachycardia
Fatigue	Hypertension
Restlessness	Hypotension
Euphoria	Cardiac arrhythmias
Hallucinations	Postflight syncope
Decreased G tolerance	Decreased exercise capacity
Gastrointestinal disturbance	Reduced blood volume
Urinary retention	Reduced plasma volume
Diuresis	Dehydration
Muscular incoordination	Weight loss
Muscle atrophy	Infectious illnesses

Dietlein, 1977.

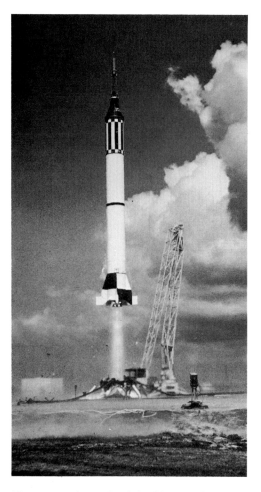

Figure 1-1. Launch of the Mercury-Redstone 3 carrying Alan Shepard, America's first man in space.

space and returning him safely to Earth was accomplished in just 3 years of program effort (Kleinknecht, 1963).

During preparation for the first manned Mercury launch, many problems were faced by biomedical scientists. One of the first was to establish criteria according to which a corps of astronauts could be formed. As this problem was being addressed, President Eisenhower directed that all astronaut candidates be recruited from the ranks of military test pilots. An important factor was the demonstrated capability of this group to meet threatening

situations in the air with accurate judgment, quick decisions, and refined motor skills. There were 100 test pilots among the applicants who fully met all requirements (Link, 1965). These individuals were given interviews, psychiatric examinations, and a complete medical evaluation, including medical stress tests. The purposes of the protracted and extensive medical evaluation were to discover any hidden medical problems, establish the physical fitness level, and, of considerable importance, compile a medical data base for each individual against which any changes brought about by later space missions might be measured and quantified. Selection criteria were taken almost directly from those used in military aviation; the challenge remained for physicians and biomedical personnel to identify those medical parameters that would be most useful in assessing man's adjustment to space.

Project Mercury required a life support system which would operate without failure under the conditions of orbital space flight. The technology to develop such a system was already established, as demonstrated in the successful balloon flight of Air Force flight surgeon David R. Simons in 1957, which attained a record altitude of 30,942 meters and lasted for 32 hours. Translating this technology into a space system, however, was a difficult undertaking for engineers and biomedical scientists. The human requirements for protection, proper breathing atmosphere, maintenance of pressure, provision of food and water, removal of metabolic by-products, and thermal control had to be considered in light of severe constraints on reliability, size, weight, power, and operation under conditions of thermal extremes, acceleration, and weightlessness. The system as finally designed functioned flawlessly.

Project Mercury, designed specifically to prove man's ability to survive in the space environment, lasted from May 1961 to May 1963. Two suborbital and four orbital missions were undertaken, including one which lasted for 34 hours and completed 22 orbits of the Earth.

The six Mercury astronauts returned in satisfactory health condition. These flights were as valuable for the many medical concerns which were dispelled as for those which were verified. The principal findings were weight loss due primarily to dehydration, and some impairment of cardiovascular function. Cardiovascular data from the final and longest Mercury flight showed orthostatic intolerance and dizziness on standing, as well as hemoconcentration (Dietlein, 1977). From the behavioral point of view, it was found that astronauts could perform well under conditions of weightlessness.

PROJECT GEMINI

Planning for Project Gemini began in May 1961, just after successful completion of the first suborbital Mercury mission. Design of the two-man Gemini capsule, built upon experience gained from Project Mercury, allowed for new capabilities such as extravehicular activity and the study of the limits of astronaut endurance in order to support more sophisticated future activities. A comprehensive Gemini objective was to conduct the development and testing necessary to: (1) demonstrate the feasibility of long-duration space flight for at least that period required to complete a lunar landing mission; (2) perfect the techniques and procedures for orbital rendezvous and docking of two spacecraft; (3) achieve precisely controlled reentry and landing capability; (4) establish capability in extravehicular activity; and (5) enhance the less obvious, but no less significant, flight and ground crew proficiency (Mueller, 1967).

Project Gemini successfully completed ten manned space missions, encompassing many notable accomplishments. The first U.S. extravehicular activity was performed in the Gemini 4 mission (Figure 1-2). The first rendezvous and docking maneuver was completed by Gemini 8 crewmembers. Of particular interest to medical scientists are the Gemini 4, 5, and 7 missions, lasting for 4, 8, and 14 days, respectively. A number of inflight experiments were conducted on these missions, as well as preflight and postflight studies.

A major concern in the Gemini medical investigations was the evaluation of the changes in cardiovascular function noted in Mercury. Cardiovascular changes seen in Gemini crewmembers were regarded as an adaptive response due to intravascular fluid losses resulting from exposure to the weightlessness of space flight. The key question was whether the observed cardiovascular deconditioning was a self-limiting adjustment.

Project Gemini reinforced the medical conclusion that humans can live and work in space, certainly for the time required for the forthcoming Apollo missions. A number of new changes such as bone mineral loss were noted, as shown in Table 1-2, but none were considered of real consequence for mission durations on the order of 2 weeks.

Gemini, though providing answers to some medical questions, left other issues unresolved. The program's biomedical findings served to structure and guide experiments designed for later missions of longer duration. Such experiments would be needed to determine the physiological basis and time course of the observed changes.

PROJECT APOLLO

The goal of the Apollo Program was singular and straightforward—to land a man on the moon and return him safely to Earth. President John F. Kennedy directed,

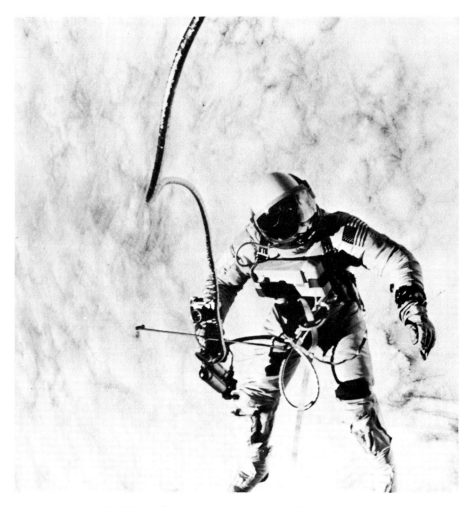

Figure 1-2. Astronaut Ed White (Gemini 4) carries out the first American extravehicular activity.

in 1961, that this goal be achieved "before this decade is out." A lunar landing was in fact achieved in 1969, with the Apollo 11 mission. The program included 29 astronauts, 12 of whom spent time on the lunar surface (Figure 1-3). The Apollo landings are among man's greatest achievements in science, engineering, and exploration.

The Apollo Program was supported by a broad biomedical effort, with three distinct goals (Johnston, 1975):

1. **Ensure the Safety and Health of Crewmembers.** The Apollo flights highlighted health issues which had not been addressed earlier. Foremost among these was the potential for inflight illness. During orbital flight it was possible to recover an astronaut within a reasonable time in the event of an inflight emergency. For a lunar mission, this is impossible, because the trajectory of the flight requires circumnavigation of the moon. Therefore, it was necessary to develop a program to minimize the likelihood of inflight illness, and allow a reasonable measure of emergency treatment should an illness occur.

TABLE 1-2

SIGNIFICANT BIOMEDICAL FINDINGS IN THE GEMINI PROGRAM

Loss of red cell mass (ranging 5–20% from baseline)

Postflight orthostatic intolerance in 100% of crews

Loss of exercise capacity compared with preflight baseline

Loss of os calcis bone density (7% from baseline)

Sustained loss of bone calcium and muscle nitrogen

Higher than predicted metabolic cost of extravehicular activity

2. **Prevent Contamination of Earth by Extraterrestrial Organisms.** The lunar landing raised for the first time the possibility of contamination of the moon by terrestrial microorganisms or, even more intriguing, the possibility of unknown microorganisms being introduced to Earth from lunar samples or exposed crewmembers. In order to ensure that unwanted microorganisms were not transported in either direction, strict quarantine and decontamination procedures were implemented before and after each mission. A special Lunar

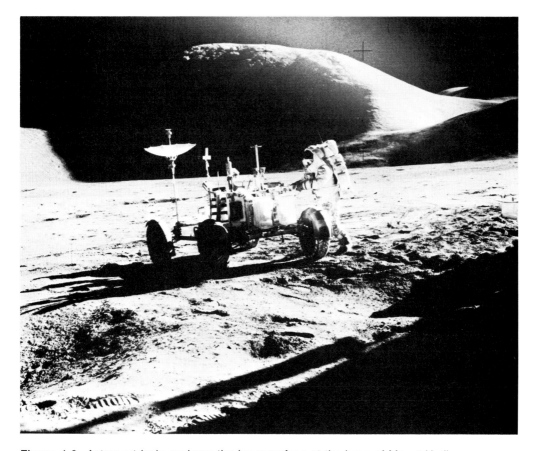

Figure 1-3. Astronaut Irwin explores the lunar surface at the base of Mount Hadley.

Receiving Laboratory was constructed at the NASA L.B. Johnson Space Center to house astronauts and lunar samples for appropriate observation and research.

3. **Study Specific Effects of Exposure to Space.** A number of physiological changes, such as cardiovascular deconditioning and bone demineralization, were identified during the Gemini Program. The longer-duration Apollo flights provided an opportunity to study these problems more closely and develop improved measurement techniques for assessing change. Although the operational complexity and rigorous demands of the Apollo Program limited the time available for biomedical experiments, the studies conducted provided a considerable amount of information. Predominant were cardiovascular, metabolic balance, and microbial load studies. In addition, limited biological experiments were conducted, including an investigation of radiation effects on the pocket mouse, and a study of the effects of heavy nuclei of galactic cosmic radiation on a number of biological systems.

Biomedical observations on Apollo added vestibular disturbances to the inventory of significant biomedical findings incident to space flight (Dietlein, 1977). No U.S. astronaut had reported motion sickness symptoms prior to the Apollo flights, although Soviet cosmonauts reported manifestations of vestibular dysfunction in flight as early as 1961 (Titov on Vostok 2). In Apollo, this problem was labeled "space motion sickness." In the Apollo 8 and 9 flights, five of the six crewmembers suffered some degree of motion sickness, ranging from stomach awareness to actual sickness. In one case, the severity of the vestibular disturbance required postponement of portions of the flight plan.

Other significant biomedical findings from the Apollo Program confirmed Gem-ini results and helped to characterize these responses in further detail (Table 1-3). Of special interest was the absence of microorganisms in the materials returned from the lunar surface.

PROJECT SKYLAB

The Skylab Program offered the first opportunity to study problems of habitability and physiological adaptation in space over an extended period of time. Comprised of a number of components, Skylab was more than simply a space vehicle; it was a space habitat and inflight laboratory. The Orbital Workshop provided the primary on-orbit living and working quarters for crewmembers. Built from the structure of an S-IVB stage, the third stage of the Saturn V booster rocket, the workshop was equipped to house three astronauts for up to 3 months. Cylindrical in shape, the workshop was 6.7 meters in diameter and 14.6 meters long: huge (approximately 294 m^3) in comparison with the cabin volume of earlier Mercury, Gemini, and Apollo spacecraft (approximately 1-8 m^3). The additional room allowed astronauts to enjoy a lifestyle somewhat closer to Earth standards, with a radical improvement in freedom of movement.

TABLE 1-3

SIGNIFICANT BIOMEDICAL FINDINGS IN THE APOLLO PROGRAM (PRE- VS. POSTFLIGHT)

Vestibular disturbances
Less than optimal food consumption (1260–2903 kcal / day)
Postflight dehydration and weight loss (recovery within 1 week)
Decreased postflight orthostatic tolerance (tilt / LBNP* tests)
Reduced postflight exercise tolerance (first 3 days)
Apollo 15 cardiac arrhythmias (frequent bigemini)
Decreased red cell mass (2–10%) and plasma volume (4–9%)

* Lower body negative pressure.

A second feature of importance in Skylab was the duration of the missions. Skylabs 2, 3, and 4 lasted for 28, 59, and 84 days, respectively. This allowed the physiological changes seen in astronauts during earlier space programs to be studied in greater detail: it was possible to establish the time course of physiological adaptation to the weightless environment of space.

Skylab once again demonstrated the value of the human crewmember in space systems. Without direct human intervention, the Skylab vehicle would have been uninhabitable because of a thermal problem caused by the loss of the micrometeoroid shield and failure of the solar array wing to deploy properly (Belew, 1977). After rendezvous and survey of the damage, the Skylab Commander and Scientist Pilot spent nearly 4 hours in EVA, attempting one of the most difficult and hazardous of all orbital repair jobs (Figure 1-4). The extent of the damage was unknown, the outcome was uncertain, and there were no special provisions to facilitate EVA. Guided by ground personnel, the Skylab team successfully released the solar wing and rectified the problem to the extent possible. The Scientist Pilot, incidentally, was Dr. Joseph P. Kerwin, the first physician to fly as part of an American space crew (Figure 1-5).

Skylab demonstrated that, with suffi-cient attention to such issues as food service, waste management, and sleep arrangements, a spacecraft can provide satisfactory living and working quarters for long periods of time. The expanded area of the Skylab Orbital Workshop provided an opportunity to investigate a number of spacecraft habitability issues. By previous standards, only minor problems were experienced. For example, sleeping compartments were not sufficiently isolated from each other and from the waste management compartment for optimum noise control. It also was learned that, in the zero-gravity environment, mobility and restraint systems are major factors in perceived habitability.

Skylab crewmen were monitored closely for signs of space motion sickness (Graybiel, 1981). In the first mission, none of the astronauts became motion sick, although one crewmember did take medication immediately after entry into orbit. During the intense extravehicular activity required of this crew to repair Skylab damage before they could enter the Orbital Workshop, no decrements in performance were noted.

The second Skylab crew, however, experienced severe motion sickness symptoms. These crewmembers did not take medication prophylactically and entered the workshop on the first day of orbit,

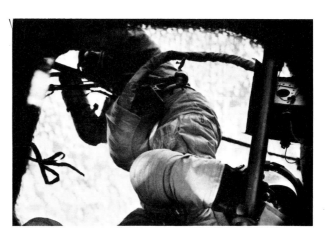

Figure 1-4. Skylab 2 crewmembers Charles Conrad and Dr. Joseph Kerwin repairing the Orbital Workshop's damaged solar array system.

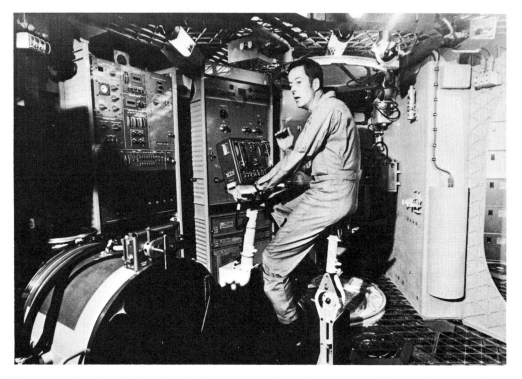

Figure 1-5. Dr. Joseph Kerwin, scientist-pilot on Skylab 2, checks out the bicycle ergometer.

immediately undertaking a full work schedule. In one case, motion sickness appeared within an hour after insertion into orbit, while the crewmember was removing his space suit. This is the earliest appearance on record of motion sickness in orbital flight (Graybiel, 1981).

The third Skylab crew took a number of special precautions, including flying aerobatic maneuvers on the day prior to the mission and following a planned schedule for anti-motion sickness medication during the early days of the mission. Two crewmembers experienced motion sickness, with symptoms for one astronaut persisting well into the fourth day of flight.

Based on subjective reports of the three Skylab crews and vestibular experiments conducted during flight, it was concluded that space motion sickness cannot be predicted by the usual ground-based tests, and can be alleviated somewhat by the prophylactic administration of medications. However, it has remained a problem through the Space Shuttle era. The search for the optimum medication and schedule of administration continues.

Particular attention was given in Skylab to cardiovascular deconditioning, since earlier space missions showed a consistent change in cardiovascular function under space flight conditions. The parameters most closely observed were orthostatic tolerance, electrical activity, and changes in heart size. During Skylab, the response of astronauts to orthostatic stress was examined for the first time in flight. Crewmen were tested using a lower body negative pressure device before, during, and after all Skylab missions. This device imposes orthostatic stress for a period of 5 minutes, through the application of a negative 50 mmHg pressure. Again, the customary indices of a reduction in cardiovascular efficiency were obtained.

However, the observed cardiovascular deconditioning was found to stabilize after a period of 4 to 6 weeks, with no apparent impairment of crew health or performance (Dietlein, 1977). The change appears to be a self-limiting adaptation to the reduced cardiovascular load imposed by weightlessness.

Other topics of concern in Skylab were bone mineral loss and mineral balance. Again, preflight measurements of bone mineral content, using a photon absorptiometric technique, were compared with similar measurements taken at varying intervals postflight. No mineral losses were observed in the upper extremities, but some bone loss was noted in the lower extremities, specifically the os calcis (Smith et al., 1977). Data from the 84-day Skylab 4 mission led to the conclusion that the mineral losses incurred are comparable to those observed in bed rest studies (Dietlein, 1977). No evidence was found during these missions that the loss of bone mineral is self-limiting.

Skylab metabolic studies showed a significant increase in the excretion of urinary calcium during flight for all crewmen measured. The loss continued throughout the period of flight, with no evidence of abatement during later stages. Significant losses of nitrogen and phosphorus also occurred, presumably associated mainly with muscle tissue loss (Whedon et al., 1977). Other evidence of muscle loss was obtained from stereometric analyses of body form in Skylab crewmembers. These analyses showed marked loss in leg volume, much of it restored within 4 days following mission completion. About one-third of the loss was attributed to partial atrophy of the leg muscles due to disuse in zero gravity, with the remainder due to a body fluid deficit (Whittle et al., 1977).

Skylab provided a wealth of biomedical data concerning the health and physiological responses of humans performing normal work activities during long-term space missions. Skylab data were particularly useful in differentiating those physiological changes which appear to be self-limiting from those which seem to continue throughout the period of exposure to weightlessness. This information provided guidance both for subsequent ground-based research and inflight studies seeking to characterize and understand human responses to the stresses of space.

THE APOLLO-SOYUZ TEST PROJECT

The Apollo-Soyuz Test Project (ASTP) was conducted jointly by the United States and the Soviet Union as a means of promoting international cooperation in space ventures. The primary mission objective was to test rendezvous and docking systems that might be needed during international space rescue missions. This required a proven ability to transfer crews between two spacecraft with dissimilar atmospheres. A second objective was to conduct a program of scientific experiments and technology applications. Both the Apollo and Soyuz spacecraft used in ASTP were identical to those flown previously (Figure 1-6). A docking module for crew transfer was constructed specially for the mission.

The ASTP lasted for 9 days, and the rendezvous and docking maneuver was successfully completed. The two spacecraft remained docked for 2 days, while the crews exchanged visits. During the recovery phase, the U.S. crew was exposed to toxic gases, mostly nitrogen tetroxide, from inadvertent firing of the reaction control system during descent. Toxic gases entered the command module through a cabin pressure relief valve opened during the landing sequence. All crewmembers developed chemical pneumonitis as a result of exposure to nitrogen tetroxide and required intensive therapy and hospitalization at the Tripler Army Medical Center, Honolulu, Hawaii (Nicogossian et al., 1977). Because of this exposure and the

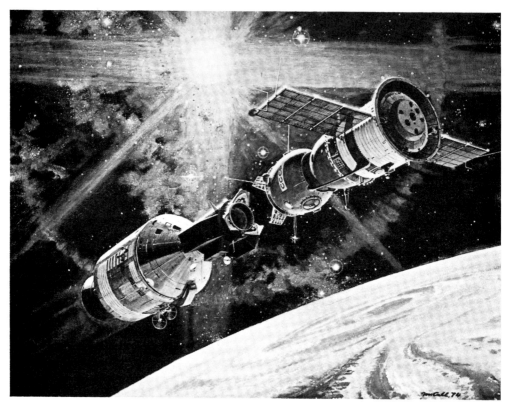

Figure 1-6. The joint U.S./U.S.S.R. Apollo-Soyuz Test Project. The Apollo capsule (left) is shown docked with the Soyuz vehicle (right).

altered postflight health condition, it was necessary to drop most of the planned postflight medical experiments and focus on clinical examination and treatment of the astronauts. Even so, considerable information was obtained concerning the human reaction to space flight conditions.

Electromyographic analyses of skeletal muscle function in leg extensor and arm flexor muscles showed that the muscle dysfunction characteristics found after 59 days of exposure to weightlessness in the Skylab 3 mission were also present after only 9 days of exposure (LaFevers et al., 1977). It was also shown that short-term exposure results in greater fatigue in muscle tissue, particularly in anti-gravity muscles.

Generalized hyperreflexia was reported following Skylab flights. Measurements

were made of the Achilles tendon reflex duration during ASTP (Burchard and Nicogossian, 1977). The reflex was measured within 2 hours after recovery and compared with preflight measurements. As in Skylab, two crewmembers showed a decrease in the reflex duration. In addition, all three crewmembers showed significant fine tremor, which it was felt might reflect the effects of inhalation of nitrogen tetroxide vapor.

SPACE TRANSPORTATION SYSTEM

The first successful orbital flight of the Space Shuttle on April 12, 1981, initiated a new era in manned space activities (Figure 1-7). The Space Shuttle is the principal component of the Space Transportation

System (STS), and the world's first reusable spacecraft.

The Space Shuttle vehicle consists of four components: a reusable orbiter mounted on an expendable, liquid propellant tank, externally mounted; and two reusable solid rocket boosters. The Shuttle is launched in the conventional manner, and, on orbit, operates as a spacecraft. Upon reentry into the atmosphere, the orbiter sails like a glider to the designated landing site. Crewmembers experience a maximum gravity load of 3-g during launch, and less than 2-g during reentry: about one-third the acceleration levels experienced on previous manned flights. Many other features of the Space Shuttle, such as a standard sea level atmosphere, make space flight more comfortable for the astronauts.

The capability of the Shuttle to support crew-managed and free flyer research in low-Earth orbit signals new possibilities for science in space. For the first time, experiments can routinely be conducted on orbit, to further explore the effects of the space environment (e.g., microgravity and radiation) on human physiology under a controlled set of conditions that cannot be duplicated in laboratories on Earth. Changes in vestibular and cardiovascular function, hematological indices, the impact of space radiation, along with the effects of gravity on basic biological processes, are issues that are studied through complementary ground-based and flight research. Flight experiments have expanded our understanding of operant basic mechanisms, and will establish the time course of biological and biomedical changes during exposure to microgravity.

Through continuous inflight observation of space crews and testing and refining of countermeasures, requirements are established for human safety, health, and productivity in space. Assurance of astronaut health and productivity in turn provides sound foundations for a broader segment of the population to participate in space missions. The long-term clinical significance of risk factors possibly associated with repeated exposure to the space environment is consistently monitored and studied after flight.

Physiological changes observed on Shuttle missions have been similar to those observed in the Apollo and Skylab Programs. Cephalad fluid shifts have invariably occurred. Accelerated heart rates on launch and reentry were similar in magnitude to those recorded in previous flights. Space motion sickness was observed in approximately 50 percent of crewmembers flown. Orthostatic intolerance was exhibited by those crewmembers who were not subjected to countermeasures. Hormonal, electrolyte, and immunological changes specific to space flight were again observed upon return to Earth. Manifestation of immediate postflight responses ranged from a few hours to several days postflight, and most parameters returned to preflight baseline by the third to fifth day postflight. No significant residual physiological decrements have been detected postflight.

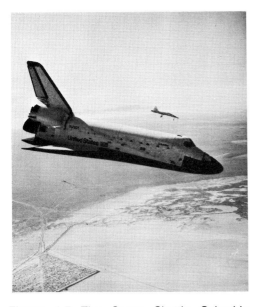

Figure 1-7. The Space Shuttle Columbia glides toward landing.

Some processes, such as the vestibular reactions, are displayed immediately, but then readjust to a new zero-gravity norm. Other responses, such as fluid and electrolyte loss, cardiovascular deconditioning, and loss of red blood cell mass adjust slowly to new zero-gravity states, while bone mineral and muscle mass loss continues with time.

A key feature of the Shuttle is the pressurized Spacelab module, a manned space laboratory in which scientists, engineers, and technicians can conduct experiments in Earth orbit. The Spacelab concept proceeded from the idea of equipping the orbiter's cargo bay with a laboratory facility where the crew could operate instruments and perform experiments in a shirtsleeve environment. Provided by the European Space Agency (ESA), Spacelab consists of a pressurized, cylindrical laboratory with an external equipment pallet. The result is a highly flexible carrier system that can be used in combinations tailored to the requirements of each mission (Figure 1-8). The Spacelab module houses most life sciences experiments, although some experiments are carried in the middeck as well.

Life Sciences missions fall into three general categories. The first is the fully dedicated mission, where the payload specialists are life scientists. While Spacelabs 1, 2, 3, and D-1 demonstrated Spacelab's capability to support multidisciplinary research, it is recognized that emphasis on single discipline missions can enhance research capability and scientific yield. The second category consists of missions with shared payloads, where various scientific disciplines are represented by onboard ex-

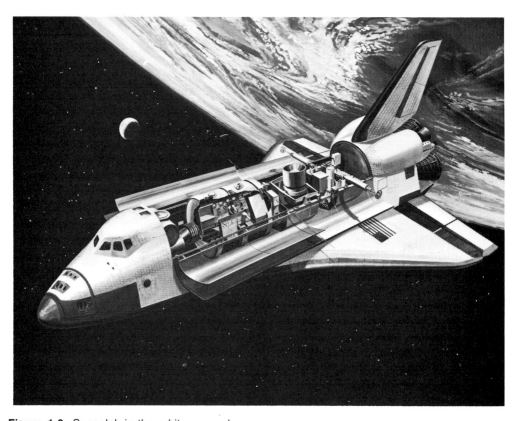

Figure 1-8. Spacelab in the orbiter cargo bay.

periments. The third category consists of small payloads that can be loaded into Spacelab or the orbiter middeck before launch, with minimal interfaces with the vehicle.

Functioning as an orbiting research laboratory, especially when carrying the Spacelab, the Space Shuttle has led to a more sophisticated scientific approach to the study of physiological adaptation and testing of countermeasures, with more experiments planned. The Space Shuttle and Spacelab are of great importance, both for the practice of space medicine and the conduct of life sciences research. Results of various completed studies are described in greater detail in the chapters ahead.

The Space Shuttle truly opened a new area in the space exploration and utilization programs. Many firsts were accomplished during the initial 5 years of the Space Shuttle Program. Multiple satellites were launched. Others were repaired on orbit and their service was extended beyond their projected lifetimes. Ailing satellites were retrieved and brought back to Earth for repair and subsequent launch. Multiple extravehicular activities were conducted on the same missions, each lasting up to 6 hours. Largest complements of crewmembers were accommodated on single missions. Eight women crewmembers performed complex on-orbit payload operations and deployments and conducted extravehicular activities. International crewmembers from many nations participated in Space Shuttle activities (Table 1-4). Scientists from universities and industry participated for the first time in investigations in space. Finally, the Space Shuttle was the first space vehicle to be launched from and landed at the same spaceport. The amount of scientific data obtained as a result of the Space Shuttle missions surpassed anything that any nation had accomplished in the past.

After 24 successful Space Shuttle flights, on January 28, 1986, the Space Shuttle Challenger was destroyed at liftoff by the explosion of a malfunctioning rocket booster, taking the lives of all seven crewmembers on board. This tragedy resulted in a hiatus of nearly 3 years in the U.S. manned space program, with a total redesign of many components of the launch vehicles and provision of an escape system for the crews. On September 29, 1988, the space shuttle Discovery was launched carrying five crewmembers and a communications satellite. During a 5-day flight, biomedical and material sciences experiments were conducted. Early in December, the 27th mission was carried out by the space shuttle Atlantis. Individual accomplishments of the U.S. and U.S.S.R., as well as other nations, are presented by mission in Table 1-5. Extravehicular activities are presented in Table 1-6.

TABLE 1-4

INTERNATIONAL ASTRONAUTS FLOWN ON THE U.S. SPACE SHUTTLE

Launch Date	Astronaut	Affiliation / Country	Mission
11-28-83	Ulf Merbold	ESA	STS-9
10- 5-84	Marc D. Garneau	Canada	41-G
6-17-85	Patrick Baudry	France	51-G
6-17-85	Prince Sultan Al-Saud	Saudi Arabia	51-G
10-30-85	Ernst Messerschmid	DFVLR	61-A
10-30-85	Reinhard Furrer	DFVLR	61-A
10-30-85	Wubbo Ockels	ESA	61-A
11-26-85	Rudolpho Neri-Vela	Mexico	61-B

TABLE 1-5

SUMMARY OF U.S. AND U.S.S.R. MANNED SPACE FLIGHT EXPERIENCE

Launch Date	Astronaut(s)/ Cosmonaut(s)	Mission	Length of Flight	Points of Biomedical Interest
12 April 1961	Gagarin	Vostok 1	1 hr 48 min	First manned orbital flight.
5 May 1961	Shepard	Mercury MR-3	15 min	Suborbital flight.
21 July 1961	Grissom	Mercury MR-4	16 min	No significant physiological problems noted.
6 August 1961	G. Titov	Vostok 2	25 hr 18 min	First reports of motion sickness, relieved by restriction of head and body movements.
20 February 1962	Glenn	Mercury MA-6	4 hr 55 min	First U.S. manned orbital flight.
24 May 1962	Carpenter	Mercury MA-7	4 hr 56 min	No significant physiological effects noted.
11 August 1962	Nikolayev	Vostok 3	94 hr 22 min	First dual mission.
12 August 1962	Popovich	Vostok 4	70 hr 57 min	Objective to study human capabilities to function as an operator in space.
3 October 1962	Schirra	Mercury MA-8	9 hr 13 min	First episode of orthostatic intolerance noted postflight.
15 May 1963	Cooper	Mercury MA-9	34 hr 20 min	
14 June 1963	Bykovskiy	Vostok 5	119 hr 6 min	
16 June 1963	Tereshkova	Vostok 6	70 hr 50 min	First flight of a woman in space. Labile cardiovascular responses inflight.
12 October 1964	Komarov Feoktistov Yegorov	Voskhod 1	24 hr 17 min	Crew operated in "shirtsleeve" environment. First medical examination in space by a physician (Yegorov). Better characterization of vestibular dysfunction.
18 March 1965	Belyayev Leonov	Voskhod 2	26 hr 2 min	First U.S.S.R. extravehicular activity (EVA). Neurovestibular function studies performed.
23 March 1965	Grissom Young	Gemini GT-3	4 hr 53 min	Cardiopulmonary monitoring inflight utilizing ECG, blood pressure, respiration rate measurements.

Date	Crew	Mission	Duration	Remarks
3 June 1965	McDivitt, White	Gemini GT-4	97 hr 48 min	First U.S. extravehicular activity (EVA). Overheating inside the EVA suit.
21 August 1965	Cooper, Conrad	Gemini GT-5	190 hr 59 min	Comprehensive medical evaluations.
4 December 1965	Borman, Lovell	Gemini GT-7	13 days 18 hr 35 min	
15 December 1965	Schirra, Stafford	Gemini GT-6	25 hr 51 min	First U.S. rendezvous flight.
16 March 1966	Armstrong, Scott	Gemini GT-8	10 hr 42 min	First docking in space with a target satellite.
3 June 1966	Stafford, Cernan	Gemini GT-9	72 hr 22 min	Two hour, seven minute walk in space performed. EVA suit visor fogging.
18 July 1966	Young, Collins	Gemini GT-10	70 hr 46 min	EVA performed without heat or work rate problems.
12 September 1966	Conrad, Gordon	Gemini GT-11	71 hr 17 min	High and exhausting work loads during EVA due to suit life support design.
11 November 1966	Lovell, Aldrin	Gemini GT-12	94 hr 34 min	Extravehicular activity included astronauts working with tools. No biomedical problems encountered during EVA.
23 April 1967	Komarov	Soyuz 1	27 hr	Reentry braking system failed. Vehicle destroyed, resulting in death of cosmonaut.
11 October 1968	Cunningham, Schirra, Eisele	Apollo 7	260 hr 9 min	Crew experienced symptoms of upper respiratory viral infection inflight.
26 October 1968	Beregovoy	Soyuz 3	94 hr 51 min	First Soviet attempt to manually dock in space with an unmanned target, Soyuz 2. Consistently high heart rates during flight.
21 December 1968	Borman, Lovell, Anders	Apollo 8	147 hr	First circumnavigation of the moon. First U.S. report of symptoms of motion sickness. Two-week preflight crew health stabilization program (HSP) instituted.
14 January 1969	Shatalov	Soyuz 4	71 hr 14 min	
15 January 1969	Volynov, Khrunov, Yeliseyev	Soyuz 5	72 hr 46 min	Spacecraft docked for approximately four hours. Two cosmonauts transferred to Soyuz 4 utilizing EVA procedures.

TABLE 1-5 (Continued)

SUMMARY OF U.S. AND U.S.S.R. MANNED SPACE FLIGHT EXPERIENCE

Launch Date	Mission	Astronaut(s) / Cosmonaut(s)	Length of Flight	Points of Biomedical Interest
3 March 1969	Apollo 9	McDivitt Scott Schweickart	241 hr 1 min	Launch postponed for three days because of viral infection. Flight plans for EVA revised because of symptoms of motion sickness.
18 May 1969	Apollo 10	Stafford Cernan Young	192 hr 3 min	Fiberglass insulation produced skin, eyes, and upper respiratory passages irritation. No impact on mission functions.
16 July 1969	Apollo 11	Armstrong Aldrin Collins	195 hr 18 min	The first walk on the moon. Occurrence of bends reported by one crewman. Lunar quarantine instituted postflight. Three weeks of HSP initiated for this and subsequent missions.
11 October 1969	Soyuz 6	Shonin Kubasov	118 hr 42 min	First mission with multiple crews. The intent was to study human performance capabilities inflight, welding of metals in space, feasibility of building a manned space station.
12 October 1969	Soyuz 7	Filipichenko Volkov Gorbatko	118 hr 41 min	
13 October 6	Soyuz 8	Shatalov Yeliseyev	118 hr 41 min	
14 November 1969	Apollo 12	Conrad Bean Gordon	244 hr 36 min	Contact dermatitis from biosensor electrolyte paste. Lunar quarantine postflight.
11 April 1970	Apollo 13	Lovell Haise Swigert	142 hr 52 min	Forced to return to Earth because of explosion in service module. Circumnavigation of moon completed. Urinary tract infection occurred due to the combined effects of cold, dehydration, and prolonged wearing of the urine collecting device.
1 June 1970	Soyuz 9	Nikolayev Sevastyanov	424 hr 59 min	Extensive biomedical investigations to determine cardiovascular and musculoskeletal responses. Test of different exercise regimen. Protracted recovery period postflight.

Date	Spacecraft	Crew	Duration	Remarks
2 February 1971	Apollo 14	Shepard, Roosa, Mitchell	216 hr 1 min	
22 April 1971	Soyuz 10 (Salyut 1)	Shatalov, Yeliseyev, Rukavishnikov	48 hr	Docked with Salyut 1 for 5 1/2 hours.
6 June 1971	Soyuz 11 (Salyut 1)	Dobrovolskiy, V. Volkov, Patsayev	552 hr	Docked with Salyut 1. During return to Earth, pressure leak in Soyuz vehicle hatch resulted in decompression and death of all three crewmen. Focal areas of atrophy in antigravity muscles noted.
26 July 1971	Apollo 15	Scott, Worden, Irwin	295 hr 12 min	Cardiac arrhythmias and extrasystoles observed during flight. Postflight lunar quarantine discontinued. First use of Lunar Rover vehicle.
16 April 1972	Apollo 16	Mattingly, Duke, Young	254 hr 51 min	Study of light flash phenomenon.
7 December 1972	Apollo 17	Cernan, Evans, Schmitt	301 hr 51 min	Record stay on the lunar surface (75 hours) and 34 km travel utilizing the Lunar Rover vehicle.
25 May 1973	Skylab 2	Conrad, Kerwin, Weitz	672 hr 49 min	First detailed metabolic studies. First U.S. physician as a crewmember.
28 July 1973	Skylab 3	Bean, Garriott, Lousma	59 days	Reversal of red cell mass loss noted in flight.
27 September 1973	Soyuz 12	Lazarev, Makarov	2 days	Spacecraft modified to hold two crewmen in space suits rather than three in coveralls.
16 November 1973	Skylab 4	Carr, Gibson, Pogue	84 days	Apparent beneficial effects of vigorous exercise in minimizing cardiovascular deconditioning postflight. First inflight determination of lung vital capacity changes.
19 December 1973	Soyuz 13	Klimuk, Lebedev	8 days	Test of countermeasures for cardiovascular deconditioning: anti-g suits, loading suits, bungee exercises. Studies of cerebral circulation utilizing rheography.

TABLE 1-5 (Continued)

SUMMARY OF U.S. AND U.S.S.R. MANNED SPACE FLIGHT EXPERIENCE

Launch Date	Astronaut(s)/Cosmonaut(s)	Mission	Length of Flight	Points of Biomedical Interest
4 July 1974	Popovich Artyukhin	Soyuz 14 (Salyut 3)	16 days	
26 August 1974	Sarafanov Demin	Soyuz 15	2 days	Failed to dock with Salyut 3.
2 December 1974	Filipichenko Rukavishnikov	Soyuz 16	7 days	Test flight to verify Soyuz systems prior to the joint U.S./U.S.S.R. ASTP mission.
9 January 1975	Gubarev Grechko	Soyuz 17 (Salyut 4)	30 days	
5 April 1975	Lazarev Makarov	Soyuz X	Aborted	Cosmonauts suffered injuries and exposure. No fatalities.
25 May 1975	Klimuk Sevastyanov	Soyuz 18 (Salyut 4)	63 days	Docked with Salyut 4. Continuation of studies to test human endurance to weightlessness.
15 July 1975	Kubasov Leonov	Soyuz 19 (ASTP)	6 days	First international manned space mission. U.S./ U.S.S.R. joint space flight experiment. Cosmonauts and astronauts transferred from respective spacecrafts. U.S. crewmen exposed to nitrogen tetroxide accidentally.
	Stafford Brand Slayton	Apollo-Soyuz Test Project	9 days	
6 July 1976	Volynov Zholobov	Soyuz 21 (Salyut 5)	48 days	
15 September 1976	Bykovskiy Aksenov	Soyuz 22	8 days	U.S.S.R./G.D.R. joint experiments.
14 October 1976	Zudov Rozhdestvenskiy	Soyuz 23	2 days	Failed to dock with Salyut 5.
7 February 1977	Gorbatko Glazkov	Soyuz 24 (Salyut 5)	18 days	Docked with Salyut 5. Evaluation of medical countermeasures to prevent deconditioning in long duration missions. Space processing.
9 October 1977	Kovalenok Ryumin	Soyuz 25	2 days	Failed to dock with Salyut 6 space station.

Date	Crew	Spacecraft	Duration	Notes
10 December 1977	Romanenko Grechko	Soyuz 26 (Salyut 6)	96 days	First prime crew of Salyut 6. Significant cardio-vascular deconditioning postflight.
10 January 1978	Dzhanibekov Makarov	Soyuz 27 (Salyut 6)	6 days	First visiting crew to Salyut 6.
2 March 1978	Gubarev Remek (Czechoslovakia)	Soyuz 28 (Salyut 6)	8 days	Second visiting and first international crew of Salyut 6.
15 June 1978	Kovalenok Ivanchenkov	Soyuz 29 (Salyut 6)	140 days	Second prime crew of Salyut 6. New EVA suit with minimum prebreathing requirements introduced.
27 June 1978	Klimuk Hermaszewski (Poland)	Soyuz 30 (Salyut 6)	8 days	Physical effort measured during exercise to develop exercise program.
26 August 1978	Bykovskiy Jaehn (G.D.R.)	Soyuz 31 (Salyut 6)	8 days	
25 February 1979	Lyakhov Ryumin	Soyuz 32 (Salyut 6)	175 days	Third prime crew of Salyut 6. First reports of recurrence of vestibular symptoms inflight and postflight.
9 April 1979	Rukavishnikov Ivanov (Bulgaria)	Soyuz 33	2 days	Fourth international flight. Failed to dock with Salyut 6.
9 April 1980	Popov Ryumin	Soyuz 35 (Salyut 6)	185 days	Routine use of "Chibis" vacuum suit. Audio, taste, and time perception experiments.
26 May 1980	Kubasov Farkash (Hungary)	Soyuz 36 (Salyut 6)	8 days	Intellectual and motor performance studies.
5 June 1980	Malyshev Aksenov	Soyuz T-2 (Salyut 6)	5 days	Docked with Salyut 6. Manned test of a new orbital transfer vehicle.
22 July 1980	Gorbatko Tuan (Vietnam)	Soyuz 37 (Salyut 6)	8 days	
17 September 1980	Romanenko Mendez (Cuba)	Soyuz 38 (Salyut 6)	8 days	Support experiment utilizing "Cuban Boot," EEG experiments. Anthropometry studies.
27 November 1980	Kizim Makarov Strekalov	Soyuz T-3 (Salyut 6)	13 days	Demonstration of 3-man capability of Soyuz T. Repair work on Salyut.
12 March 1981	Kovalenok Savinykh	Soyuz T-4 (Salyut 6)	75 days	Last prime crew onboard Salyut 6 space station. Extensive use of mechanical countermeasures for motion sickness and cardiovascular deconditioning.

TABLE 1-5 (Continued)

SUMMARY OF U.S. AND U.S.S.R. MANNED SPACE FLIGHT EXPERIENCE

Launch Date	Astronaut(s) / Cosmonaut(s)	Mission	Length of Flight	Points of Biomedical Interest
22 March 1981	Dzhanibekov Gurragcha (Mongolia)	Soyuz 39 (Salyut 6)	9 days	Demonstration of "Mongolian collar" device as motion sickness countermeasure.
12 April 1981	Crippen Young	STS-1	54 hr 21 min	First demonstration of successful man-piloted hypersonic flight. First experience with G_z forces on reentry. First runway landing.
14 May 1981	Popov Prunariu (Romania)	Soyuz 40 (Salyut 6)	8 days	Last use of original Soyuz vehicle. Last visiting crew to Salyut 6.
12 November 1981	Engle Truly	STS-2	54 hr 13 min	
22 March 1982	Fullerton Lousma	STS-3	8 days	Expanded manned test of the STS vehicle.
14 May 1982	Berezovoy Lebedev	Soyuz T-5 (Salyut 7)	211 days	Enhanced Salyut 7 space station. Detailed health maintenance studies.
24 June 1982	Dzhanibekov Ivanchenkov Chretien (France)	Soyuz T-6 (Salyut 7)	8 days	Visiting international crew (French) to Salyut 7. First inflight cardiovascular measurements utilizing echocardiography.
27 June 1982	Mattingly Hartsfield	STS-4	7 days	
19 August 1982	Savitskaya Popov Serebrov	Soyuz T-7 (Salyut 7)	8 days	Second woman in space.
10 November 1982	Brand Overmyer Lenoir Allen	STS-5	5 days	First launch of 4-man crew. Entirely manual reentry and landing.
4 April 1983	Weitz Bobko Peterson Musgrave	STS-6	5 days	EVA into cargo bay. Electrophoresis experiment. Studies of orthostatic intolerance during reentry.

Date	Crew	Mission	Duration	Notes
20 April 1983	V. Titov, Strekalov, Serebrov	Soyuz T-8	2 days	Aborted at rendezvous.
18 June 1983	Crippen, Hauck, Fabian, Ride, Thagard	STS-7	6 days	Physician Astronaut (Thagard). Space adaptation medical experiments. First American woman in space.
27 June 1983	Lyakhov, Aleksandrov	Soyuz T-9 (Salyut 7)	150 days	Tavriya–flu virus electrophoresis (1000 hours of visual observations). Six-hour, 2-man EVA.
30 August 1983	Truly, Brandenstein, Gardner, Bluford, Thornton	STS-8	6 days	Biomonitoring of crew leg volume changes. Animal Enclosure Module tests. Extensive medical studies by Thornton.
27 September 1983	V. Titov, Strekalov	Soyuz T-X		Launch explosion (crew unharmed).
28 November 1983	Young, Shaw, Garriott, Parker, Merbold (ESA), Lichtenberg	STS-9	10 days	Spacelab 1. Vestibular, cardiovascular, fluid and electrolyte changes, radiation experiments, biological experiments.
3 February 1984	Brand, Gibson, McCandless, Stewart, McNair	41-B	8 days	Manned Maneuvering Units tested during 5-hour EVA. Pre-breathe time shortened. Cabin pressure dropped to 10.2 psi.
8 February 1984	Kizim, Solovyev, Atkov	Soyuz T-10 (Salyut 7)	237 days	Second Soviet physician (Atkov). Echocardiograph in flight. DNA separation in space. Study of adaptation and efficacy of countermeasures.
4 April 1984	Malyshev, Strekalov, Sharma (India)	Soyuz T-11 (Salyut 7)	7 days	First Indian in space. Vectorcardiograph experiment. Special cuffs tested to slow fluid shift.

TABLE 1-5 (Continued)

SUMMARY OF U.S. AND U.S.S.R. MANNED SPACE FLIGHT EXPERIENCE

Launch Date	Astronaut(s) / Cosmonaut(s)	Mission	Length of Flight	Points of Biomedical Interest
6 April 1984	Crippen Scobee G. Nelson Hart Van Hoften	41-C	7 days	First on-orbit repair of crippled satellite (Solar Max). MMU used to dock with satellite during 6-hour EVA.
17 July 1984	Dzhanibekov Savitskaya Volk	Soyuz T-12 (Salyut 7)	12 days	First woman in EVA.
30 August 1984	Hartsfield Coats Hawley Mullane Walker Resnik	41-D	6 days	Continuous flow electrophoresis sample processing.
5 October 1984	Crippen McBride Sullivan Ride Leestma Garneau (Canada) Scully	41-G	8 days	First mission to include seven crewmembers. First EVA by an American woman. Space Adaptation Syndrome experiments. Radiation studies.
8 November 1984	Hauck Walker Fisher Allen Gardner	51-A	8 days	Two satellite retrievals. Radiation studies.
24 January 1985	Mattingly Shriver Onizuka Buchli Payton	51-C	3 days	Aggregation of red blood cells experiment.

Date	Mission	Crew	Duration	Description
12 April 1985	51-D	Bobko Williams Seddon Hoffman Griggs Walker Garn (U.S. Senator)	7 days	Continuous flow electrophoresis pharmaceutical experiment. American Echocardiograph, motion sickness tests.
29 April 1985	51-B	Overmyer Gregory Lind Thagard Thornton Vandenberg Wang	7 days	Spacelab 3. Autogenic feedback training, experiment, research animal holding facility, and Rodent Sample Bank program.
6 June 1985	T-13 (Salyut 7)	Dzhanibekov Savinykh	Dzhanibekov and visiting cosmonaut Grechko returned to Earth Sept. 26. Dzhanibekov spent 115 days in space. Savinykh remained in Salyut with remaining T-14 crew.	Repair of damaged Salyut 7 space station. Five-hour EVA August 2. First handover of station to new crew without shutting down and reactivating (Sept. 26).
17 June 1985	51-G	Brandenstein Creighton Nagel Fabian Lucid Baudry (France) Al-Saud (Saudi Arabia)	7 days	French Echocardiograph experiment, French postural and eye-movement experiments.
29 July 1985	51-F	Fullerton Bridges Henize England Musgrave Acton Bartoe	8 days	Spacelab 2. Vitamin D metabolite study.
27 August 1985	51-I	Engle Covey Lounge Fisher Van Hoften	7 days	Two EVAs to repair Syncom (Leasat) IV-3 satellite. Initial EVA longest in history of U.S. Space Program (7 hr., 8 min.). MMU not used.

TABLE 1-5 (Continued)

SUMMARY OF U.S. AND U.S.S.R. MANNED SPACE FLIGHT EXPERIENCE

Launch Date	Astronaut(s)/Cosmonaut(s)	Mission	Length of Flight	Points of Biomedical Interest
17 September 1985	Grechko A. Volkov Vasyutin	T-14 (Salyut 7)	Vasyutin and Volkov spent 64 days, 22 hours aboard the Salyut 7/T-14/Cosmos 1686 complex, with Savinykh logging 168 days, 4 hours.	Joined T-13 crew. Dzhanibekov and Grechko returned to Earth Sept. 26, leaving Savinykh, Volkov, and Vasyutin aboard Salyut 7. The three cosmonauts returned to Earth 21 November 1985 due to illness of Vasyutin.
3 October 1985	Bobko Grabe Stewart Hilmers Pailes	51-J	4 days	
30 October 1985	Hartsfield Nagel Dunbar Buchli Bluford Messerschmid Furrer (DFVLR) Ockels (ESA)	61-A	7 days	Spacelab D-1. Vestibular sled tests, cognitive behavior experiments, studies of central venous pressure, intraocular pressure, body impedance, and blood analyses.
26 November 1985	Shaw O'Connor Cleave Spring Ross Walker Neri (Mexico)	61-B	7 days	Innoculation of bacteria experiment, internal equilibrium tests, leg volume and fluid shift measurements, rate of medication absorption tests, CFES hormone purification, electropuncture and biocybernetics studies.
12 January 1986	Gibson Bolden G. Nelson Hawley Chang-Diaz Cenker C. W. Nelson (U.S. Congressman)	61-C	6 days	Blood storage and sedimentation studies, protein crystal growth, sensory-motor and cardiovascular system adaptation studies, fluid shift, electrolyte balance and pharmacokinetic experiments. Payload specialist exhibited pharyngitis.

Date	Flight	Crew	Duration	Remarks
28 January 1986	51-L	Scobee Smith McNair Onizuka Resnik Jarvis McAuliffe	73 sec.	Crew of 7 perished following explosion 73 seconds into flight.
13 March 1986	Soyuz T-15 (Salyut 7 / Mir)	Kizim Solovyev	125 days	Cumulative (career) time in space for Kizim: over 1 year. Transfer EVA from Mir to Salyut 7. Cumulative (career) EVA time for both cosmonauts: over 24 hours.
6 February 1987	Soyuz TM-2 (Mir)	Romanenko Laveikin	160 days (Laveikin) 326 days (Romanenko)	Manned flight of modified Soyuz-TM vehicle to Mir. EVA to remove obstruction from Astrophysics module docking seal (3 hr, 40 min.). Two EVAs to erect solar panels (3 hr., 15 min.; 1 hr., 53 min.). Laveikin exhibited abnormal ECG and returned to Earth with two visiting crewmembers 30 July.
22 July 1987	Soyuz TM-3 (Mir)	Aleksandrov Viktorenko Faris (Syria)	8 days (Vitorenko and Faris) 160 days (Aleksandrov)	First visiting crew to Mir. Laveikin returned to Earth July 30 with Viktorenko and Faris. Aleksandrov took prime crew duty.
21 December 1987	Soyuz TM-4 (Mir)	Titov (prime) Manarov (prime) Levchenko (visit)	8 days (Levchenko)	Successful crew rotation. Levchenko flew an airplane immediately after return to Earth. Titov and Manarov stayed on board Mir to assume prime crew duty.
7 June 1988	Soyuz TM-5 (Mir)	Solovyev Savinykh Aleksandrov (Bulgaria)	10 days	Visiting crew. Evaluation of human work capacity.
29 August 1988	Soyuz TM-6 (Mir)	Lyakhov Polyakhov Mohmand (Afghanistan)	10 days (Lyakhov and Mohmand)	Third Soviet Physician (Polyakhov) remained with prime crew Titov and Manarov.
29 September 1988	STS-26	Hauck Covey Lounge Hilmers G. Nelson	5 days	Pre- and postflight echocardiography, protein crystal growth experiments, pharmacokinetic studies, total body water measurements, otolith experiments.

TABLE 1-6

SUMMARY OF U.S. AND U.S.S.R. EXTRAVEHICULAR ACTIVITY (EVA)

Year	Mission	EVA Date	Astronauts / Cosmonauts Participating in EVA	Duration
1965	Voskhod 2	March 18	Aleksey Leonov	24 min
	Gemini 4	June 6	Edward White[a,b]	36 min
1966	Gemini 9-A	June 5	Eugene Cernan[a]	2 hr 7 min
	Gemini 10	July 19	Michael Collins[a]	49 min
		July 20	Michael Collins[a]	38 min
	Gemini 11	Sep. 13	Richard Gordon[a]	33 min
		Sep. 14	Richard Gordon[a,b]	2 hr 8 min
	Gemini 12	Nov. 12	Edwin Aldrin[a,b]	2 hr 29 min
		Nov. 13	Edwin Aldrin	2 hr 6 min
		Nov. 14	Edwin Aldrin[a,b]	55 min
1969	Soyuz 4/5	Jan. 16	Yevgeniy Khrunov[c] Aleksey Yeliseyev	1 hr
	Apollo 9	March 6	Russell Schweickart	1 hr 7 min
		March 6	David Scott[b]	1 hr 1 min
	Apollo 11	July 21	Neil Armstrong[d] Edwin Aldrin	2 hr 48 min
	Apollo 12	Nov. 19	Charles Conrad[d] Alan Bean	4 hr
		Nov. 20	Charles Conrad[d] Alan Bean	3 hr 46 min
1971	Apollo 14	Feb. 5	Alan Shepard[d] Edgar Mitchell	4 hr 48 min
		Feb. 6	Alan Shepard[d] Edgar Mitchell	4 hr 35 min
	Apollo 15	July 30	David Scott[e]	33 min
		July 31	David Scott[d] James Irwin	6 hr 33 min
		Aug. 1	David Scott[d] James Irwin	7 hr 12 min
		Aug. 2	David Scott[d] James Irwin	4 hr 50 min
		Aug. 5	Alfred Worden[f]	38 min
		Aug. 5	James Irwin[f,b]	38 min
1972	Apollo 16	Apr. 21	John Young[d] Charles Duke	7 hr 11 min
		Apr. 22	John Young[d] Charles Duke	7 hr 23 min

TABLE 1-6 (Continued)

SUMMARY OF U.S. AND U.S.S.R. EXTRAVEHICULAR ACTIVITY (EVA)

Year	Mission	EVA Date	Astronauts/Cosmonauts Participating in EVA	Duration
1972	Apollo 16	Apr. 23	John Young[d] Charles Duke	5 hr 40 min
		Apr. 25	Thomas Mattingly[f] Charles Duke[f]	1 hr 24 min
	Apollo 17	Dec. 11	Eugene Cernan[d] Harrison Schmitt	7 hr 12 min
		Dec. 12	Eugene Cernan[d] Harrison Schmitt	7 hr 37 min
		Dec. 13	Eugene Cernan[d] Harrison Schmitt	7 hr 15 min
		Dec. 17	Ronald Evans[f]	1 hr 6 min
		Dec. 17	Harrison Schmitt[f]	1 hr 6 min
1973	Skylab 2	May 25	Paul Weitz[b]	35 min
		June 7	Charles Conrad Joseph Kerwin	3 hr 23 min
		June 19	Charles Conrad Paul Weitz	1 hr 36 min
	Skylab 3	Aug. 6	Owen Garriot Jack Lousma	6 hr 31 min
		Aug. 24	Owen Garriot Jack Lousma	4 hr 30 min
		Sep. 22	Owen Garriot Alan Bean	2 hr 41 min
	Skylab 4	Nov. 22	Edward Gibson William Pogue	6 hr 34 min
		Dec. 25	Gerald Carr William Pogue	7 hr 3 min
		Dec. 29	Edward Gibson Gerald Carr	3 hr 29 min
1974	Skylab 4	Feb. 3	Edward Gibson Gerald Carr	5 hr 19 min
1977	Salyut 6–Soyuz 26	Dec. 20	Georgiy Grechko[g]	1 hr 28 min
1978	Salyut 6–Soyuz 29	July 29	Vladimir Kovalenok Aleksandr Ivanchenkov	2 hr 5 min
1979	Salyut 6–Soyuz 32 (crew launched in Soyuz 32; Soyuz 34 at station time of EVA)	Aug. 15	Vladimir Lyakhov Valeriy Ryumin	1 hr 23 min
1982	Salyut 7–Soyuz T-5	July 30	Anatoliy Berezovoy Valentin Lebedev	2 hr 33 min

TABLE 1-6 (Continued)

SUMMARY OF U.S. AND U.S.S.R. EXTRAVEHICULAR ACTIVITY (EVA)

Year	Mission	EVA Date	Astronauts / Cosmonauts Participating in EVA	Duration
1983	STS-6	Apr. 7	F. Story Musgrave Donald Peterson	4 hr 17 min
	Salyut 7–Soyuz T-9	Nov. 1	Vladimir Lyakhov Aleksandr Aleksandrov	2 hr 50 min
		Nov. 3	Vladimir Lyakhov Aleksandr Aleksandrov	2 hr 55 min
1984	41-B	Feb. 7	Bruce McCandless[h] Robert Stewart	5 hr 30 min
		Feb. 9	Bruce McCandless Robert Stewart	6 hr
	41-C	Apr. 8	George Nelson James Van Hoften	3 hr
		Apr. 11	George Nelson James Van Hoften	6 hr
1984	Salyut 7–Soyuz T-10 (crew launched in Soyuz T-10; Soyuz T-11 at station at time of EVA)	Apr. 23	Leonid Kizim Vladimir Solovyev	4 hr 15 min
	Salyut 7–Soyuz T-10 (crew launched in Soyuz T-10; Soyuz T-11 at station at time of EVA)	Apr. 26	Leonid Kizim Vladimir Solovyev	5 hr
	Salyut 7–Soyuz T-10 (crew launched in Soyuz T-10; Soyuz T-11 at station at time of EVA)	Apr. 29	Leonid Kizim Vladimir Solovyev	2 hr 45 min
	Salyut 7–Soyuz T-10 (crew launched in Soyuz T-10; Soyuz T-11 at station at time of EVA)	May 4	Leonid Kizim Vladimir Solovyev	2 hr 45 min
	Salyut 7–Soyuz T-10 (crew launched in Soyuz T-10; Soyuz T-11 at station at time of EVA)	May 18	Leonid Kizim Vladimir Solovyev	3 hr 5 min
	Salyut 7–Soyuz T-12 (Soyuz T-10/T-11 crew there also)	July 25	Svetlana Savitskaya Vladimir Dzhanibekov	3 hr 35 min
	Salyut 7–Soyuz T-10 (crew launched in Soyuz T-10; Soyuz T-11 at station at time of EVA)	Aug. 8	Leonid Kizim Vladimir Solovyev	5 hr
	41-G	Oct. 11	Kathryn Sullivan David Leestma	3 hr 29 min
	51-A	Nov. 12	Joseph Allen Dale Gardner	6 hr
		Nov. 14	Joseph Allen Dale Gardner	5 hr 42 min

TABLE 1-6 (Continued)

SUMMARY OF U.S. AND U.S.S.R. EXTRAVEHICULAR ACTIVITY (EVA)

Year	Mission	EVA Date	Astronauts / Cosmonauts Participating in EVA	Duration
1985	51-D	Apr. 12	Jeff Hoffman David Griggs	3 hr 7 min
	Salyut 7–Soyuz T-13	Aug. 2	Vladimir Dzhanibekov Victor Savinykh	5 hr
	51-I	Aug. 31	James Van Hoften William Fisher	7 hr 8 min
		Sep. 1	James Van Hoften William Fisher	4 hr 32 min
	61-B	Dec. 1	Jerry Ross Sherwood Spring	5 hr 32 min
		Dec. 3	Jerry Ross Sherwood Spring	5 hr 42 min
1986	Soyuz T-15 (Transfer from Mir to Salyut 7)	May 28	Leonid Kizim Vladimir Solovyev	3 hr 50 min
1987	Soyuz TM-2 (Mir)	Apr. 12	Aleksandr Laveikin Yuri Romanenko	3 hr 40 min
		June 12	Aleksandr Laveikin Yuri Romanenko	3 hr 15 min
		June 16	Aleksandr Laveikin Yuri Romanenko	1 hr 53 min
1988	Soyuz TM-4 (Mir)	Feb. 26	Vladimir Titov Musa Manarov	4 hr 25 min

[a] The duration for the Gemini EVAs is the time from hatch opening to hatch closing. For Apollo and Skylab, both space and lunar EVAs are computed from the time cabin pressure reached 3.0 psi during depressurization and repressurization. The durations presented for the two-person EVAs are the amount of time spent by each person.
[b] Stand-up EVA.
[c] Y. Khrunov and A. Yeliseyev were launched on Soyuz 5 and transferred to Soyuz 4 via EVA.
[d] Lunar surface EVA.
[e] Stand-up EVA from lunar module on lunar surface.
[f] Cis-lunar or deep-space EVA.
[g] Y. Romanenko remained in the depressurized compartment during G. Grechko's EVA. Western sources do not consider or list this as an EVA although some Soviet sources do.
[h] First untethered EVA.

THE EUROPEAN MANNED SPACE PROGRAM

The European Space Agency (ESA) was founded in 1975 by the merger of the European Space Research Organization (ESRO) and the European Launcher Development Organization (ELDO). The Headquarters of the ESA is located in Paris. Thirteen countries are participating members of the ESA (with Canada having "observer" status and Finland having "associate member" status). ESA is supported by specialized development centers such as the European Space Research and Technology Center, European Space Operations Center, European Tracking and Data Acquisition Network, and European Space Research Institute. Between 1968 and 1983 NASA launched 11 ESA scientific satellites. In 1973, ESA began the development of a multipurpose manned space laboratory (Spacelab) for the Space Shuttle. So far, four Spacelab missions have flown in space—Spacelabs 1, 2, 3, and the Deutsch-1. The latter was outfitted by the Federal Republic of Germany. Spacelab proved to be a significant capability for life sciences investigations in space. France and the Federal Republic of Germany have embarked on ambitious manned space programs in the area of life sciences, and have contributed to the development of unique instrumentation for biomedical investigations in space.

ESA has perfected a launch vehicle for unmanned operations called Ariane, which made its debut in December, 1979. Plans are underway to develop a multipurpose laboratory called "Columbus" for the International Space Station "Freedom" era, and to complete the manned launch reusable space plane "Hermes," to be operational before the end of the 20th century.

THE JAPANESE MANNED SPACE PROGRAM

The Japanese National Space Development Agency (NASDA) was established on October 1, 1969. NASDA is also supported by several development centers, with most of its research activities partitioned in the university and industry sectors. The main unmanned launch vehicle is designated as H-I with plans to develop a more powerful booster, H-II, by early 1990. NASDA is preparing for its microgravity and life sciences mission, Spacelab-J, early in the 1991 time frame. NASDA has selected

three astronauts. Like ESA, NASDA has undertaken the development of a multipurpose laboratory to be operated in conjunction with the Space Station Freedom, and a reusable manned space shuttle to be operational in the early 21st century. Over the last several years, NASDA has significantly expanded its technological base in support of space missions.

THE SOVIET PROGRAM

SPUTNIK

The launch of Sputnik 1 in October, 1957, heralded the beginning of the space age. The Soviets launched Sputnik 2 one month later, carrying a dog named Laika. Laika's cabin contained air regeneration and thermal regulation systems, and equipment for monitoring respiration, blood pressure, and heart rate activity. Environmental and physiological parameters were telemetered back to Earth throughout the 1-week flight. This historic flight offered the first evidence that a higher vertebrate, fairly similar to man physiologically, could withstand the rigors of launch and remain alive in space.

Subsequently, a series of five Korabl Sputnik flights served as precursors to the first manned mission. Korabl Sputnik-2, launched on August 10, 1960, carried two dogs, forty mice, two rats, a number of flies, and a variety of plants into orbit and back to Earth. This was the first time that living organisms were flown in space and safely returned. Instrumented manikins and live television transmissions supplemented the substantial amount of biomedical data that Soviet investigators obtained regarding the effects of space flight on living organisms (DeHart, 1974).

VOSTOK PROGRAM

On April 12, 1961, 27-year-old Air Force Senior Lieutenant Yuri Gagarin completed a single orbit in a flight lasting 108 minutes. His spacecraft, Vostok-1, consisted of a near spherical capsule containing life support systems, instrumentation, and an ejection seat, plus a conical service module containing gas bottles, batteries, rockets, and support equipment. After reentry, Gagarin ejected from the cabin and completed the final portion of his descent by parachute.

The presence of a human in the spacecraft focused the efforts of Soviet scientists on four problems (Prishchepa, 1981):

1. Assuring the safety of the cosmonaut in case of launch malfunction
2. Protecting the cosmonaut against the space environment and ensuring normal functions during orbital flight
3. Ensuring reliable operation of equipment in space
4. Ensuring safe and accurate reentry and descent.

Most of these were technical and engineering issues. However, a critical question dealt not with mere survival, but with human performance in space. Previous animal experiments indicated that normal physiological function could be maintained, but confidence was by no means complete. Consequently, Gagarin was monitored by video camera for signs of distress or disorientation. The flight program included (in addition to the first human observations of the Earth and stars from space) the intake of food and water. Medical parameters monitored during the brief flight included continuous heart rate, pneumography, ECG, seismocardiography, electroencephalography, electrooculography, thermography, electromyography, and galvanic skin response. These parameters have been monitored on all subsequent Soviet missions, although the emphasis has varied for each flight (Dodge, 1976).

Gagarin showed no inflight deviations from normal psychological and physiological function. Nearly 4 months later, Air Force Major Gherman Titov completed 17 orbits in Vostok-2. During this 1-day flight, the cosmonaut experienced spatial disorientation and motion sickness. This first indication of what would become the most persistent problem in the initial period of short-duration space flights prompted a strong emphasis on the vestibular system in cosmonaut selection and training. Titov was also the first human to sleep in space, and the first to exercise autonomous spacecraft control. His vital signs were reported to be within normal ranges.

Subsequent Vostok missions were paired flights of two vehicles launched a day or so apart. The first pair was co-orbited so that the two spacecraft approached to less than 4 miles of each other. This was a test of both the feasibility of rendezvous in space (as a prelude to later dockings) and the ground control coordination necessary for such maneuvers. The influence of identical conditions of space flight could also be observed; in the 3- and 4-day flights, no significant biomedical problems were reported. The second pair of flights, Vostok-5 and -6, were noted for a manned flight duration record of 5 days, and the first space flight by a woman, pilot Valentina Tereshkova, a 26-year-old textile factory worker who did not have the usual military aviation background (Smith, 1976).

VOSKHOD PROGRAM

The second-generation spacecraft, Voskhod, differed from the Vostok craft primarily in the removal of the ejection seat to afford room for a three-man crew. Due to the success of the previous series, the crew wore coveralls rather than the cumbersome pressurized suits. In October, 1964, Voskhod-1 flew the first crew of three. Inclusion of the first physician in space (Yegorov) on this mission allowed a more comprehensive body of medical data to be gathered in flight. The flight also included onboard studies of hearing, pulmonary function, the vestibular apparatus, and muscle strength in weightlessness. In March of 1965, Voskhod's second (and last) flight was launched with two cosmonauts on board. With the aid of an accordion-like external airlock and a self-contained life support system, Aleksey Leonov completed mankind's first "space walk." The EVA consisted of 12 minutes outside the spacecraft and 10 minutes in the depressurized, inflatable airlock (OTA, 1983).

Due to a failure of the automatic reentry system, the crew of Voskhod-2 also accomplished the first manually controlled reentry. They landed in a dense, snowy forest hundreds of miles north of the target and spent the night in their capsule, awaiting recovery.

SOYUZ PROGRAM

After a pause of nearly 2 years, during which the American Gemini Program completed many successful flight operations, the Soviets embarked in 1967 on what was to be their most ambitious and long-running program of manned missions. The initial version of the Soyuz vehicle contained two passenger compartments: a work compartment (or orbital module) and a command (or reentry) module in which the spacecraft was piloted. The two compartments, connected by an airlock, had a total volume of about 9 m³. A docked unit was optional, and the Soyuz craft could be outfitted with one, two, or three seats. Unlike the Vostok/Voskhod ships,

which had a ballistic trajectory on reentry, the Soyuz reentry module employed aerodynamic lift to permit a controlled reentry and more precise landing. The load on reentry was thus reduced from 8–10-g (in the previous series) to between 5 and 7 g.

The objective of the Soyuz program was to provide a multi-purpose spacecraft which could be employed in connection with an orbital space station: as a base for assembly, as a supply and transport ship, and as a vehicle for conducting additional, independent studies of space. The ship was designed for broad maneuverability, a docking capability, and the support of long-duration flight—in essence, the Soyuz was intended as a combination transport ship and orbital station (Malyshev, 1981).

The first trial of this new and more sophisticated vehicle, in April, 1967, ended in tragedy. A loss of attitudinal stability on reentry resulted in a spin about the longitudinal axis; the parachute system became tangled and failed to deploy fully, resulting in the death of cosmonaut Vladimir Komarov upon impact.

Soyuz-3, the next manned flight, was delayed for 18 months. During this 4-day mission the pilot twice approached to within a few feet of the unmanned Soyuz-2, in what were apparently unsuccessful attempts at docking (Smith, 1976). In the following missions (Soyuz-4 and -5), rendezvous and docking of two spacecraft was successful, forming an experimental orbital space station. Soyuz-6, -7, and -8 tested the simultaneous command and control of three spacecraft for rendezvous in space and the performance of tasks (welding) in the space vacuum.

None of the cosmonauts participating in these Soyuz missions demonstrated unusual or unexpected physiological changes. The typical cardiovascular response was an increase in pulse rate during launch and orbital insertion, and an increase in pulse rate variability over much or all of the flight. ECGs were normal, except for an occasional depression of the S-T segment. Respiration rate ordinarily increased during launch and insertion, and both respiration and cardiac contraction rates increased during performance of complex work tasks and EVAs.

Medical monitoring of Soyuz cosmonauts was specifically intended to assess the effects of weightlessness. In addition to cardiorespiratory measurements, extensive pre- and postflight examinations addressed the central nervous system, metabolism, blood chemistry, and fluid-electrolyte balance. The primary objective of Soyuz-9 was the examination of physiological stresses associated with space flight. Pre- and postflight exercise studies of cardiorespiratory response were carried out. The exercise program in this mission was extensive, with each cosmonaut exercising for two 1-hour periods per day. Chest muscle expanders, isometric exercises, elastic tension straps, and an early version of the "Penguin" constant body compression suit were employed. Other tests assessed pain sensitivity, hand strength, mental capability, and vestibular function.

The two cosmonauts demonstrated pronounced orthostatic intolerance after this 18-day flight, and had to be carried from the spacecraft. Postflight readaptation to gravity took at least 11 days. This anomalous experience (in view of the absence of similar responses in subsequent, longer missions) sparked renewed concern about the outlook for long-term manned missions, prompting a vigorous search for countermeasures to physiological deconditioning in the next phase of the Soviet manned space program.

THE SALYUT ERA

Work began on the first Salyut orbital station in 1969, after technical problems associated with rendezvous and docking had been solved. The station was conceived as a long-term habitat for rotating crews, with a power plant, extensive onboard systems, and scientific equipment. Provisions for maintenance and housekeeping were incorporated, as well as facilities for eating, sleeping, hygiene, and physical exercise.

As developed, the basic Salyut station is cylindrical, with an overall length of about 21 m, a maximum diameter of 4.2 m, and a total internal volume of 100 m^3 (Smith, 1976). The Soyuz craft is used as a transfer vehicle; its use for independent missions was virtually eliminated with the construction of Salyut.

Salyut-1 was launched into orbit unmanned on April 19, 1971 and first used by the three-man crew of Soyuz-11, which remained on board for 23 days, conducting a comprehensive program of geographical, space, and biomedical research. However, during the return, a valve malfunctioned in the Soyuz upon separation of the reentry module from the work module, resulting in rapid depressurization. The three crewmembers died of dysbarism.

This tragedy forced a lengthy delay, while stronger measures to ensure crew safety were formulated. After 2 years, Salyut-2 was launched, but it was evidently damaged by explosion of the carrier rocket's upper stage upon entry into orbit, and was abandoned. The next manned mission, Soyuz-12, was not flown until September, 1973. The Soyuz vehicle was by then modified to hold two crewmembers wearing pressure suits, rather than three who previously wore coveralls.

The second successful Soviet space station, Salyut-3, was launched in June 1974 and remained on orbit for 7 months. Improvements included movable solar panels, more efficient life support systems, and a more "homelike" interior design and decoration. On the 15-day Soyuz-14 mission to this station, extensive physical exercise was again employed to assess the efficacy of physical conditioning with regard to eventual readaptation to gravity. A combined treadmill and improved Penguin suit provided a universal trainer that could simulate walking, running, jumping, and weightlifting. Some evidence of readaptation to simulated gravity was seen (Dodge, 1976). Medical experiments included studies of blood circulation in the brain and blood velocity in the arteries. A regular daily schedule consisted of 8 hours sleep, 8 hours work, and 8 hours for exercise and administrative/housekeeping duties.

Launched in December 1974, Salyut-4 functioned on orbit for more than 2 years. This model featured larger solar panels that could be individually and automatically rotated to produce 4 kilowatts of power. The first mission to the new space station was the 30-day flight of Soyuz-17. For the first time, the "Chibis" lower body negative pressure suit was used to reduce the volume of headward fluid shifts. This variant of a lower body negative pressure device is worn during exercise and for extended periods during normal activity in an effort to reduce cardiovascular deconditioning postflight. A swivel chair similar to that later used on Skylab was installed for the study of vestibular reactions. A bicycle was included, in addition to the treadmill. Another new approach to physical conditioning was electrical stimulation of various muscle groups by means of the "Tonus" apparatus. With this flight, the exercise program began to assume the appearance of a standard regimen: 3 days of regulated exercise (three times per day, 2.5 hours total) followed by a fourth day on which exercise was optional.

The follow-on Soyuz-18 mission (63 days) continued these programs. A high-salt diet and forced intake of water to increase body fluid volume were combined with physical exercise during the final 10 days of the flight to facilitate readaptation to gravity. This extended preparation period was an innovation, first instituted on

the Salyut-4 space station; the prescribed combination was found to be successful (Smith, 1976). Similar measures were taken on 49- and 18-day missions to Salyut-5, which flew for over a year during 1976 and 1977.

With increasing mission duration, the logistical problem of resupply of consumables became more pressing. Limitations on weight and volume meant that life support system reserves which could support a two-man crew could be carried for no more than 120 days. Each crewmember requires over 10 kg of consumables per day. Fuel reserves needed to be replenished periodically, and fresh storage batteries had to be supplied. The Soyuz transport craft alone was unable to ferry enough additional cargo to meet these needs. In addition, in case of malfunction or damage to the docked Soyuz vehicle, there was no place for a reserve ship to dock with the station (Feoktistov and Markov, 1982).

These and other concerns led to the development of a second-generation orbital station, Salyut-6 (Figure 1-9). Its main structural difference was an additional docking unit at the opposite end of the station. To provide an expanded resupply capability, an unmanned "Progress" cargo ship was developed (actually a modified Soyuz). This vehicle is automatic and nonreturnable, and delivered about 2,300 kg of cargo to the Salyut on each trip. It allowed not only longer missions, but more extensive and versatile scientific and technical programs, since additional scientific equipment could be ferried to and from the station to accommodate varying requirements. The station itself had provisions for expanded maintenance by the crew, and additional amenities, such as a shower. These capabilities meant that the Salyut station was now indeed a full-scale orbiting research laboratory, and the Soviets made full use of its capabilities.

Over its four and one-half years of active manned operation between September

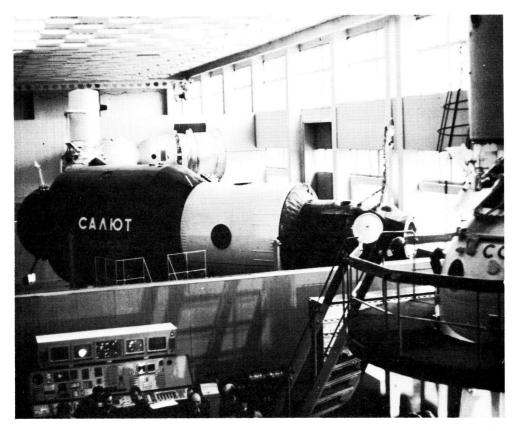

Figure 1-9. A mockup of the Salyut station, which was used for cosmonaut training in Star City.

1977 and June 1981, Salyut-6 was visited by 27 cosmonauts participating in 15 separate missions. Six of these individuals made two flights to the station, and seven spent more than 100 days in space. During this period cosmonauts from Czechoslovakia, Hungary, Mongolia, Romania, Vietnam, Cuba, GDR, Poland, and Bulgaria participated as crewmembers on shorter-duration flights. More than 1,600 experiments were conducted in areas of Earth resources, materials processing, and biomedical and biological research.

A total of five prime crews visited Salyut-6 for 96, 140, 175, 185, and 75 days. Due to an accident to a trainee, one member of the 175-day crew, Valeriy Ryumin, returned to the station nearly 8 months after his flight to participate in the 185-

day mission, thus becoming, at that time, the world's record-holder for time in space, with nearly a year.

In order to maximize physiological and psychological adaptation to space flight, Soviet medical specialists instituted on board Salyut-6 a sleep-wake-work cycle keyed to normal Moscow time, with a 5-day work week and 2-day weekend. A "psychological support program" was also implemented, which included not only monitoring for performance and mood changes, but morale boosters such as frequent two-way communications with families, access to radio and television, and delivery of gifts, letters, and news. These measures were reported to ease the stress of long-term confinement.

The final addition to the Salyut-6 program was a new model of the Soyuz ferry craft, designated Soyuz-T. This is essentially a three-seat version of the old Soyuz. The first manned flight of the new craft, T-2, took place in June 1980. Subsequently, it was used to transport the crew of the final long-term mission to Salyut-6. It has now completely replaced the old Soyuz, which was last flown in the Soyuz-40 mission.

In April, 1982, a new Salyut station (Salyut-7) was launched. With two docking ports, one of which had been modified to accommodate larger spacecraft, this version was similar in size and shape to Salyut-6. Station operations were further automated and the Salyut-7 was made more habitable. Windows were specially coated against ultraviolet radiation, the color schemes were changed to improve the appearance, and a refrigerator was installed. New medical examination and diagnostic systems extended the range of biomedical parameters that could be monitored, either by the cosmonauts or remotely from the ground.

The Soyuz T-5 transported the first crew to the Salyut in May, 1982. The crew of two performed about 300 experiments and set a new endurance record for space flight: 211 days. A visiting crew of three from Soyuz T-6 included a French Spationaute, Jean-Loup Chretien, who performed cardiovascular and vestibular studies utilizing echocardiography "Ace du Coeur" and "Posture" equipment. On a separate occasion, Soyuz T-7 carried another crew of three, including the second woman cosmonaut, Svetlana Savitskaya.

In April, 1983, Soyuz T-8 failed to dock with Salyut-7, causing the mission to be aborted. Two months later, the Soyuz T-9 successfully docked, carrying cosmonauts Lyakhov and Aleksandrov. The crew carried out many scientific experiments during their lengthy flight of 150 days (Dubbelaar, 1986). In the course of two EVAs totaling 5 hours 45 minutes, Lya-

hov and Aleksandrov installed additional solar batteries on the station.

An attempt to fly a two-man replacement crew in September was aborted by a launch pad explosion, from which the cosmonauts escaped unharmed. On February 9, 1984, the crew of the third main expedition, Soyuz T-10, comprised of cosmonauts Kizim, Solovyev, and Atkov (inflight physician), began work on board the space station. Galactic cosmic radiation was measured and medical studies by Dr. Atkov evaluated cosmonauts' health, fitness, and work capacity. Cardiovascular activity was monitored by ultrasound equipment. A serum analytical device designated the "Glyukometr" enhanced biochemical investigations in the area of carbohydrate and mineral metabolism. The "Sport" experiment was conducted to determine an optimum set of physical exercises and increase their effectiveness in space flight.

On April 3, 1984, the Soyuz T-11 carried a visiting crew comprised of Malyshev, Strekalov, and Sharma (India) to the Salyut-7. This was the first time six cosmonauts worked together on board the space station. During their stay, the crew completed medical studies to study countermeasure effectiveness.

July 17 of the same year marked the launch of Soyuz T-12, carrying another visiting crew: cosmonauts Dzhanibekov, Savitskaya, and Volk. One outstanding event during their 12-day visit was the space walk of Svetlana Savitskaya, the first by a woman. During the 3 hours and 35 minutes of her EVA she performed a variety of manual tasks (spraying coatings, welding) (Canby, 1986). The mission of the primary crew was completed on October 2, 1984, after 237 days.

On June 6, 1985, the Soviet Union launched two cosmonauts on board the Soyuz T-13 spacecraft. Savinykh and Dzhanibekov efficiently carried out a series of difficult repairs and reactivation operations on the station, which had completely shut down after the crew had returned home (Canby, 1986).

Soyuz T-14, with a visiting crew consisting of Vasyutin, Grechko, and Volkov, was launched September 17 to dock with the orbital complex Salyut-7/Soyuz T-13. Dzhanibekov and Grechko returned to Earth in the Soyuz T-13, leaving Savinykh with the new crew to complete the experiments. On November 21, the flight was terminated when Vasyutin became ill and had to be returned to Earth for hospital treatment.

The return of Savinykh, Vasyutin, and Volkov essentially ended the "Salyut era." The Salyut program contributed a substantial body of information on human function for long periods of time in space. The next step was the development of a third-generation space station, "Mir."

THIRD-GENERATION SPACE STATION: MIR

The construction of a multi-modular space complex, designated the Mir ("Peace"), represents a third-generation space station. The core of the Mir was launched February 20, 1986, the first stage of the modular complex. The space station contains six docking ports for manned or unmanned capsules traveling to and from Earth. Two axial ports can accommodate Soyuz vehicles or Progress resupply ships. Dedicated laboratory modules docked to the core will enable inflight studies in such areas as astrophysics, materials processing, biomedical research, and geophysics. This space station also features improved crew facilities: private quarters, better quality materials in the windows, improved communications, an upgraded life support system, expanded galley and food heating system with high quality dehydrated foods, and increased station automation.

Unlike Salyut, the core module serves mainly as the crew habitat, as most of the work stations are located in the dedicated laboratory modules. The habitable crew area is much more spacious than on previous stations. The main computer complex, also located in the core, is more sophisticated and capable of running the space station autonomously (Soviet Aerospace, 1986).

On March 13, 1986, cosmonauts Kizim and Solovyev (who set an endurance record of 237 days in space in 1984 on Salyut-7) were launched in the Soyuz T-15 vehicle to become Mir's first occupants.

On May 6, the cosmonauts returned to the Salyut to perform several tasks left unfinished when the last crew left quickly in November, 1985. This was the first flight between space stations. The Soyuz T-15 docked with Salyut-7 after leaving the Mir. The transfer was regarded as a major accomplishment, opening new possibilities for servicing space stations in the future (Aviation Week and Space Technol., 1986).

While docked with Salyut-7, the cosmonauts performed an EVA on May 28 to construct a pylon in space. This 3-hour, 50-minute space walk brought the cumulative EVA time to over 24 hours for each individual. The cosmonauts spent a total of 125 days in orbit before returning to Earth.

Soyuz TM-2 (an improved version of the Soyuz T) was launched February 6, 1987, carrying cosmonauts Romanenko and Laveikin—the Mir's second crew. The first dedicated module, an astrophysics module designated "Kvant," was launched March 31. After two failed docking attempts, the module finally docked with the core unit April 12, after the cosmonauts removed a foreign object during a 3-hour, 40-minute EVA (Soviet Aerospace, 1987).

In July, 1987, the prime crew received a visiting crew consisting of a representative from Syria (Faris) and two Soviet cosmonauts (Aleksandrov and Vitorenko). Laveikin, however, had exhibited an abnormal ECG during treadmill exercise, and the decision was made to return him to Earth with two of the visiting crewmembers (Faris and Vitorenko), leaving Aleksandrov to finish prime crew duties with Romanenko.

The crew received its replacement on December 23, 1987: Titov and Manarov (with an additional crewmember, Levchenko, visiting for 1 week). On December 29, Romanenko, Aleksandrov, and Levchenko returned to Earth. Romanenko had spent 326 days in space, breaking the previous record of 237 days.

Over the course of their year-long flight, the new prime crew, Titov and Manarov, received three visiting crews which included cosmonauts from Bulgaria, Afghanistan, and France. With the second visiting crew, the flight of the third Soviet physician, Polyakhov, took place. Polyakhov remained on board the Mir with the prime crew. The third visiting crew included veteran spationaute Jean-Loup Chretien, who remained on board for almost a month. The French biomedical experiments emphasized the cardiovascular and neurosensory systems and continued the biomedical research carried out during the earlier flight of Chretien in 1982. The flight also included an EVA—the first by a spationaute.

SPACE MEDICINE TODAY

Both in the U.S. and U.S.S.R., problem and research areas have been defined, identified on the basis of experience from 28 years of space flight. These include microgravity effects on the body, such as:

- Space motion sickness
- Cardiovascular deconditioning
- Hematological/immunological changes
- Bone mineral loss
- Muscular deconditioning

Other occupational issues in space medicine are directly related to the types of missions planned for the future. Preceding flight programs have helped define areas of biomedical consequence and illustrate the co-evolution of support requirements with mission objectives and durations. Tracing the history of manned missions— and projecting the development of one of the most ambitious spacecraft, the Space Station "Freedom," and possibly advanced missions to the moon or Mars—the following issues emerge as important in space medicine:

- Selection of space personnel
- Medical training of flight crews
- Inflight medical care
- Life support, especially bioregenerative systems to produce food
- Extravehicular activity
- Postflight rehabilitation and therapy
- Radiation protection
- Habitability/toxicology
- Artificial gravity
- Countermeasures to deconditioning
- Human factors considerations in man/ machine interface
- Psychology/group dynamics

Space medicine is beginning to mature. New problems, both medical and physiological, will be identified as the number of flights, length of stay time, and population of individuals exposed to weightlessness increase. Some problems may require unique solutions, and the practice of space medicine will take shape in space as experience is gained in Earth orbit and beyond.

REFERENCES

Air et Cosmos. "Experience Sovietique de Simulation d'apesanteur pendant un an." No. 1137, April 4, 1987.

Aviation Week and Space Technology. "Cosmonauts Complete Transfer between Mir and Salyut 7." Page 28, May, 1986.

Belew, L.F. (Ed.). Skylab, our first space station (NASA SP-400). U.S. Government Printing Office, Washington, D.C., 1977.

Burchard, E.C., and Nicogossian, A. E. Achilles tendon reflex. In: The Apollo-Soyuz Test Project medical report (NASA SP-411). Edited by A.E. Nicogossian, National Technical Information Service, Springfield, VA, 1977.

Canby, T. A generation after Sputnik: Are the Soviets ahead in space? National Geographic. pp. 420-459, Oct., 1986.

DeHart, R. Biomedical aspects of Soviet manned space flight (ST-CS-13-373-75). Defense Intelligence Agency, Washington, D.C., 1974.

Dietlein, L.F. Skylab: A beginning. In: Biomedical results from Skylab (NASA SP-377). Edited by Johnston, R.S., and Dietlein, L.F. U.S. Government Printing Office, Washington, D.C., 1977.

Dietlein, L.F., and Johnston, R.S. U.S. manned space flight: The first twenty years. A biomedical status report. Acta Astronautica, 8(9-10):893-906, 1981.

Dodge, C.H. The Soviet space life sciences. In: Soviet space programs, 1971-1975: Overview, facilities, and hardware, manned and unmanned flight programs, bioastronautics, civil and military applications, projections of future plans (Vol. 1). Library of Congress, Science Policy Research Division, Congressional Research Service, Washington, D.C., 1976.

Dubbelaar, B. The Salyut Project (English translation). Progress Publishers, Moscow, 1986.

FBIS-Sov-87-233, "Shatalov on Cosmonaut Training Mission Problems." (PM021627 Moscow Nedelya, in Russian, 14 Oct. 1987). 41:7-9, 4 Dec. 1987.

Feoktistov, K.P., and Markov, M.M. Evolution of Salyut orbital stations. JPRS, USSR Report: Space, 15:1-11, 29 March 1982.

Graybiel, A. Coping with space motion sickness in Spacelab missions. Acta Astronautica, 8(9-10):1015-1018, 1981.

Johnston, R.S. Introduction. In: Biomedical results of Apollo (NASA SP-368). Edited by Johnston, R.S., Dietlein, L.F., and Berry, C.A. U.S. Government Printing Office, Washington, D.C., 1975.

Kleinknecht, K.S. Preface. In: Project Mercury, a chronology (NASA SP-4001). Edited by Grimwood, J.M. U.S. Government Printing Office, Washington, D.C., 1963.

LaFevers, E.V., Nicogossian, A.E., Hursta, W.N., and Baker, J.T. Electromyographic analysis of skeletal muscle. In: The Apollo-Soyuz Test Project medical report (NASA SP-411). Edited by A.E. Nicogossian. National Technical Information Service, Springfield, VA, 1977.

Link, M. Space medicine in Project Mercury (NASA SP-4003). U.S. Government Printing Office, Washington, D.C., 1965.

Lovelace, W.R., II. Introduction. In M. Link, Space Medicine in Project Mercury (NASA SP-4003). U.S. Government Printing Office, Washington, D.C., 1965.

Malyshev, Yu. Evolution of the Soyuz spacecraft. JPRS, USSR Report: Space, 9:8-13, 2 March 1982.

Mueller, G.E. Introduction. In: Gemini summary conference (NASA SP-138). U.S. Government Printing Office, Washington, D.C., 1967.

Nicogossian, A.E., LaPinta, C.K., Burchard, E.C., Hoffler, G.W., and Bartelloni, P.J. Crew health. In: The Apollo-Soyuz Test Project medical report (NASA SP-411). Edited by A.E. Nicogossian. National Technical Information Service, Springfield, VA, 1977.

Office of Technology Assessment: "Salyut: Soviet Steps Toward Permanent Human Presence in Space," OTA-TM-ST1-14, GPO no. 052-003-00937-4, Washington, D.C., December, 1983.

Prishchepa, V.I. Twentieth anniversary of Gagarin's flight: A collection of articles. JPRS, USSR Report: Space, 7-10, 13 October 1981.

Smith, M.S. Program details of man-related flights (Ch.3). In: Soviet space programs, 1971-1975: Overview, facilities, and hardware, manned and unmanned flight programs, bioastronautics, civil and military applications, projections of future plans (Vol.1). Library of Congress, Science Policy Research Division, Congressional Research Service, Washington, D.C., 1976.

Smith, M.C., Jr., Rambaut, P.C., Vogel, J.M., and Whittle, M.W. Bone mineral measurement-experiment M078. In: Biomedical results from Skylab (NASA SP-377). Edited by Johnston, R.S., and Dietlein, L.F. U.S. Government Printing Office, Washington, D.C., 1977.

Soviet Aerospace. "Press Conference with Soyuz T-15/Mir/Salyut 7 Cosmonauts," Washington, D.C., August, 1986.

Soviet Aerospace. "Cosmonauts Rescue Kvant—Enter Module to Begin Work." Washington, D.C., 13 April 1987.

von Beckh, H.F. The space medicine branch of the aerospace medical association. Aviat., Space, and Envir. Med., 50(5):513-516, 1979.

Whedon, G.D., Lutwak, L., Rambaut, P.C., Whittle, M.W., Smith, M.C., Reid, J., Leach, C.S., Stadler, C.R., and Sanford, D.D. Mineral and nitrogen metabolic studies-experiment M071. In: Biomedical results from Skylab (NASA SP-377). Edited by Johnston, R.S., and Dietlein, L.F. U.S. Government Printing Office, Washington, D.C., 1977.

Whittle, M.W., Herron, R., and Cuźzi, J. Biostereometric analysis of body form. In: Biomedical results from Skylab (NASA SP-377). Edited by Johnston, R.S., and Dietlein, L.F. U.S. Government Printing Office, Washington, D.C., 1977.

Zemlya i Vselennaya, "A physician on the flight crew." 5:49-57, 1985.

THE SPACE ENVIRONMENT

section II

2 Orbital Flight

ARNAULD E. NICOGOSSIAN

D. STUART NACHTWEY

It is important that life scientists, just as astronomers and physical scientists, understand the nature of space. The continued success of manned space missions requires this understanding in order to properly design crew living quarters, personal protective systems, work procedures, and, indeed, all aspects of space systems which support human survival and performance.

For the foreseeable future, the U.S. space program calls for increasing manned missions. As the U.S. Space Station is developed, a larger force of space workers can follow a variety of pursuits, and crewmembers will remain in space for considerably longer periods. During the period of growth and change in manned space missions, there is one feature which will remain constant: all manned missions and activities in this century will most likely be undertaken in Earth orbit. Taking a longer-range view, however, it seems inevitable that man will eventually return to the Moon and visit more distant parts of the solar system. Therefore, it is important for practitioners of space medicine to understand the environment of orbital space,

and begin to consider interplanetary environmental issues as planning begins for 21st century missions.

TRANSITION TO NEAR-EARTH ORBITAL SPACE

The gaseous envelope that forms our atmosphere is acted upon principally by two forces: the terrestrial gravitational force that binds it to Earth, and solar thermal radiation, which causes its gases to tend to expand into near-Earth space. Because these two forces are in relatively constant balance, the atmosphere exhibits a distinct vertical profile of density and pressure. As distance from Earth increases, the density of the gaseous medium decreases (Figure 2-1). The border of the **atmosphere** is defined as the point where collisions between air molecules become immeasurably infrequent (about 700 km above the Earth's surface). Above this level is the **exosphere,** a zone of free-moving air particles that gradually thins out into true space. Even

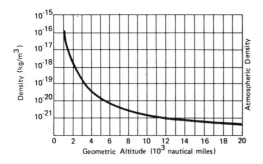

Figure 2-1. Atmospheric density as a function of altitude. The rapid decrease in density is correlated with decreases in atmospheric pressure and partial pressure of oxygen. (Adapted from Air Force Surveys in Geophysics).

in space, however, the density of gas particles is about 1–10 particles per cubic centimeter.

The transition zone from the atmosphere to space contains two points of particular interest for spacecraft design. At an altitude of approximately 80 km, the so-called von Karman line is encountered. This is the maximum altitude at which aircraft control surfaces are aerodynamically effective. Above this line, orientation of space vehicles is controlled by reaction jets. At about 180 to 200 km, air resistance

becomes insignificant; this is considered to be the mechanical border between the atmosphere and space. These and other significant transition altitudes are shown in Table 2-1.

Manned flight in near-Earth orbit takes place at altitudes on the order of 240 to 500 km, below the region defined as "true space." However, even at these altitudes a space vehicle is well beyond the functional limits of the atmosphere. Designers of manned space vehicles must account for the new operating environment (weightlessness), the lack of a life-supporting atmosphere, and specific problems such as radiation and the danger of collision with small objects (micrometeoroids, space debris).

FORCE FIELDS

The inertial or rotational forces acting on an astronaut in space are a key feature of this environment, since these forces can affect productivity, health, and even compromise survival. Two kinds of issues must

TABLE 2-1

SIGNIFICANT ALTITUDES IN THE TRANSITION FROM THE EARTH'S ATMOSPHERE TO SPACE

Boundaries	Approximate Altitude		
	(km)*	(St mi)[†]	(Naut mi)[§]
Oxygen limit—maximum altitude for sustained O_2 breathing through a pressure mask	13	8	7
Tropopause—upper limit for most atmospheric weather effects	15	9	8
Physiological limit—space suit or cabin a requirement for protection of human body	20	12	11
Von Karman line—aerodynamic control no longer effective	80	50	43
Mechanical boundary—air resistance becomes negligible	200	125	108
Collision limit—"space vacuum" achieved with essentially no collisions between air molecules	700	435	378

* Kilometers   [†] Statute miles   [§] Nautical miles.

be considered with respect to the force environment encountered in an orbital mission. The first is the acceleration or deceleration experienced as a space vehicle is launched or reenters the atmosphere at the completion of a mission. The second is the absence of the normal gravitational force. This loss of gravity, or "weightlessness," occurs when the gravitational force vector is exactly counterbalanced by the centrifugal force imparted to a spacecraft as it travels tangentially to the Earth's surface.

Launch and reentry acceleration forces in space flight have been well within the tolerance limits established for healthy, well-conditioned subjects. Indeed, as new craft are developed, imposed acceleration loads have decreased. Figure 2-2 shows the acceleration profile during the launch phase of a manned flight in the Mercury Program, where for a brief period acceleration reached an 8 G_x value (chest to back). Reentry forces also were high, reaching a value greater than 6 G_x during the peak period of deceleration during atmospheric reentry. These values contrast with those experienced during Space Shuttle missions. Measures taken during the launch of the first Space Shuttle orbital

mission (STS-1) showed an acceleration profile typical of previous spacecraft launches, but with a maximum of only +3.4 G_x. The programmed reentry profile, with acceleration forces acting on a different line due to the changed orientation during reentry (Figures 2-3 and 2-4), shows only nominal forces of +1.2 G_z (head to foot). While these forces are considerably less than those for earlier missions, they operate over a much longer period of time (17-20 minutes), and this has significant implications for the cardiovascular system.

ZERO GRAVITY

The most striking environmental feature of orbital flight is weightlessness. Living and working in an environment in which there is no gravity is an experience characterized by its novelty, but one with a broad range of important medical and behavioral consequences. The novelty aspects are apparent in Figure 2-5, in which two Skylab astronauts illustrate the ease with which heavy objects can be manipulated in weightlessness.

The dynamics of human evolution have been continuously shaped by the pervasive one-gravity force. Every conscious movement is made in a manner which accounts for gravity. Even a simple motor act such as leaning forward involves a number of muscle systems which control the movement of the body as the center of the gravitational effect also moves. Ordinarily, these highly skilled acts require no conscious thought. On exposure to weightlessness, however, each movement and act is subject to the implications of the new environment, and a period of relearning is required. Fortunately, problems of relearning have not proven as difficult as some predicted. Dr. Joseph Kerwin, in recounting his experience as a Skylab 2

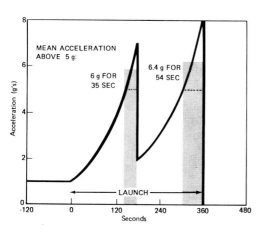

Figure 2-2. Acceleration profile of launch phase of the manned Mercury-Atlas 6 orbital flight. (Waligora, 1979).

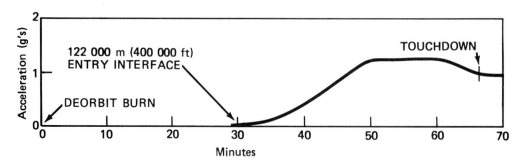

Figure 2-3. Acceleration profile of the Space Shuttle vehicle as a function of time. (Waligora, 1979).

crewmember, noted that "the primary theme was one of pleasant surprise at all the things that didn't change, at all the things that were pleasant and easy to do" (Kerwin, 1977).

Following whatever relearning is necessary, the zero-gravity environment can be employed in a beneficial manner. Berry (1971), summarizing the early Apollo experiences, noted that the absence of gravity could represent a bonus for locomotion, since motion requires much less work than on Earth. Movement is accomplished with

minimal effort, frequently in a swimming manner. Acrobatic maneuvers, such as rolling, tumbling, and spinning, are performed with ease. Additionally, inflight activities frequently are aided by the easy capability to impart minimal velocities to objects to be moved.

Effects of the zero-gravity environment on the physiological function of major body systems are less obvious, but of greater medical consequence. On entry into space, there is an immediate redistribution of body fluids. The function of the

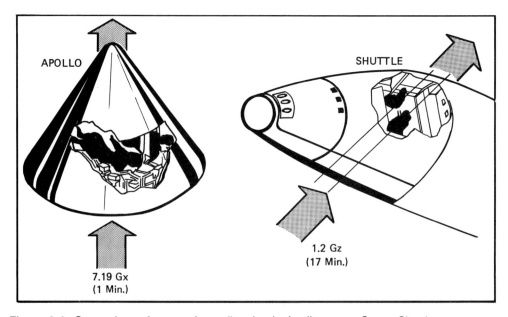

Figure 2-4. Comparison of reentry force direction in Apollo versus Space Shuttle.

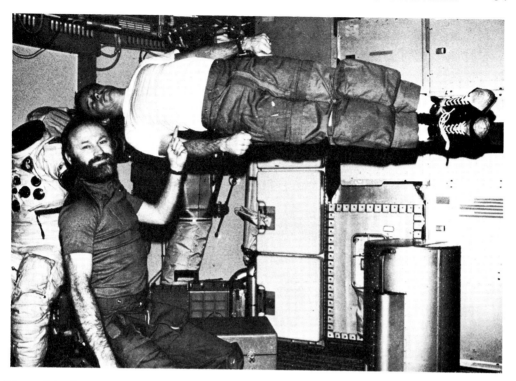

Figure 2-5. Skylab 4 astronauts demonstrate the effect of zero gravity on weight.

vestibular system, which is uniquely sensitive to gravity, is disturbed. Other systems begin a slow process of adaptation to the altered environment. For example, the cardiovascular system adjusts to a new set point in which the demands placed on it are greatly decreased. The result is a system which functions appropriately for life in weightlessness but, having become "deconditioned" by Earth standards, encounters real difficulty in the sudden readjustment to one gravity. Later chapters in this book address in detail the physiological changes brought about by long-term exposure to zero gravity.

MICROMETEOROIDS

A number of solid objects (meteoroids) regularly penetrate the orbital environment of the Earth. Meteors, or "shooting stars," appear on occasion as long streaks in the sky. These objects are heated to incandescence by friction with the atmosphere. Remnants of meteoroids that survive the passage through the atmosphere are called meteorites or micrometeorites. Micrometeorites account for most of the extraterrestrial material reaching the Earth's surface, estimated at 10,000 metric tons per day. Meteorites are of three general classes: irons—composed of 98 percent or more of nickel-iron; stoney-irons—composed of equal portions of nickel-iron and a mineral known as olivine; and stone. Sixty-one percent of meteorites are stone, 35 percent iron, and 4 percent mixed (Lundquist, 1979).

The terms "meteoroid" and "micrometeoroid" describe the individual solid objects found in interplanetary space. Micrometeoroids are often referred to as interplanetary dust particles.

The extent to which micrometeoroids represent hazards for manned space flight is not completely known. Therefore, all missions have included some means of protection for crewmembers. In some instances, protection has been provided through the shielding afforded by the spacecraft itself. During the Apollo Program, astronauts who were scheduled for periods on the lunar surface were provided with an integrated thermal micrometeoroid garment (Carson et al., 1975), a lightweight multilaminant assembly that covered the torso-limb suit assembly. Materials such as rubber-coated nylon, aluminized mylar, dacron, and teflon-coated filament Beta cloth provided the required protection. No instances of significant damage by micrometeoroids were reported during the many hours spent in lunar exploration or extravehicular activities.

The Skylab Program presented an opportunity to obtain measures over an extended period of the extent of micrometeoroids in orbital space. Since a number of these objects were expected to strike Skylab, an experiment was developed in which thin foils and polished metal plates were exposed on the exterior of the vehicle to record penetrations by micrometeoroids (Lundquist, 1979). On return to Earth, the exposed materials were studied with optical and scanning electron microscopes at magnifications of 200X and 500X. Table 2-2 shows the results of these analyses. Since the exposed plates were located at

TABLE 2-2

MICROMETEOROID IMPACTS
RECORDED DURING SKYLAB
EXPERIMENTS (EXPOSED AREA
$= 1200$ CM^2)

Sample Period	No. of Impacts
1–34 days	23
2–46 days	17
3–34 days	21

Lundquist, 1979

different positions and orientations, these figures represent an approximation of the micrometeoroid flux in orbit.

The size of the impact craters measured in the Skylab experiment showed all of the impacting particles to be quite small, with one believed to have been between 0.1 and 0.2 mm in diameter. The particles did have considerable power, as indicated by craters measured in the stainless steel surface. However, even though Skylab's micrometeoroid shield was lost during launch, the Orbital Workshop's wall, 3.18 mm thick, was not penetrated. There appears to be little if any meteoroid hazard to spacecraft in orbit with an exterior of such thickness.

SPACE DEBRIS

The abundance of space debris was unknown prior to 1957, because man had not yet ventured into Earth orbit. However, many satellites were launched in the decades that followed, and material began to collect in low Earth orbit. The amount of space debris is far greater than the meteoroid material below 2000 kilometers altitude (200 kilograms for meteoroids; 2,000,000 kilograms for space debris). Unlike meteoroids, which decrease in number exponentially with increasing size, significant space debris mass is concentrated in objects several meters in diameter (Space Station Program Office, 1986).

It is not obvious that objects at the same orbital inclination pose a danger, since the differential velocity should be minor. However, over the years, debris has spread uniformly over longitude due to even small differences in orbital period or inclination, and thus can possess large differential velocity even at the same inclination.

The North American Air Defense Command (NORAD) has tracked a total of 15,000 objects in the last few decades. Over 6,000 objects remain in low Earth orbit. The remainder deorbit due to atmospheric drag. However, the NORAD tracking system can only track objects larger than 10-20 centimeters, so smaller objects, which could be very large meteoroids, are not detected.

Figure 2-6 shows a comparison of the projected space debris flux and the meteoroid flux. This projected flux is based on NORAD measurements (sizes larger than 10 centimeters), telescope measurements (sizes larger than 1 centimeter), and

spacecraft impact measurements (sizes smaller than 0.02 centimeters), as well as projected growth rates. The average debris impact velocity is 10 kilometers per second, and mass densities are approximately equivalent to that of aluminum (2.8 gm/cm^3) for sizes smaller than 1 centimeter.

New studies of impact on returned spacecraft, such as panels from Solar Max, indicate that at sizes below 0.05 centimeters space debris such as paint flakes or aluminum oxide particles from rocket fuel comprises more than half of the impacts. This indicates that space debris may follow a curve similar to meteoroids below 1 millimeter in diameter, and that the flux shown in Figure 2-6 may need to be increased by about a factor of 10 for sizes smaller than 0.01 centimeter. This should be considered in spacecraft design studies.

Steps have been taken in the design of recent spacecraft to minimize the space debris hazard. For example, unused rocket fuel in booster rockets is burned, so that it will not explode later and create debris.

It is plausible to expect that by the year 1990 space debris will be dominant by at least a factor of 10 over the natural meteoroid flux in the millimeter and larger sizes.

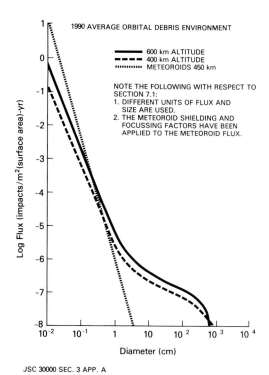

JSC 30000 SEC. 3 APP. A

Figure 2-6. Meteoroids and 1990 average environment of orbital debris. (Space Station Program Office, 1986).

RADIATION

The vacuum of space, while more perfect than any vacuum that can be achieved on Earth, nonetheless contains a great deal of matter which is of interest to planners of space missions. Biomedical scientists are particularly concerned with ionizing radiation which, when absorbed in a living cell, ionizes atoms or molecules and may result in cell death, a change in the cell leading to cancer, or other changes manifesting years after original exposure. Table 2-3 lists the ionizing radiation of concern during space flight.

Radiation encountered during orbital flight can be classed as primary galactic cosmic radiation, geomagnetically trapped radiation (Van Allen belts), and solar particle event radiation due to solar flares (Warren and Grahn, 1973). The latter two classes are important factors in determining schedules and trajectories for orbital flights. Anticipated radiation levels are always taken into account prior to a mission.

Earth's atmosphere and magnetic field shield man from virtually all types of radiation which could be damaging during space flight. In the electromagnetic spectrum, there are only two "windows" which allow radiation from the sun and deep space to penetrate to the Earth's surface. One permits the entry of visible light and portions of the ultraviolet and infrared frequencies. The other permits entry of radio frequencies of approximately 109 Hz (Olson and McCarson, 1974). All other radiation is effectively blocked. The protection afforded Earth's inhabitants means that most of the knowledge gained concerning space radiation has come from space missions and probes flown during the past 30 years.

GALACTIC COSMIC RADIATION

Galactic cosmic radiation (GCR) consists of particles which originate outside the solar system, probably resulting from earlier cataclysmic astronomical events such as the supernova explosion witnessed by Chinese astronomers in the year 1054 A.D. Measurements from space probes show that GCR particles consist of 87 percent protons (hydrogen nuclei), 12 percent alpha particles (helium nuclei), and 1 percent heavier nuclei ranging from lithium to tin. Individual particle energies are extremely high, in some instances up to 10^{19} electron volts. The high particle energies mean that GCR particles, though of very low flux density, are virtually unstoppable by passive shielding. At present, principal interest is focused on determining the extent to which periodic or continuous exposure to GCR might affect career limits for space workers.

TRAPPED RADIATION

A project team led by Dr. James Van Allen of the University of Iowa conducted experiments in 1958 in the U.S. Explorer satellite series in which they discovered the

TABLE 2-3

IONIZING RADIATION IN SPACE

Name	Charge (Z)	Location
X-rays	0	Radiation belts, solar radiation and in the secondaries from
Gamma rays	0	nuclear reactions, and by stopping electrons
Electrons	1	Radiation belts
Protons	1	Cosmic rays, inner radiation belts, solar cosmic rays
Neutrons	0	Produced by nuclear interactions; found near the planets, sun, and other matter
Alpha particles	2	Cosmic rays, solar particle events
Heavy ions	>3	Cosmic rays

Adapted from Johnson and Holbrow, 1977.

existence of bands of geomagnetically trapped particles encircling the Earth. Electrons and protons of the solar wind are trapped by the Earth's magnetic field, leading to a period of oscillation along the lines of magnetic force. The trapped particles follow the magnetic field completely around the Earth (Figure 2-7).

There are two portions to the Van Allen belts, with effects evident at altitudes as high as 55,000 kilometers. The inner belt begins at an altitude of roughly 300 to 1,200 kilometers, depending on latitude. The outer belt begins at about 10,000 kilometers, with its upper boundary dependent upon solar activity.

In the low Earth orbits of Space Shuttle missions, radiation doses from the Van Allen belts are low. However, there is an irregularity in the Earth's geomagnetic field in the southern hemisphere, known as the South Atlantic Anomaly, which extends from about zero to 60 degrees west longitude and 20 to 50 degrees south latitude. In this region, trapped proton intensity for energies more than 30 MeV is the equivalent at 160-320 kilometers altitude to that at 1,300 kilometers altitude elsewhere (Warren and Grahn, 1973). Almost all radiation received by Space Shuttle crews in a low-Earth, low-inclination orbit would result from passes through the South Atlantic Anomaly. With the $28\frac{1}{2}°$ orbit used for most Shuttle flights, about six orbital rotations per day pass through the South Atlantic Anomaly, while about nine per day do not. On these nine, there is essentially no radiation exposure. Extravehicular activities thus can be scheduled at a time in the orbital trajectory when radiation will not pose a problem.

SOLAR PARTICLE EVENTS

Solar particle events (SPE), which sometimes accompany solar flares, are possibly the most potent of the radiation hazards. The sun follows approximately an 11-year cycle of activity. When activity peaks, disturbances on the surface of the sun can be spectacular, as seen in Figure 2-8. Solar

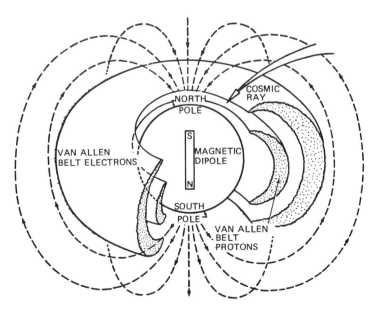

Figure 2-7. Solar wind electrons and protons are trapped by the Earth's magnetic field, forming the Van Allen belts.

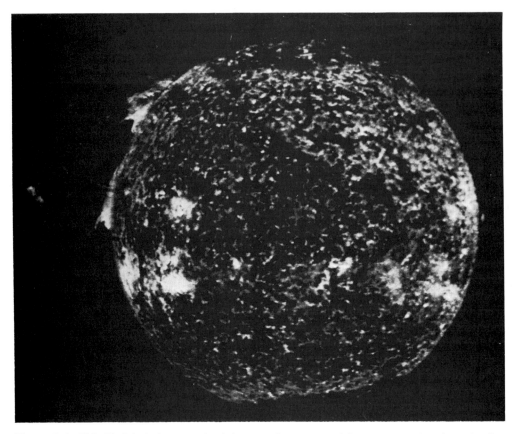

Figure 2-8. This Skylab 4 photograph of the sun shows one of the most spectacular solar flares ever recorded (upper left).

flares result from solar magnetic storms, which build up over several hours and persist for several days. While their occurrence cannot be forecast, buildup can be detected. As the flare builds, there are increases in visible light, X-rays, and radio-frequency radiation. The principal problem, however, is with the high-energy protons ejected from the sun toward Earth. These protons are further energized by interaction with the sun's magnetic field, so that by the time the "cloud" reaches Earth's vicinity, the energy ranges from about 10 MeV to about 500 MeV (Olson and McCarson, 1974). The flux also may be quite high.

The largest solar flares appear to occur either just before the peak of a sunspot cycle or on the downward limb of the measured solar activity. Figure 2-9 shows the correspondence between high-energy protons, measured from Earth, and solar activity as reflected in number of sunspots. Note that the largest proton flux yet recorded occurred in August 1972, during a period of decline of solar activity. This would have represented a particularly dangerous time for the conduct of extra-vehicular activity, with a real possibility of an astronaut receiving a lethal dose. However, at low-inclination, low-Earth orbits, the geomagnetic field protects space

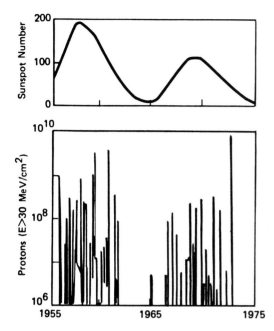

Figure 2-9. Increases in sunspot activity (top) produce corresponding increases in solar flare proton flux (bottom) (From Nachtwey, 1982).

crews; the August 1972 event would not be detectable at 28½° orbit.

NEUTRON FLUX

Skylab provided an opportunity to evaluate yet another radiation hazard in space, the energetic neutron. Neutrons were known as one component of space radiation before Skylab, but their magnitude and, in particular, their source were not well understood. Neutrons are of biomedical importance because, upon colliding with a hydrogen nucleus (a proton), there is a high probability of energy exchange (Lundquist, 1979). Since the human body contains an abundance of hydrogen-rich compounds such as protein, fat, and especially water, neutron exposure could cause considerable damage. It is therefore necessary to understand ambient neutron flux within a space vehicle.

It is known that free neutrons are not stable. With a half-life of 11 minutes, neutrons decay into a proton and an electron. This means that neutrons detected in a space vehicle must be generated either within the spacecraft or within the Earth's atmosphere, and must represent products of nuclear reactions caused by strikes of primary radiation. Skylab measurements showed that neutron flux within a spacecraft is higher than had been predicted. This flux was too high to be attributed to solar neutrons, Earth albedo neutrons, or even neutrons induced by cosmic rays in Skylab materials (Lundquist, 1979). It was concluded that the neutrons were produced through bombardment of spacecraft material by trapped protons in the Van Allen belt. However, the flux level was not high enough to be considered a biological hazard for crewmembers.

REFERENCES

Air Force Surveys in Geophysics, AFCRL, No. 115, August, 1959.

Berry, C.A. Biomedical findings on American astronauts participating in space missions: Man's adaptation to weightlessness. Paper presented at the Fourth International Symposium on Basic Environmental Problems of Man in Space, Yerevan, Armenia, U.S.S.R., 1–5 October 1971.

Carson, M.A., Rouen, M.N., Lutz, C.C., and McBarron, J.W., II. Extravehicular mobility unit. In: Biomedical results of Apollo (NASA SP-368). Edited by R.S. Johnston, L.F. Dietlein, and C.A. Berry. U.S. Government Printing Office, Washington, D.C., 1975.

Johnson, R.D., and Holbrow, C. (Eds.). Space settlements—a design study (NASA SP-413). U.S. Government Printing Office, Washington, D.C., 1977.

Kerwin, J.P. Skylab 2 crew observations and summary. In: Biomedical results from Skylab (NASA SP-377). Edited by R.S. Johnston and L.F. Dietlein. U.S. Government Printing Office, Washington, D.C., 1977.

Lundquist, C.A. (Ed.). Skylab's astronomy and space sciences (NASA SP-404). U.S. Government Printing Office, Washington, D.C., 1979.

Nachtwey, S. Radiation exposure, detection, and protection. Paper presented at the 53rd Annual Scientific Meeting of the Aerospace Medical Association, Bal Harbour, FL, May 10–13, 1982.

Olson, R.E., and McCarson, R.D., Jr. (Eds.). Space handbook (Tenth Revision) (AU-18). Maxwell Air Force Base, AL, Air University Institute for Professional Development, July 1974.

Page, L.W., and Page, T. Apollo-Soyuz pamphlet no. 6: Cosmic ray dosage (9-part set). U.S. Government Printing Office, Washington, D.C., 1977.

Space Station Program Office. Natural environment definition for design. JSC 30000, sec. 3 App. A., 1986.

Waligora, J.M. Physical forces generating acceleration, vibration, and impact. In: The physiological basis for spacecraft environmental limits (NASA RP-1045). National Aeronautics and Space Administration, Scientific and Technical Information Branch, Washington, D.C., November 1979.

Warren, S., and Grahn, D. Ionizing radiation. In: Bioastronautics data book (2nd ed.) (NASA SP-3006). Edited by J.F. Parker, Jr., and V.R. West. U.S. Government Printing Office, Washington, D.C., 1973.

3 Manned Planetary Exploration

MICHAEL B. DUKE

The Apollo Program transformed Earth's moon from an object of astronomical interest to one directly accessible to human exploration and investigation. Subsequently, automated spacecraft missions to every major planet in the solar system have provided a level of understanding of those planets to some extent equivalent to our pre-Apollo understanding of the moon. The new photographs and remote sensing of chemical and physical characteristics of the planets constitute a rich base for the emerging science of planetology, which has as its objectives the understanding of the present physical and chemical state of the planets, the mechanisms that shaped their development, and the processes by which they originally came into existence as solid or gaseous bodies. The science of planetology now extends beyond the study of the nine planets to their satellites, asteroids, comets, and interplanetary dust.

Much remains to be learned about the moon and planets. Even now, after intense study of lunar samples and data from the Apollo experiments, there is no fully acceptable hypothesis for the origin of the moon. Intensive study of the planets by sophisticated spacecraft, detailed laboratory study of materials collected by automated probes, and, in some cases, human expeditions will be instrumental in achieving an understanding of the solar system's development and evolution, and resolving whether life is a phenomenon unique to Earth.

Often for reasons of cost, and because the environments of some planets are quite inhospitable to humans, much of the exploration of the solar system will be carried out by sophisticated probes. The unmanned planetary exploration program has provided enough information to allow speculation on the most suitable solar system targets for manned exploration. This chapter reviews current knowledge of the planets and considers the possibility of human exploration. This review is offered as a means of identifying problems that will have to be faced and solved, if the humanization of the solar system is to be undertaken.

At the current level of technological development, humans are limited to relatively brief sojourns beyond Earth's protective envelope of gravity and atmospheric shield against radiation. Humans have been to the moon, and missions approaching 1 year have been completed in low Earth orbit. Within the limitations and capabilities of the ballistic rockets that form the Space Transportation System, human crewmembers are probably limited to trips within the inner solar system (the moon, Mars, possibly Venus) within the next 25 years. Beyond that, development of new propulsion technology (such as nuclear electric propulsion), power sources (such as fusion reactors), shielding, and spacecraft life support capabilities (e.g., closed ecological life support systems and artificial gravity) may open the outer solar system to human expeditions. Human missions to the giant planets, or to the boundaries of the solar system, may become possible within the next 100 years.

THE MOON

The moon is the only extraterrestrial body to have been explored directly by man. Between 1969 and 1972, six Apollo missions transported 12 astronauts to the lunar surface, where they deployed instruments, explored the surface, and collected 380 kg of sample materials for study on Earth. Through orbital instruments, including cameras and sensors, the Lunar Orbiter Program and Apollo constructed a fair map of most of the lunar surface and a rudimentary picture of the chemical composition of about 20 percent of the area directly under the Apollo ground track. The polar regions of the moon remain poorly mapped, as do some portions of the lunar farside. During and following the Apollo explorations, the Soviet Union conducted lunar surface investigations with an automated roving vehicle and returned

small amounts of samples from three locations near the eastern rim of the lunar nearside.

Before Apollo, a wide range of views of the probable origin of the moon competed within the scientific community. Some considered the moon a well-preserved, pristine chunk of the matter that originally constituted the solar system. Others accepted the view that the moon was once a part of the Earth, spun off by tidal action when the planet was young and still hot. In fact, the moon has proven to be a world in its own right, with a unique history. Lunar samples revealed the close relationship of the moon and the Earth, consisting largely of the same elements, with the same isotopic ratios of important elements such as oxygen (the ratio of $^{16}O/^{17}O/^{18}O$ are identical for the two bodies, whereas the same ratios in all meteorites are different). However, the moon's composition is most like Earth's mantle, the portion outside the planet's core. Although spinning the moon off the Earth by tidal action could explain the compositional relationship, this explanation fails on dynamical grounds. A new hypothesis has taken hold in recent years (Hartmann, 1986), which states that the moon was the result of a major collision between the Earth and a body of the size of Mars after the Earth's core had separated from the mantle. This hypothesis is currently undergoing serious investigation, as it apparently accounts for all existing data on the chemical, physical, and geological characteristics of the moon.

The moon, shortly after it formed, was apparently molten throughout at least the uppermost several hundred kilometers. A lunar crust was formed by the flotation of less dense silicates toward the surface. During this time, much of the volatile material that may have been present initially was lost to space. Thus, the moon has virtually no atmosphere, and the rocks at the surface are free of volatile compounds, such as water. Small and large impacts cratered the moon's surface and created huge basins (the largest of these, Mare Imbrium, is about 1050 km in diameter) which were later filled by the volcanic rocks that form the dark lunar maria. Today, the moon appears to be a "dead" planet, with no observable internal volcanic activity and a lifeless surface where high-energy radiation from space maintains a sterile environment (Figure 3-1).

The issue of indigenous lunar life has been settled. No life forms were discovered in the lunar samples, despite intensive examination in a specially constructed Lunar Receiving Laboratory which served as a quarantine facility for lunar samples for the first three Apollo missions. When it was determined that lunar materials posed no threat to terrestrial life forms, the strict quarantine was discontinued for later missions (although additional tests for organically active materials continued). Highly sensitive analyses for organic compounds, such as amino acids, were conducted on special samples which had been protected from any possibility of terrestrial contamination. Small amounts of carbon, nitro-

gen, and hydrogen compounds formed from nuclei implanted by the solar wind were found in all lunar surface soil samples, but no evidence of indigenous complex organic compounds was discovered (Bibring et al., 1974). Even organic compounds known to survive in some meteorites were absent from the lunar soil.

The lunar surface has been bombarded throughout time by micrometeoroids, as well as cosmic rays. Most of the surface is covered by several meters of powdered soil. Astronaut David R. Scott (1973) observed that "a dark-grey moon dust—its consistency seems to be somewhere between coal dust and talcum powder—mantles virtually every physical feature of the lunar surface. Our boots sink gently into it as we walk; we leave sharply chiseled footprints" (Figure 3-2).

Although the moon has been more thoroughly studied than any planet except Earth, there is more to be learned not only about its origin, but the early history of planets, because the absence of a lunar atmosphere, hydrosphere, and plate tectonics has preserved early lunar features. The

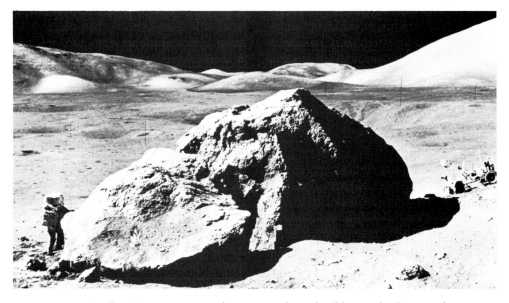

Figure 3-1. An Apollo 17 astronaut stands next to a huge boulder on the lunar surface.

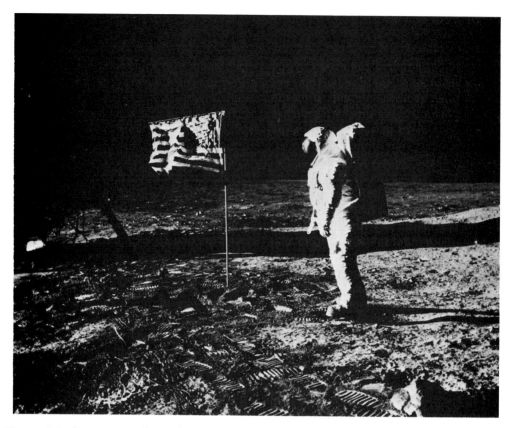

Figure 3-2. Astronaut on the surface of the moon, with the Lunar Module at the left.

youngest rocks on the moon were formed at a time before the oldest rocks found on Earth, providing a unique view into Earth's earliest history. The lunar surface layers contain evidence of crustal formation processes, and have retained a record of cosmic ray and asteroidal and cometary impact for the last 4 billion years, and possibly longer. This will provide an invaluable window into the moon's and the Earth's past, once the record is unraveled.

The next step will be to obtain a global map of the surface chemical composition, which can be achieved with instruments on board a polar orbiter spacecraft, and more detailed information on the moon's internal structure, obtained through seismometers and further experiments. Further lunar exploration may lead to the first permanent human outpost on another solar system body. A NASA Study Group (Johnson and Holbrow, 1977) concluded: "Space colonization appears to offer the promise of near limitless opportunities for human expansion, yielding new resources and enhancing human wealth. The opening of new frontiers, as it was done in the past, brings a rise in optimism to society." More recently, Mendell (1985) collected a large set of papers describing the benefits and significance of a permanent base on the moon.

Among the attractions of a lunar base, aside from scientific uses, is access to resources that can be used in space, with greatly reduced transportation cost due to the lower gravity field of the moon and the absence of an atmosphere, both of which make it easier to launch rockets from the lunar surface. The highest effectiveness is gained if all propellants can be manufactured from lunar materials (for example, cryogenic hydrogen and oxygen, or aluminum and oxygen), or if alternative means of propulsion which require no expendable propellants, such as electromagnetic launchers, can be developed (Arnold et al., 1979). Under these conditions, lunar materials should be deliverable for use in space for $\frac{1}{20}$ th or less than the energy and possibly the cost of the equivalent delivery from Earth. Thus, provision of bulk materials, such as liquid oxygen, for use in rocket systems, or materials for space construction or shielding could become a major activity of a lunar settlement (Duke et al., 1985). Essentially all of the common major elements on Earth—oxygen, silicon, aluminum, magnesium, iron, titanium—and most of the minor elements are present in lunar surface materials. Some of the latter may be found in concentrated deposits when lunar exploration is resumed. Except for iron, which exists in the metallic state in small amounts, extraction of metals and oxygen requires substantial quantities of energy. The volatile elements hydrogen, carbon, and nitrogen are rather scarce on the moon, contained primarily in the soil; however, they should be easily extracted by heat, and the total lunar inventory is substantial.

The principal hazard to the first lunar settlers, aside from the hard vacuum conditions, is the solar and galactic radiation flux. As the moon has no magnetic field, particulate radiation strikes the surface with unabated intensity. For extended stays, it will be necessary to provide habitats with shielding equivalent to about 2 meters of lunar soil, with adequate shelters to protect against solar particle events (flares). Settlers will also have to adapt to days and nights equivalent to 14 Earth days, and surface temperatures that range from as low as −178°C in the dark to 110°C

in direct sunlight. These restrictions, and the one-sixth gravity of the lunar surface, will control the architecture of lunar development. Clever engineering approaches will be necessary to develop self-sufficient and comfortable habitats. Nevertheless, the moon will be the testing ground for these new technologies, which will be needed elsewhere, for example on Mars. Humans cannot expect to gain footholds beyond Earth unless means of utilizing indigenous materials can be developed and conservation-minded approaches to scarce resources undertaken.

MERCURY

Of the other planets, Mercury, closest to the sun, seems most like the moon. Mariner 10 flew by the planet twice—in September 1974 and again 6 months later, obtaining images of approximately half its surface. These images showed a heavily cratered surface of lunar-like appearance (Figure 3-3). It is known that the bulk density of Mercury, however, is much higher than that of the moon, indicating a higher content of iron, possibly concentrated in a sizeable core. Like the moon, Mercury has essentially no atmosphere; however, recent telescopic studies indicate a tenuous, extended atmosphere containing sodium atoms (Potter and Morgan, 1985). Mercury's period of rotation on its axis is equivalent to 58.65 Earth days, and its period of revolution around the sun is 88 days, yielding a solar day on Mercury that is equal to 176 Earth days. During periods of illumination, the surface temperature rises as high as 690°C when Mercury is closest to the sun, while at Mercurian night the uppermost surface cools rapidly to about −180°C. The large difference in temperature between unlit and lit regions measured by Mariner 10 indicates low thermal conductivity on the surface. Like the moon, Mercury is prob-

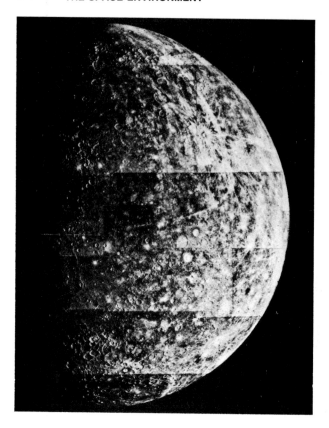

Figure 3-3. Mosaic of the planet Mercury, obtained by Mariner 10.

ably covered by a blanket of insulating silicate dust.

Whether humans will ever journey to Mercury is a matter for conjecture at this time. It is possible to envision a suitably protected installation which could house humans through the Mercurian night, although the temperature under the thermally insulating blanket of dust must remain in the vicinity of 150°C, even at night. There is currently no clear rationale for establishing a human presence on Mercury, although the association of material resources of the solid planet with the energy-rich environment of the near-sun region (solar radiation flux at Mercury is approximately 7 times that in the vicinity of Earth) may eventually attract development.

Exploration of Mercury has a modest scientific priority in NASA's planetary exploration program. The next step would be a long-duration Mercury polar orbiter, which would map the chemical composition of the planet, photograph the entire surface, determine the nature of the magnetic field and study its interaction with solar radiation. Instruments emplaced by automated landers could determine internal seismic activity, internal structure, and perhaps surface mineralogy, and provide important information on the evolution and present state of the planet. Currently, Mercury missions are on the limit of performance of space transportation technology, so further exploration will be dependent upon development of solar electrical propulsion, advanced propulsion technology, or clever orbital mechanics applications.

VENUS

Venus has been the target for more automated spacecraft missions than any other planet, for a variety of reasons. First, it is the nearest planet to Earth and more Earth-like in its bulk properties than any other. Its proximity (and associated relatively short mission duration) made it a logical early target, following the moon, for both U.S. and Soviet space programs. Venera 1 was launched by the Soviet Union in 1961 and passed within 100,000 km of the planet. Mariner 2 was flown by the United States in 1962, passing within 35,000 km of the planet, and was the first mission to return data from Venus. Although the Mariner program became more diverse in its objectives, the Soviet Union concentrated its efforts toward Venus, sending spacecraft at each opportunity starting in 1965. This concentrated effort probed the atmosphere, landed cameras and experiments on the surface, and obtained spectacular radar images of the planet. The U.S. explored Venus with Mariner 5 and Mariner 10 (which flew on to Mercury), and the Pioneer-Venus mission. In addition, orbits utilizing Venus gravity assists are important in conducting missions to other planets. The Soviet VEGA (Venus-Halley Comet mission) used a Venus swingby as part of its orbital mechanics, as did the later Phobos mission to Mars.

Venus is obscured by clouds, which have been shown to contain sulfuric acid aerosols suspended in an atmosphere largely composed of carbon dioxide. Water vapor, nitrogen, and sulfur dioxide have been detected in the atmosphere. Atmospheric pressure at the surface is equivalent to about 100 Earth atmospheres. Although the atmosphere of Venus reflects 75 percent of the incoming solar energy, the high carbon dioxide content traps essentially all the rest, bringing the temperature at ground level to approximately 500°C. The rotation of Venus on its axis is somewhat slower than that of its circuit around the sun, causing a retrograde rotation (sunrise in the west rather than the east). Equatorial winds are strong at high altitudes

(100 meters/second), but measured wind velocities are slight at the surface, on the order of 1 meter/second. The temperature difference between day and night at the planet's surface also appears to be slight. Lightning storms have been detected in the Venusian atmosphere and may contribute to the night glow observed with satellite instruments.

Pioneer Venus Radar Altimetry (Fimmel et al., 1983) discovered three classes of physiographic features on the Venusian surface—ancient crust (about 65 percent of the surface area) lying at intermediate elevations, relatively smooth lowland plains (about 25 percent of the surface area), and complex continental highlands (Figure 3-4). Plateaus and mountains are as high as those on Earth, but the lowlands are only one-fifth the maximum depth of the Earth's oceanic basins. Soviet orbital radar images are now filling in a picture which shows a complex and poorly understood surface structure. Current scientific opinion is that volcanic activity was important in shaping the continental masses, but that plate tectonics have not shaped the present surface morphology. The crust is quite rigid and supports the continental masses, suggesting that it is either quite thick, quite dry, or both.

The Soviet Venera spacecraft were the first to survive landing on the planet's surface. Venera 9 transmitted black and white photographs to Earth in 1975, showing a Venusian landscape with sharp rocks indicating little erosion. Since then, several landers have added imagery and compositional analyses of the surface, which indicate that basaltic volcanic rocks may underlie the landing sites. There has been speculation that active volcanism continues on Venus. Additional study of the solid body properties of Venus are planned by the U.S. in its Venus Radar Mapper Mission (Magellan), to be launched in 1989. The Soviet Union, in 1986, apparently turned away from Venus, to focus its future planetary program on Mars.

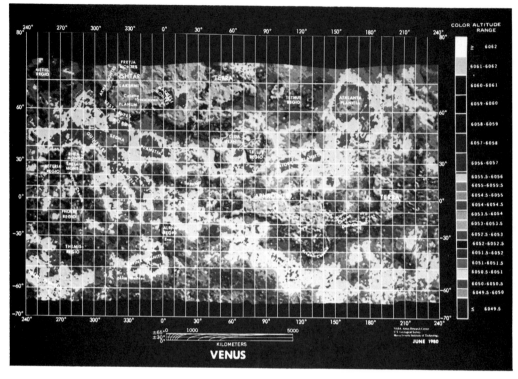

Figure 3-4. This global view of Venus was taken by the radar altimeter of the Pioneer-Venus spacecraft, so that the planet's cloud cover is eliminated. The large feature at the top of the picture is Venus' northern "continent," Ishtar.

Venus has no intrinsic magnetic field to shield it from the solar wind, which strikes the upper atmosphere unimpeded. There is an ionosphere, derived from the interaction of solar ultraviolet radiation with the atmosphere, which acts as an obstacle to the solar wind, and ends abruptly at an altitude of a few hundred kilometers. The induced magnetic field at this "ionopause" transmits solar wind pressure to the ionosphere, which causes the ionopause to move in and out according to the intensity of the solar wind, particularly to day/night fluctuations.

Venus is not expected to represent a target for manned missions, due to the high surface pressure and temperature. However, flybys of manned spacecraft are possible, because some trajectories from Earth to Mars use Venus swingbys to achieve the proper orbital characteristics. It would be possible for long-lived floating stations to exist in the atmosphere—such balloons have been developed by the French for Soviet Venus missions. Eventually, such floating facilities could perhaps become laboratories where initial experiments might investigate long-term modification of the atmosphere of the planet.

MARS

Throughout the past two centuries, the red planet has been a source of inspiration for astronomers and science fiction writers alike. Space age explorations, particularly Mariner 4, Mariner 9, and Viking, have shown Mars to be a dry and currently lifeless planet, with an intriguing geological past. Early spacecraft observations suggested a moon-like history of early crustal formation, followed by an intense impact bombardment. Subsequent data have shown that this history is much more complex. Huge shield volcanos, one as large as the state of New Mexico, are among the youngest features. Great chasms in the crust, within which Earth's Grand Canyon would practically disappear, testify to internal forces that wrenched the planet's crust in ancient times. In addition, many canyons and other sculpted features suggest past fluvial erosion, which raises questions about past climatic conditions, as the current atmospheric pressure is so low that liquid water would not be stable at the surface. Other features suggest widespread subsurface permafrost poleward of 30° latitudes. The polar caps consist of frozen carbon dioxide and water ice, and can be observed (from Earth) to migrate with the Martian seasons.

The U.S. Viking Program was a blend of science and advanced technology that for the first time carried an automated scientific laboratory to a soft landing on the surface of another planet. Viking 1 landed on Mars on July 20, 1976, and was followed by Viking 2 on September 3. These spacecraft traveled through space as a unit, separating in Mars orbit after appropriate landing sites had been selected. The orbiter then served as a scientific satellite and radio relay for data from the surface. Landing sites for Viking 1 and 2 were carefully chosen in the smoothest, least boulder-strewn areas that could be identified from orbital data. Despite this, it was seen that both had landed in boulder-strewn terrains (Figure 3-5) and a good deal of luck was involved in their safe descent to the surface. The Viking orbiters yielded many images of the planet's surface and, at the close of the mission, were lowered in altitude to obtain a small number of very-high-resolution pictures of the surface.

Mars, like Earth, has produced basaltic

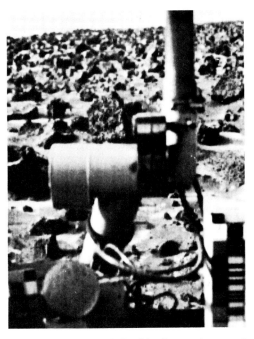

Figure 3-5. View of the Martian surface and sky taken by Viking 1. Color reconstruction showed that orange-red surface materials (probably iron oxides) overlie darker bedrock, and that the sky is pinkish-red.

volcanos, suggesting that volcanism is a general property of planets. The Viking experiments provided some information on the chemical properties of the Martian surface; however, an unknown portion of the material analyzed was ubiquitous surface dust. Deconvolution of compositional data suggests that the younger volcanics are composed of iron-rich basalts, similar to those found among the Shergottite meteorites. This finding reinforces recent investigations showing these meteorites to contain trapped gases similar to the Martian atmosphere composition determined by Viking. This has strengthened the hypothesis that the Shergottite meteorites are actually Martian rocks expelled by large impacts. The discovery in Antarctica of fragments of lunar rocks, which fell to Earth as meteorites, also supports that hypothesis.

The Martian atmosphere, in contrast to

that of Venus, is extremely thin, with surface pressures measured by Viking landers in the range from 6.5 to 7.5 millibars, less than one percent of the sea-level atmospheric pressure on Earth. Like Venus, the atmosphere is composed principally of carbon dioxide, with significant amounts of nitrogen, argon, neon, oxygen, and small amounts of water vapor. Mars rotates once on its axis in a little over one Earth day, and atmospheric circulation bears some resemblance to that of Earth. Viking photographed small clouds near the peaks of the highest volcanos and surface frosts in the vicinity of the landers. Dust storms have been known to exist for some time, and the Mariner 9 spacecraft which orbited Mars in late 1971 photographed a planet-wide dust storm that persisted for a 2-month period before the atmosphere cleared. Dust particles lifted by the thin Martian atmosphere must be quite small (a few microns) to be transported around the planet.

A prime objective of Viking was to search for evidence of life with three automated experiments in the Biology Instrument Package (Klein, 1977). These experiments did not detect any life forms. Instead, they demonstrated that the Martian soil contains highly reactive agents, possibly superoxides, which have apparently oxidized any organic materials. Most scientists are of the opinion that carbon-based life forms do not presently exist on Mars. However, evidence for the past presence of liquid water suggests that life could have developed earlier in Mars' history. The search for evidence of ancient life will be a significant part of future Mars missions.

Mars has two small satellites, Phobos and Deimos, which may be captured asteroids. They appear to be of rather low density, and their reflectance properties suggest that they may consist of materials like those in the carbonaceous meteorites. According to astronomical observations of asteroid reflectance spectra, similar materials are located in the outermost regions of the asteroid belt that lies beyond Mars.

Mars remains an attractive target for human exploration. Although distant, the planet contains the fundamental materials—water, oxygen, nitrogen, carbon—which, with appropriate controlled environment facilities, could sustain life. Because the thin atmosphere is insufficient to filter out high-energy cosmic radiation, long-term habitation would be largely underground. However, surface and immediate subsurface temperatures are moderate, and daytime surface activities should be sustainable. Although the solar energy flux is about one-fourth that at Earth's surface, sufficient solar energy may be available to support a human outpost. Studies have concluded that manned missions will be feasible toward the end of the 20th century; however, they will represent significant operational challenges, primarily because of the $2\frac{1}{2}$–3 years required for a round trip mission, and the cost of early missions will be quite high (Duke and Keaton, 1986). Nevertheless, the development of the indigenous resources of Mars and its satellites, Phobos and Deimos, could hasten the establishment of a permanently manned human outpost there, and an increase in Earth-Mars trips in the first or second quarter of the 21st century. In the meantime, automated spacecraft will continue to probe Mars and its moons. The Soviet Union plans a mission to Mars and Phobos in 1988, the U.S. will launch a Mars Orbiter (Mars Observer Mission) in 1990, and plans have been laid for the automated return of Martian samples in a mission to be carried out before the end of the 20th century.

ASTEROIDS

Between Mars and Jupiter lies the asteroid belt. Once thought to be remnants of a

isotope could be the fuel of choice for nuclear fusion reactors in the next century, but has not been considered due to its absence on Earth. It has been argued that ^{3}He from the moon, and later from Jupiter, could provide limitless energy for use in space and on Earth. As human trips to Jupiter may require both nuclear propulsion and nuclear power supplies, this may become a logical development objective. In the meantime, exploration of the Jupiter system will be carried out by automated spacecraft. The Galileo mission, a Jupiter orbiter and atmospheric probe, will be launched by the U.S. to continue this exploration.

SATURN

Saturn, a large "gaseous" planet like Jupiter, is distinguished by its rings, which are the most prominent of any in the solar system (Jupiter and Uranus also have thin rings). First discovered by Galileo, three distinct rings can be observed from Earth; however, it remained for Pioneer 11 (1979) and Voyagers 1 and 2 (1980–1981) to elucidate the complex ring structure and dynamics. These missions also carried out an intensive study of the planet and many of its satellites (Figure 3-7), and demonstrated that spacecraft could safely tra-

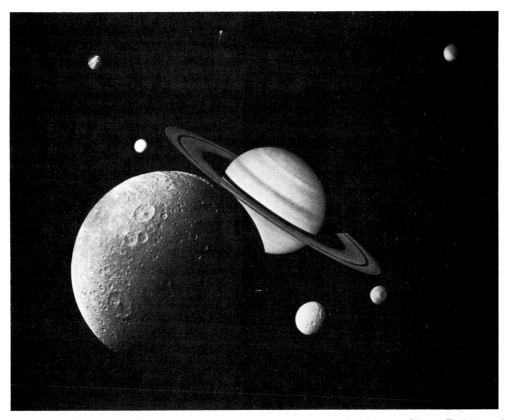

Figure 3-7. Montage of Saturn and its principal moons. In the forefront is Dione. Tethys and Mimas are at the right of Saturn, Enceladus and Rhea are off the rings to the left, and at the upper right is Titan.

verse the ring plane, which was a concern of mission planners.

Saturn's mass is 95 times that of Earth, and is largely composed of liquid molecular hydrogen and helium. A region of liquid metallic hydrogen may be present below this, and a solid rocky core may constitute 25 percent of the planet's mass (Ingersoll, 1981). Like Jupiter, Saturn apparently converts internal gravitational energy to heat, which flows toward the surface. Above the liquid surface, an atmosphere similar to that of Jupiter is present, containing dark belts, white-banded zones, and circulating storm regions. A red spot similar to Jupiter's and believed to be a manifestation of atmospheric convection is about 11,250 km in length, and appears to have long-term stability (Smith, 1980). Maximum wind speeds at the equator can reach 1,600 km/hr. Auroral emissions were observed near the poles, but no lightning has been detected.

The rings of Saturn are believed to consist of rocks and ice having the appearance of "dirty snowballs" (Smith, 1980). Particle sizes range from microns to meters. The well-known A, B, and C rings were found to consist of hundreds of ringlets, some of which are elliptical in shape. The F ring is more complex, and may consist of three interwoven rings bounded by two "shepherding" satellites. "Spokes" observed in the B ring may be due to fine electrically charged particles above the ring, perhaps resulting from lightning occurring in the ring. Within the ring system many small satellites have been observed, the most recent total rising to above 25. With the exception of Titan, all of Saturn's moons are covered with ice, probably water ice (Stone and Miner, 1981). The larger satellites show evidence of heavy cratering.

Voyager 1 passed within 7,000 km of Titan, the second largest moon in the solar system (behind Ganymede). It has a measurable atmosphere, found to consist largely of nitrogen, with lesser amounts of methane, ethane, acetylene, ethylene, and hydrogen cyanide. The atmosphere is three times as dense and ten times as deep as that of Earth. The atmosphere down to the planet's surface is quite cold, with a near-surface temperature of −182°C. The surface, which is not visible through the atmosphere, may be liquid methane or liquid nitrogen.

Saturn remains a major target for future solar system exploration. Many interesting questions persist about the properties of its atmosphere, interior, and rings, and Titan represents a unique solar system body that may have experienced internal evolution similar to that of the inner terrestrial planets. It is likely that only one more automated Saturn system mission will be possible in the remaining years of the 20th century. The mission most widely discussed is a Saturn orbiter/Titan probe, similar to the Galileo mission in its objectives. This has been considered as a possible collaborative mission between the U.S. and the European Space Agency, under the name Titan-Cassini. Manned missions must wait for the next century or beyond, depending on new developments in propulsion, power, and life support systems. Although farther from the sun than Jupiter, Saturn's radiation environment is much more benign. It may be the best location for an outer planet human outpost, from which important scientific observations can be made and interstellar flights launched or fueled.

URANUS

The Voyager 2 flyby in January 1986 found Uranus to be as fascinating and enigmatic as the other planets. In addition to the five previously known moons, Voyager 2 discovered 10 previously undetected satellites; two of them are shepherd satellites within a system of rings, which are darker than those of Jupiter and Saturn.

One of the newly discovered small satellites which was imaged at close range appeared irregular in shape and dark. Perhaps the surface is rich in carbonaceous materials, such as are believed to constitute comets and other primordial solar system material. The other new satellites, not observed closely, are also dark. The five previously known larger satellites are each unique, with different geological histories. All have an upper icy layer; however, underlying geologic activity is indicated by fault lines and other linear features. Impact craters have interplayed with the underlying activity and flowage within the ice layers to give each satellite a different appearance. The satellites appear to have larger ratios of rock to ice than would have been expected from previous solar system origin models.

The planet itself is a nearly featureless green ball, surrounded by an atmosphere principally consisting of hydrogen. The axis of rotation of Uranus lies nearly in the plane of its rotation around the sun, whereas the axes of the other planets are approximately perpendicular to their rotational planes and the ecliptic. The planet rotates on this axis every 17.24 hours. Voyager discerned clouds in the atmosphere, concentric around the south pole (which at this time is the sunward pole and in 44 years will point away from the sun). The winds blow from east to west, as they do on Venus, Earth, Jupiter and Saturn, and blow faster than the planet's rate of rotation. Uranus was also found to have an internal magnetic field which, unlike that of the Earth, is tilted markedly with respect to the axis of rotation. The explanation of this phenomenon is unclear.

COMETS AND INTERSTELLAR SPACE

The interstellar media consists largely of hydrogen and helium formed at the creation of the universe, some 13–15 billion years ago, and augmented by gas, dust, and energetic radiation produced in the processes of star formation and dispersed in supernovae. A wide variety of organic compounds has been detected primarily by radio wave observations. Complex molecules such as cyanogen and formaldehyde have also been detected, which are of interest as possible precursors of living matter. Portions of the interstellar media are in the form of dust particles, characterized by infrared spectral observations. Perhaps some of these interstellar particles are constituents of comets, which represent primordial matter that formed on the boundary of the solar system. Others surely entered the solar system, where it is conceivable that large dust detectors perhaps deployed on the Space Station will one day distinguish and characterize them with respect to the solar system dust background.

The study of presolar materials has been invigorated by the discovery of peculiar isotopic anomalies in certain primitive meteorites such as the Allende carbonaceous chondrite. These isotopic effects are interpreted by some to be the result of the injection of supernova materials into the solar system at the time of initial condensation of its matter. Because tentative evidence links carbonaceous chondrites to comets, there is much interest in the possibility of further comet missions. The successful investigations of Comet Halley by the U.S.S.R. VEGA and the ESA Giotto missions in 1986 provided the bases for the proposed U.S. Comet Rendezvous Asteroid Flyby mission, which could be carried out in the 1990's, and a subsequent Comet Sample Return mission, which may be possible in the late 1990's.

Another research effort currently taking shape is the study of planets around other stars, made possible by advances in astrometry. Within the next 10 years, it should become possible, using a Space Station astrometric telescope, to distinguish Jupiter-sized and perhaps smaller planets around the sun's nearest neighbors in the galaxy.

Finally, serious efforts are underway in NASA's Search for Extraterrestrial Intelligence (SETI) Project to determine whether coherent radio signals emanate from other solar systems, signals that might indicate the presence of intelligent life. There are a large number of potential abodes for life in the universe, and current investigations may be able to place limits on the possible distribution of life in the galaxy.

These and other future investigations will be aimed at determining humanity's place in the cosmos. Positive results from the astrometry or SETI programs could provide new impetus to future interstellar travel. This would be a very long-term goal for humanity, as it would require acceleration to high velocities and very long trip times. Hazards of the interstellar media would have to be countered and new levels of system autonomy and reliability would have to be achieved. However, the initial tentative explorations of the 20th century will pave the way for future, grander human missions.

REFERENCES

Arnold, W.H., Bowen, S., Fine, K., Kaplan, D., Kolm, M., Kolm, H., Newman, J., O'Neill, G.K., and Snow, W.R. Mass Drivers I: Electrical Design. Space Resources and Space Settlements (NASA SP-428). Edited by Billingham, J. and Gilbreath, W. U.S. Government Printing Office, Washington, D.C. pp. 87–100, 1979.

Bibring, J.P., Burlingame, A.L., Chaumont, J., Langevin, Y., Maurette, M. and Wszolek, P. Simulation of lunar carbon chemistry: I. Solar wind contribution: Proc. Fifth Lunar Conference, Geochim. et Cosmochim. Acta, Supplement 5, 2:1747–1762, 1974.

Duke, M.B. and Keaton, P.W. Manned Mars Missions (NASA M-001), Marshall Space Flight Center, Huntsville, AL, 1986.

Duke, M.B., Mendell, W.W., and Roberts, B.B. Toward a Lunar Base Programme, Space Policy, 1(1):49–61.

Fimmel, R.O., Colin, L., and Burgess, E. Pioneer Venus, (NASA SP-461), U.S. Government Printing Office, Washington, D.C., 1983.

Gaffey, M.J., Helin, E.F., and O'Leary, B. An Assessment of Near-Earth Asteroid Resources. In: Space Resources and Space Settlements, (NASA SP-428). Edited by Billingham, J. and Gilbreath, W. U.S. Government Printing Office, Washington, D.C. pp. 191–204, 1979.

Hartmann, W.K. moon origin: The impact-trigger hypothesis. In: Origin of the moon. Edited by Hartmann, W.K., Phillips, R.J., and Taylor, G.J. Lunar and Planetary Institute, Houston, TX, pp. 579–608, 1986.

Ingersoll, A.P. Jupiter and Saturn. Scientific American, 245(6):90–108, 1981.

Johnson, R.D., and Holbrow, C. Space Settlements—A Design Study (NASA SP-413), U.S. Government Printing Office, Washington, D.C., 1977.

Klein, H.P. The Viking Biological Investigation: General Jour. Geographical Res., (82)28:4677–4680, 1977.

Mendell, W. Lunar Bases and Space Activities of the 21st Century. Lunar and Planetary Institute, Houston, TX, 1985.

Morrison, D., and Samz, J. Voyager to Jupiter (NASA SP-439), U.S. Government Printing Office, Washington, D.C., 1980.

Potter, A. and Morgan, T. Discovery of Sodium in the Atmosphere of Mercury. Science (229): 651–653, 1985.

Scott, D.R. What is it like to walk on the moon? National Geographic, 144(3):326–329, 1973.

Shoemaker, E.M., and Helin, E.F. Populations of Planet-Crossing Asteroids and the Relation of Apollo Objects to Main-Belt Asteroids and Comets. Internat. Astron. Union Trans. Colloq. 39, 1977.

Smith, B.A. Voyager 1 finds answers, new riddles. Aviation Week and Space Technology, 133(2):16–20, 1980.

Stone, E.C., and Miner, E.D. Voyager 1 encounter with the Saturnian System. Science, 212(4491):159–162, 1981.

Wittenberg, L.J., Santarius, J.F., and Kulcinski, G.L. Lunar Source of ^{3}He for Commercial Fusion Power, Fusion Technology, 10(2), 1986.

SPACE
FLIGHT
SYSTEMS
AND
PROCEDURES

section III

4 Space Vehicles for Manned Programs

ARNAULD E. NICOGOSSIAN
JAMES F. PARKER, JR.
VICTORIA GARSHNEK

THE UNITED STATES

During the first two decades of manned space flight, the vehicles designed to house and protect astronauts during their ventures into space basically followed a linear course of development. From the conical "tin can" of Project Mercury, through the Gemini program, and over the course of the Apollo and Skylab missions, the external configuration of the manned vehicle changed little. However, internal configuration and systems design were altered, often considerably, to accommodate increasing mission complexity, duration, crew size, and changing objectives. These changes were essentially elaborations upon the basic requirements for life support and instrumentation necessary for spacecraft control and task performance. Apart from the Skylab Orbital Workshop, which was designed for habitation rather than transportation, it was not until the advent of the Space Shuttle that American space vehicles underwent a fundamental change in design and appearance. The following discussion reviews the design of these spacecraft and the philosophy underlying their development.

PROJECT MERCURY

In the late 1950's, U.S. leaders attached great importance to the inception of a manned space flight program. Accordingly, the approach taken in Mercury was to use existing technology and off-the-shelf equipment in conjunction with the simplest design that would be reliable. All systems would be automated, with the astronaut functioning primarily as an observer and backup operator should manual control become necessary. The design requirements for the Mercury craft (Smith, 1981) were:

- An escape system which would separate the spacecraft from the launch vehicle in the event of a prelaunch emergency
- Drag braking for reentry
- A retrorocket system for deorbit
- A water landing and recovery capability
- Provisions for manual control of spacecraft attitude by the pilot.

Figure 4-1 (Grimwood, 1963) shows the configuration of the spacecraft and escape system. The escape system was positioned over the manned capsule at launch, as shown at left in the figure. In the event of a prelaunch emergency, the escape rocket would propel the capsule away from the launch site; shortly thereafter, a tower jettison rocket would detach it from the capsule. The actual spacecraft is shown at right in Figure 4-1 and includes an an-

tenna can, a recovery compartment containing the descent parachute system, and the habitable capsule. At the base of the capsule was a retropack containing rockets for separating the spacecraft from the actual launch vehicle and retrorockets for deorbit. This retropack was jettisoned just prior to reentry.

The bottom of the cone was covered with a beryllium heat shield for the suborbital Mercury flights, and ablating fiberglass for the orbital flights. Inside the capsule, the astronaut sat upright in a couch (Figure 4-2), facing the central section of a three-piece instrument panel and a trapezoidal window. The bottom portion of the panel contained a periscope for direct observation of the Earth. Power was supplied by six batteries with 24 V DC output.

Although the Mercury spacecraft could not change its orbit, provision was made for attitude control. Of the four attitude

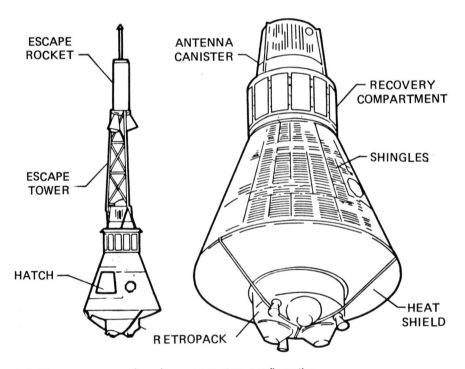

Figure 4-1. Mercury spacecraft and escape system configuration.

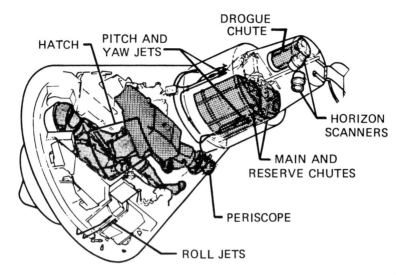

Figure 4-2. Mercury spacecraft interior layout.

control modes tested by Mercury astronauts, the most successful and frequently used was manual fly-by-wire (FBW). A three-axis control stick was located at the astronaut's right hand.

During descent, a drogue parachute was deployed at 6,700 meters for deceleration, followed by deployment of the main chute at 3,300 meters. The G-forces at splashdown were greatly reduced by a "landing-shock attenuation system" consisting of a fiberglass cushion which was inflated with air during descent.

The first two manned flights in the Mercury program were suborbital. The only significant mishap was the loss of the Mercury capsule "Liberty Bell 7" after splashdown: when a hatch blew prematurely, the vehicle filled with water and sank. The astronaut, however, was unharmed. Subsequently, four orbital missions were successfully flown, culminating in 23 orbits and a maximum mission duration of over 34 hours. During three missions, manual control of spacecraft attitude in orbit and during reentry was critical to mission success.

GEMINI PROGRAM

The Gemini Program was undertaken to extend American manned space flight capabilities in anticipation of a lunar landing (achieved in the follow-on Apollo Program). Therefore, Gemini's two most important objectives were: (1) to extend mission duration and (2) to develop and practice techniques and procedures necessary for rendezvous and docking. Secondary objectives were to precisely control reentry and landing, gain experience in extravehicular activity (EVA), and improve the proficiency of flight crew and ground control operations (Smith, 1981).

The Gemini capsule was a logical successor to that of Mercury. There were two primary functional differences: the Gemini capsule was designed to carry two astronauts, rather than one, and greatly emphasized crew control over automated systems. Care was taken to ease spacecraft maintenance, in anticipation of multiple launches and acceleration of the program timetable toward a manned lunar landing. To this end, easily replaceable modular subsystem assemblies were employed, which could be accessed from outside the spacecraft by several technicians simultaneously.

The Gemini craft was comprised of a reentry module, which included the crew cabin, and an adapter module, which was jettisoned prior to reentry (Figure 4-3). The reentry module, which was the forward or top section, was itself comprised of three separate sections. The first section (A) housed rendezvous and radar systems, parachutes, a UHF antenna, and docking mechanisms. The second section (B) contained the attitude control system used during reentry (not during orbital flight), and was one of the few fully automated systems on Gemini. The third section (C) was the cabin, which was conical in shape, with bases of 229 and 97 centimeters and a height of 190 centimeters. Above each crewmember's head was an EVA hatch which could be opened manually, with a window in each hatch (see Figure 4-3). An aft hatch beneath the crew couches opened into a compartment containing portions of the environment control system (ECS). An ablative heat shield covered the base of the reentry module.

The Gemini spacecraft's adapter module contained two sections. The first, or retrograde, section (D) housed four retrorockets for reentry or emergency abort during launch. It also contained six thrusters for the Orbital Attitude and Maneuvering System (OAMS), which permitted orbital parameter adjustment (an upgrade from Mercury). The second section, the equipment section (E), contained ten additional OAMS thrusters, fuel cells providing electricity and drinking water, part of the ECS, and supporting electronic equipment. The adapter module was also conical in shape, with a 229-centimeter top, a 305-centimeter base, and a height of 229 centimeters. The entire adapter module was jettisoned just prior to reentry.

The eight translational thrusters of the OAMS were controlled by the commander using a maneuverable joystick. Attitudinal thrusters were controlled manually by a side-arm stick mounted between the pilots. Overall, there were five separate modes for attitude, three manual and two automatic. Control and guidance systems were considerably more sophisticated in Gemini than in Mercury, since the spacecraft was designed for rendezvous and docking in orbit.

Like Mercury, the Gemini capsule was designed for a parachute-assisted ocean landing. Gemini's parachute was somewhat different, however. A drogue parachute was deployed at 15,000 meters, with the main parachute deploying from the nose at 3,300 meters. Rather than impact-

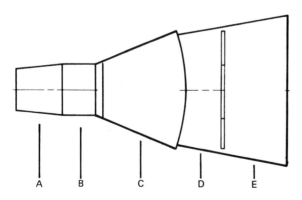
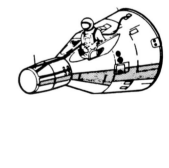

Figure 4-3. Gemini spacecraft configuration. (Functions of sections A–E are described in text.)

ing heat-shield down, the Gemini capsule was suspended at two points from the parachute, with attachments at either end of the craft, so that it landed on its side in the water. At 2,250 meters the landing attitude switch was activated, shifting the vehicle to two-point suspension.

The successful Gemini Program gave the U.S. more flexibility in space operations and garnered many important "firsts" in space. It also opened the way to the eventual realization of Apollo Program objectives. Between March 1965 and November 1966, there were ten manned Gemini flights. The progressive buildup to a 14-day Gemini VII mission removed all doubts regarding the ability of spacecraft and crews to function in space long enough to carry out a lunar landing and return. Ten rendezvous were completed, along with nine different dockings of spacecraft on orbit. EVAs were performed in five different Gemini missions. In addition, a wide variety of inflight experiments was conducted, laying the groundwork for extensive onboard research in future programs (Mueller, 1967).

APOLLO PROGRAM

Of all the scientific explorations ever undertaken by mankind, the Apollo Lunar Landing Program was the largest and most complex. The program's goal of landing the first man on the moon was accomplished in less than a year from the first manned flight test of the Apollo vehicle. The accelerated program was not, however, without mishap. A flash fire on board Apollo 1 (scheduled as the first manned Apollo flight) during prelaunch testing caused the deaths of three astronauts. An investigation eventually resulted in a number of hardware and procedural changes to further ensure crew safety. To regain lost time, the planned inflight biomedical experiments were cancelled.

A total of 11 manned Apollo flights were launched between October 1968 and December 1972; 12 astronauts worked on the lunar surface. A program of Earth-orbital flights (the Apollo Applications Program), originally planned to fly concurrently with the lunar program, was reduced in scope during the early 1970's and eventually became the Skylab Program. The Apollo spacecraft was used to transport Skylab and Apollo-Soyuz Test Project crews (Smith, 1981).

The three-man Apollo spacecraft was comprised of three modules: the Command Module and the Service Module (referred to in combined form as the Command and Service Module, or CSM), and the Lunar Module (LM). A launch escape system, similar to that used in the Mercury Program, was also present. This overall configuration (Figure 4-4) was determined by the decision to adopt lunar orbit rendezvous (LOR) as the method for accomplishing the mission (Smith, 1981). The LOR concept involved launch to lunar orbit, separation of the LM from the CSM for descent to the lunar surface, and subsequent return of the LM to lunar orbit for docking with the CSM.

The Command Module (CM) was essentially a conical pressure vessel encased in a heat shield, as shown in the top half of Figure 4-5 (Johnston and Hull, 1975). It was 3.5 meters long, with a diameter of 3.9 meters at the base. There were three sections to the CM: the forward compartment contained reaction control engines and recovery parachutes; the middle section contained crew accommodations, controls and displays, and other systems; the aft compartment housed additional reaction control engines and storage tanks for fuel, gas, and water. Overall habitable volume was 5.95 cubic meters—more than four times the size of the Gemini vehicle. The three crew couches were positioned so that seated crewmembers faced the display console, toward the apex of the cone.

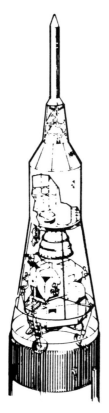

Figure 4-4. Configuration of the Apollo spacecraft at launch.

The interior of the CM was divided into nine equipment bays for compartmentalized stowage of equipment, materials, and provisions. Two hatches were present, at the side and top of the capsule. After the Apollo 1 fire, the side access hatch was reconfigured for easier opening, particularly in one gravity. Five observation windows permitted extensive outside viewing and photography.

The Service Module (SM) was a cylindrical structure 3.9 meters in diameter by 6.9 meters long. Mounted below the CM (lower portion of Figure 4-5), this part of the spacecraft contained the main propulsion system and provided stowage for most consumable supplies. The SM remained attached to the CM from launch until just before reentry, when it was jettisoned. The service propulsion system was used for midtransit maneuvers and to reduce spacecraft velocity before entering lunar orbit.

The LM (Figure 4-6) was a two-stage vehicle used to transport astronauts between the orbiting CSM and the lunar surface, and to provide living quarters and a base of operations on the moon. It had an overall height of 7 meters and a diagonal width between landing gear of 9.5 meters. An LM adapter provided an aerodynamic casing during launch, and was jettisoned shortly after the spacecraft left Earth orbit. Because it was designed to fly only in the vacuum of space, the LM was incapable of reentering Earth's atmosphere, and was jettisoned to free-fall back to the lunar surface.

The ascent stage of the LM (Figure 4-6-A) was 3.8 meters long by 4.3 meters in diameter and consisted of three sections: the crew compartment, the midsection, and the aft equipment bay. The crew compartment and midsection were pressurized. Habitable cabin volume was 4.5 cubic meters. Figure 4-6-C shows the interior of the LM cabin. The descent stage of the LM (Figure 4-6-B) was the unmanned portion of the LM. It supported the ascent stage (which would later leave the lunar surface) and contained the propulsion system used to slow the spacecraft for landing on the moon. During descent, four landing gear struts unfolded to form the landing gear. Foot pads at the ends of the legs contained sensors which signaled the crew to shut down the descent engine upon contact with the lunar surface. Four bays surrounding the descent engine contained the propellant tanks, the Modularized Equipment Stowage Assembly (TV equipment, lunar sample containers, and portable life support systems), the Lunar Roving Vehicle (LRV), and the Apollo Lunar Surface Experiment Package (ALSEP).

Of these subassemblies, the LRV merits description here. Used for the first time on Apollo 15, the fourth lunar landing operation, this battery-operated vehicle doubled the traverse radius during lunar expeditions (Johnson and Hull, 1975). It was guided with a T-shaped hand controller, and equipped with a television camera and communications system which transmitted voice and biomedical/life support data. It had a lunar payload that was several times the vehicle's own (Earth) weight.

The only major operational problem encountered during any of the 11 manned Apollo missions flown was the explosion of an oxygen tank on board Apollo 13, en route to the moon. A resulting loss of power in the CSM forced the crew to live in the LM while orbiting the moon just prior to the mission's return phase. The

fact that no ships or crews were lost in space during this complex and accelerated program is a testament to the design integrity of the vehicles and the expertise of crews and controllers.

SKYLAB PROGRAM

One of the uses originally envisioned for the Apollo spacecraft was to assist advanced research and studies in Earth orbit. Various concepts for an orbital space station had been discussed in connection with the Apollo Applications Program. By 1969, the project had taken definitive shape: a Saturn IVB rocket stage would be outfitted as a workshop on the ground, with solar

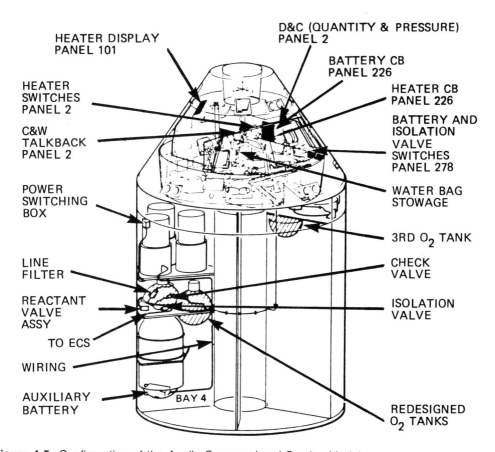

Figure 4-5. Configuration of the Apollo Command and Service Module.

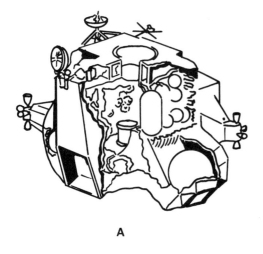

A

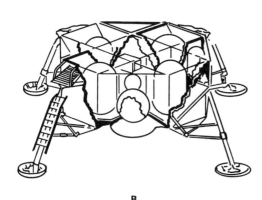

B

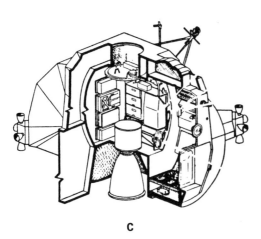

C

Figure 4-6. Lunar Module: A—ascent stage; B—descent stage; C—cabin interior.

panels for power supply, and an external Apollo Telescope Mount (ATM) for conducting solar observations. In 1970, as support for this and other NASA programs was scaled down, the Apollo Applications Program was renamed Skylab (Smith, 1981).

In manned orbital operation, Skylab consisted of five components: the Apollo ferry craft, the Orbital Workshop and, connecting the two, an Airlock Module and Multiple Docking Adapter; a fifth component was the ATM. These components are shown in launch configuration atop a Saturn V booster in the left-hand portion of Figure 4-7, and in fully deployed orbital configuration at the right (NASA, 1973).

The Apollo transport craft was identical to the lunar CSM described in the preceding section. The Skylab Orbital Workshop (SOW), which was the heart of the complex, was 14.6 meters long and 6.7 meters wide, with a habitable volume of nearly 275 cubic meters (Smith, 1981). On Earth, the fully equipped workshop weighed 35,400 kilograms. Enveloping the SOW structure was a thin, aluminum meteoroid shield intended to absorb micrometeoroid impacts and protect the workshop from direct solar radiation. (This shield broke off during launch, and was later replaced in orbit by an umbrella-like structure.) The interior of the SOW consisted of two major sections: an upper compartment for large-scale experiments, which contained two scientific airlocks; and a lower compartment containing areas for food preparation and eating, sleeping, waste management, and an experiment work area.

The habitation compartment's food system and waste management system helped to provide a living environment that simulated terrestrial conditions as closely as possible in space. The food system consisted of a wide variety of frozen, thermostabilized, and freeze-dried foodstuffs,

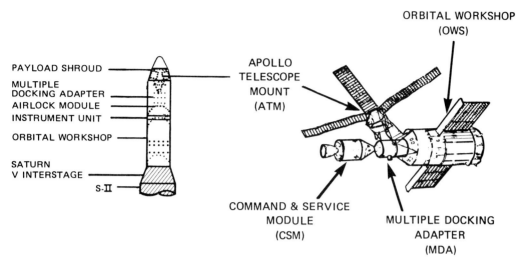

PAYLOAD SHROUD

MULTIPLE
DOCKING ADAPTER
AIRLOCK MODULE
INSTRUMENT UNIT

ORBITAL WORKSHOP

SATURN
V INTERSTAGE

S-II

APOLLO
TELESCOPE
MOUNT
(ATM)

ORBITAL WORKSHOP
(OWS)

COMMAND & SERVICE
MODULE
(CSM)

MULTIPLE DOCKING
ADAPTER
(MDA)

Figure 4-7. Skylab configuration at launch (left) and in Earth orbit (right).

and facilities for preparation and consumption. Approximately one ton of food was stored in the SOW at launch; packaged in 6-day supply increments, it was moved as needed to the galley area for preparation and eating. The galley contained a freezer, a food chiller, hot and cold water taps, and attachments for trays and diners. Food trays had accessed openings (some of which had warmers) for holding food cans. Food and water containers were designed for use in zero gravity (Johnston, 1977).

The Skylab waste management system included equipment for collection, measurement, and processing of urine and feces, as well as management of garbage. Feces were individually collected into a bag beneath a commode seat, weighed, labeled, processed, and stored. Urine was collected in a 24-hour collection bag. The volume of the bag was regularly estimated, and every 24 hours a sample was removed and frozen for postflight analysis. Trash was discarded through an airlock into a holding tank. Other provisions for personal hygiene included a shower contained

in a collapsible cloth bag; each crewman showered once per week in this device (Johnston, 1977).

Three long-term, three-man missions were flown on Skylab in 1973 and 1974, lasting 28, 59, and 84 days. The third and longest mission set a space flight endurance record that was not broken until 1978. Skylab's orbit eventually decayed, and the station reentered over western Australia in July 1979.

SPACE TRANSPORTATION SYSTEM

The Space Transportation System (STS) consists of three major components (shown in Figure 4-8): the orbiter, an external tank (ET), and two solid rocket boosters (SRBs). The orbiter is the actual spacecraft, designed to carry up to seven crewmembers and the payload to and from Earth orbit. The SRBs and the ET are part of the propulsion system which boosts the orbiter into space (Luxenberg, 1981).

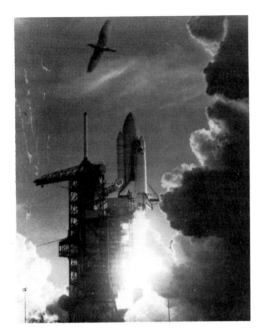

Figure 4-8. The Space Transportation System (Space Shuttle).

The Shuttle Orbiter

Figure 4-9 shows a more detailed diagram of the orbiter vehicle. It is comparable to a DC-9 in size and weighs approximately 68,000 kg. The major components and subsystems are described in Table 4-1.

The orbiter is an extremely versatile vehicle. It is designed for vertical launch, but assumes horizontal flight for an unpowered aircraft-type approach and landing after reentering Earth's atmosphere. It contains accommodations for up to seven crewmembers; although during an emergency the orbiter can carry as many as ten persons. Orbital stay capability is up to 8 days, with the potential for extension to 30 days when special power modules are developed. The orbiter can support a variety of different payloads and payload functions. For example, it can support Spacelab (the primary facility for life science experiments) or the Space Telescope, or can accommodate up to five satellites. The payload bay contains one manipulator arm as standard equipment, which can be used to retrieve satellites or place them into orbit. A second arm can be installed and controlled if required by the mission.

The aluminum hull of the orbiter is covered with thermal materials to protect the spacecraft from solar radiation and the extreme heat of atmospheric reentry. Two types of reusable surface insulation—

TABLE 4-1

COMPONENTS AND SUBSYSTEMS OF THE ORBITER

Orbiter Component	Principal Functions
Crew cabin	A two-level cabin which provides seating and living accommodations for seven crew and passengers. During emergencies, the crew cabin can accommodate as many as ten people.
Payload bay	Designed to contain one of several payloads (such as the Spacelab, the Space Telescope, up to five individual satellites, or satellites with an additional propulsion stage for insertion into higher Earth orbit or deep space).
Orbital maneuvering	Provides the thrust required for orbit subsystem insertion, orbit circularization, orbit transfer, rendezvous and deorbit after separation of the external tank. Propellants (MMH and N_2O_4) are contained in two pods, one on each side of the aft fuselage.
Reaction control	Three modules (one in the forward fuselage and Subsystem [RCS] two in the aft) containing a total of 44 thrusters, fueled by MMH and N_2O_4 in separate RCS tanks. This propulsion subsystem provides attitude control to the spacecraft during orbital insertion, orbit, and reentry.

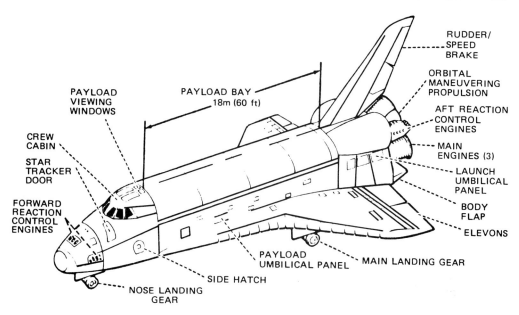

Figure 4-9. Configuration of Space Shuttle orbiter.

coated silica tiles and coated flexible sheets—cover the top and sides of the vehicle. The coatings on both types of insulation give the orbiter an off-white color with optical properties that reflect solar radiation. Silica tiles with a high-temperature coating cover the bottom of the orbiter and the leading edge of the tail. These glossy black tiles provide protection against temperatures up to 1,260°C.

Fuel Tank and Boosters

The external tank contains the propellants for the orbiter's main engines. Fluid controls and valves for the main propulsion system are located in the orbiter. The ET is jettisoned when its fuel is exhausted, shortly after separation of the SRBs, and is the only nonreusable portion of the Space Transportation System. The two SRBs, attached to the ET at launch, provide additional initial ascent thrust. After their fuel is exhausted, they separate from the ET and orbiter and deploy a system of self-contained parachutes. When the SRBs strike the water, the parachutes are jetti-

soned and the rockets are towed to port by recovery ships.

Crew and Passenger Accommodations

The orbiter cabin has a volume of about 71 cubic meters, with three levels. The upper level, or flight deck, contains the displays and controls used to pilot, monitor, and control the Shuttle vehicle and payload. The middeck contains payload specialist/passenger seating, living quarters, accommodations for hygiene and sleeping, galley, airlock, and avionics equipment compartments. The lower deck contains the environmental control equipment, and is accessible from the middeck by removable floor panels.

Like Skylab, the Shuttle orbiter is equipped with food, food storage, and food preparation facilities sufficient to accommodate from two to seven crewmembers. Food is available in dehydrated, thermostabilized, irradiated intermediate-moisture, natural, and beverage forms. The following food service facilities are provided: a water dispenser of ambient-temperature and chilled water for drinking and food reconstitution; a small, portable warmer that can simultaneously warm meals for four crewmembers; and food trays with restraints for food items and accessories (Figure 4-10). A multi-purpose meal galley is carried on most flights, mounted on the middeck floor and designed for airliner-like efficiency. It provides centralized food preparation facilities and storage of accessories. Figure 4-11 shows the food rehydration unit for operational Shuttle missions. The galley provides hot and cold water, pantry, and oven, and includes a personal hygiene station for washing. A table doubles as a dining surface and a work table during orbital operations.

The orbiter's waste collection system (WCS) is also an integrated, multi-functional system designed to collect and process biowastes from crewmembers in zero and one gravity. The system is designed to perform the following general functions:

- Collecting, storing, and drying fecal wastes, toilet paper, and emesis collection bags
- Processing wash water from the personal hygiene station
- Processing urine
- Processing water from the Extravehicular Mobility Unit in the airlock
- Transferring collected fluids to waste storage tanks in the waste management system
- Venting air and vapors from trash storage units

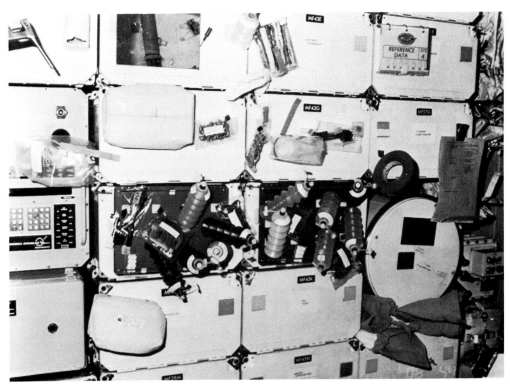

Figure 4-10. Fruit juice containers and other culinary items are shown fastened to food trays and locker doors in the orbiter galley.

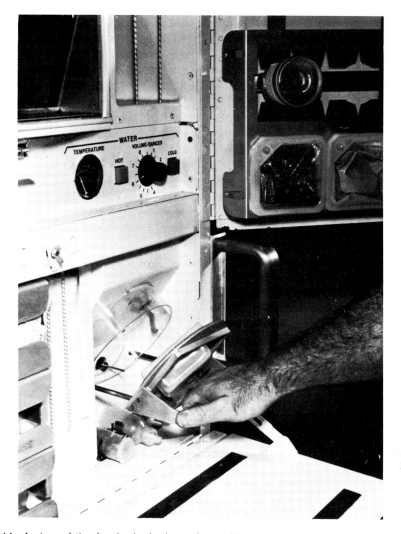

Figure 4-11. A view of the food rehydration unit used in meal preparation on board the orbiter.

• Transfer of waste water overboard, as a contingency.

The WCS station is located in a small compartment in the middeck. The unit is roughly cubical, with dimensions of 69 × 69 × 74 centimeters, and has separate assemblies for handling fluids (a cup-and-tube urinal) and solids (a commode). Various controls, filters, and fan separators are common to both assemblies.

Spacelab

Spacelab, the prime experimental facility for the Space Transportation System, is an on-orbit laboratory constructed under the direction of the European Space Agency (ESA). Components of this modular facility can be carried in the payload bay for experimental investigations in such fields as Earth observation, materials science, astrophysics, and life sciences. Spacelab is designed for maximum flexibility to reduce the costs of experiments in space, and to meet the needs of investigations in many disciplines. Figure 4-12 is an internal view of the Spacelab taken during the Spacelab D-1 mission.

Spacelab's two major components are modules and pallets (Lord, 1987). A module provides a habitable volume of variable size for the crew, biological specimens, and laboratory equipment, accessible from the cabin through a tunnel. Depending on mission requirements, a module can consist of either one (short module) or two (long module) segments, as shown in Figure 4-13. The forward segment of the long module (and the only segment of the short module) is called the core segment, and contains the electrical power, environmental control, and command and data management subsystems. Approximately 60 percent of the core segment volume is available for experimental equipment.

Pallets are rigid, U-shaped structures, 2.3 meters long, on which experiments and equipment can be mounted for direct exposure to the space environment. Pallet segments may be carried separately if no module is required for the mission. Figure 4-14 shows a diagram of a pallet mounted behind a long module.

When the orbiter is carrying both a module and pallets, the Spacelab subsystems inside the module's core segment provide the necessary power, data management, and other housekeeping equipment for the experiments mounted on the pallets. When only pallets are carried, these subsystems are contained in a cylindrical "igloo," shown in Figure 4-15.

The modular approach employed in the design of Spacelab permits a large number of mission-specific configurations (Figures 4-16 and 4-17). A long or short module can be carried with or without pallets, and pallet segments can be carried without a module.

The interior of the Spacelab module has

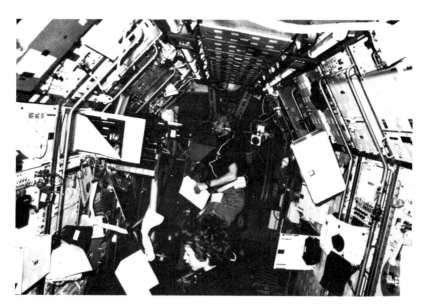

Figure 4-12. Astronaut Bonnie J. Dunbar and German Payload Specialist Reinhard Furrer conducting experiments inside the Spacelab. The concept of Spacelab is to provide a versatile laboratory in which experiments can be conducted using the unique microgravity environment of space.

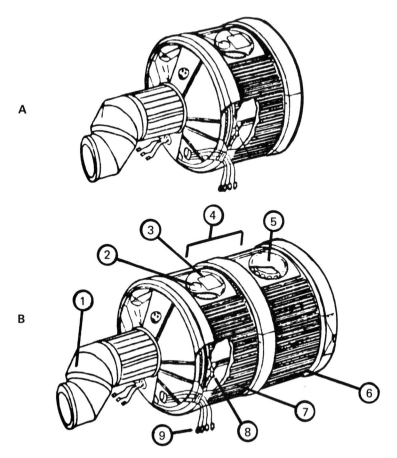

Figure 4-13. A. Short module (core segment only). B. Long module (core and experiment segments): 1—tunnel, 2—viewport, 3—optical window, 4—module, 5—airlock, 6—experiment segment, 7—core segment, 8—orbiter attach fittings, 9—utility interface.

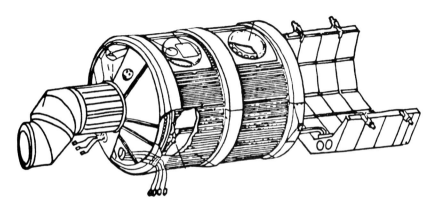

Figure 4-14. Long module with pallet.

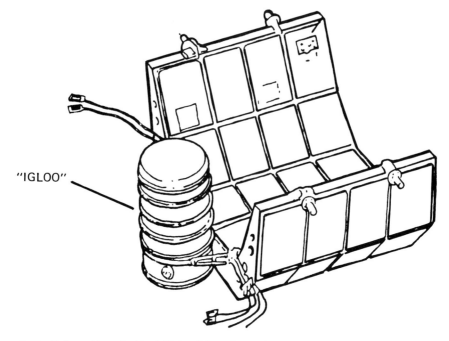

"IGLOO"

Figure 4-15. Pallet with cylindrical "igloo" housing subsystems.

been designed for maximum flexibility. It contains standard racks for experimental equipment, each of which is provided with power and data interfaces and cooling subsystems. Equipment can be stored in ceiling containers and under the floor.

Uses of Spacelab

Spacelab can be used in a number of different ways for various scientific disciplines: as an observation platform, research laboratory, test bed for equipment designed for use in space, or production facility to manufacture materials (e.g., crystals, alloys with new properties, high quality optical supplies, and improved vaccines).

In order to resolve conflicting requirements and maximize the efficiency of the time spent on orbit, most Spacelab missions focus on a cluster of related disciplines with similar operational and equipment requirements. For example, Spacelab microgravity missions can be dedicated exclusively to life science investigations. For these missions, the Spacelab module is equipped with appropriate laboratory equipment and specialized support systems, and carries from 15 to 30 life science experiments. Life science experiments can also be carried as mini-labs on multidisciplinary missions, or as self-contained experiments requiring minimum crew time.

THE SOVIET UNION

Historically, the Soviet approach to space vehicle development and to the advancement of their space program in general has been conservative and consistent. The overall goal is the development of large space habitats utilizing the best standardized vehicle prototypes.

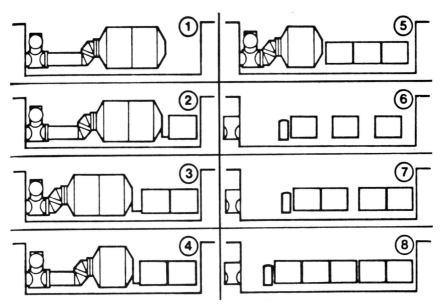

Figure 4-16. Basic configurations for Spacelab.

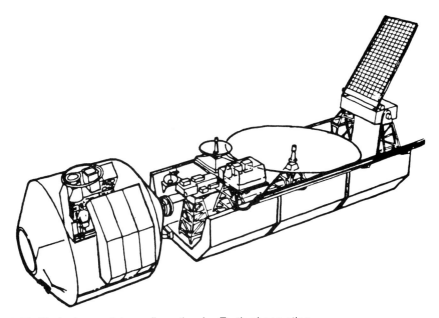

Figure 4-17. Typical spacelab configuration for Earth observation.

VOSTOK / VOSKHOD

The eight missions in these two programs served as trial runs for many basic activities eventually conducted in space, and as test flights to observe human reactions to the space environment. The principal differences between the Vostok and Voskhod vehicles were the removal of an ejection seat to provide room in Voskhod for a three-man "shirtsleeve" crew, and, in Voskhod 2, the addition of an airlock.

The Vostok/Voskhod spacecraft (Figure 4-18) consisted of two modules. A near-spherical manned cabin contained the crew couch(es), a life support system, radios, instrumentation and (in Vostok) an ejection seat apparatus for optional use. The capsule had three small portholes for exterior viewing, external radio antennas, and a covering of ablative material. The cabin was attached to a service module resembling two truncated cones joined at the bases, with a ring of gas pressure bottles on the upper cone. This module carried batteries, orientation rockets, and the retrorocket system.

In Earth orbit the spacecraft was allowed

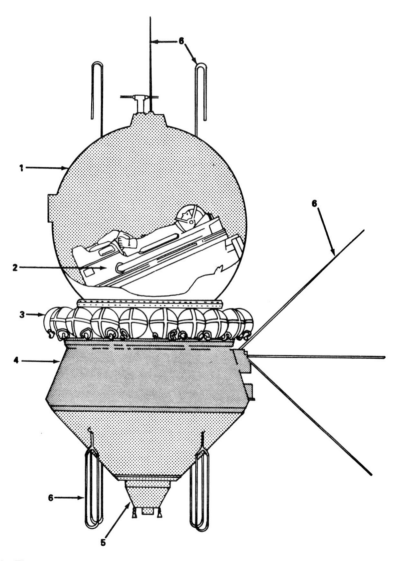

Figure 4-18. The configuration of the Vostok spacecraft (nearly identical to the later Voskhod vehicle). Labels denote: 1—ablative heat shield; 2—ejection seat; 3—oxygen and nitrogen pressure bottles; 4—service module; 5—retrorocket; and 6—antennas.

to tumble slowly to distribute the heat load evenly, but could be stabilized on command for operations such as retrofire. A key difference between this spacecraft and its American counterparts was that Vostok/Voskhod was primarily a land recovery operation. In Vostok, crews had the option of a hard landing with the parachute-slowed vehicle, or ejecting at 2,100 meters to descend independently by parachute. In Voskhod, the descent was decelerated by a final braking rocket (Smith, 1976).

SOYUZ

The workhorse of the Soviet manned space program has been the Soyuz vehicle, in almost continuous use since 1967. The Soyuz was developed to eventually ferry crews to the Soviet space stations. Like the American Apollo spacecraft, the Soyuz vehicle was larger and more versatile than its predecessors, providing expanded capability for mission activities and duration, and incorporating many design improvements based on prior mission experience. The Soyuz craft had an overall length of 8 meters and a maximum diameter of about 2.5 meters. It consisted of two modules: an orbital module which served as a work compartment, and the recoverable command module, also termed the reentry module. The two compartments were separated by an airlock, and equipment and accessories were stowed in compartments aft of the command module, where a cruise engine was also located. An outer hatch in the orbital module permitted egress for EVA.

The total volume of the two modules was about 8.5 cubic meters. Appropriately outfitted, the Soyuz could remain on orbit up to 30 days and, unlike Vostok/Vos-

khod, was capable of large orbital path adjustments and maneuvering. Some versions could fly up to a distance of 1,300 km from Earth (Smith, 1976). Over the years, the Soyuz evolved a number of variants to accommodate different needs. A ferry, or transport, version was used to carry crews and supplies to and from orbiting space stations (Figure 4-19). This version had a modest maneuvering capability and relied on batteries rather than solar panels for power. It could operate independently for about 3 days, but sometimes remained docked with a space station for up to 90 days awaiting further use. Another type of Soyuz craft was the "Progress" cargo ship (Figure 4-20) used to transport large quantities of fuel, food, equipment, and other necessities to space stations. This was essentially a stripped-down ferry vehicle outfitted with cargo bays and capable of carrying over 2,300 kilograms of payload. A third version of Soyuz had solar panels to provide power for long-term, independent research missions. In this mode, the Soyuz functioned as a sort of small-scale space station (Commit. Comm., Sci., and Transp., 1984).

Additional alterations on the Soyuz could be achieved by varying the number of crew seats (Soyuz could accommodate from one to three people in coveralls, and one or two in pressure suits) and the type of docking gear. Different types of active and passive docking units were available (as well as vehicles without a docking unit) (Commit. Comm., Sci., and Transp., 1984).

Unlike its predecessors, which followed a ballistic trajectory on reentry, Soyuz had special aerodynamic features which permitted more precisely controlled reentry and landing. Cosmonauts now remained in the cabin until they had safely landed. A drogue parachute was deployed at 9 km, and at 1 meter above the ground a gunpowder rocket fired, cushioning the impact.

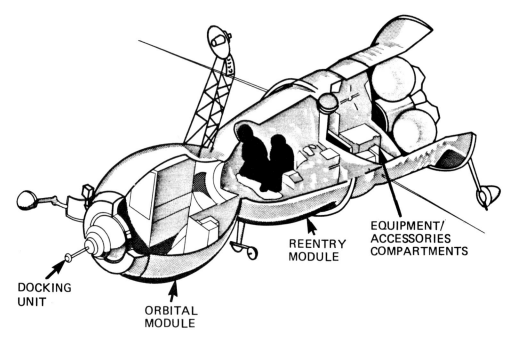

Figure 4-19. Configuration of the Soyuz used as a transport craft.

Soyuz T

The next model of the Soyuz line was first flown manned in 1980. Externally, this ship differed little from its predecessor; internally, the changes were substantial. The Soyuz T seated three crewmembers rather than two. An onboard computer complex gave the cosmonaut more control of docking and other activities (in this respect, it was similar to American spacecraft since the Apollo program). The Soyuz T also featured new instrumentation, improved radio communications and heat control systems, new life support and orientation and control systems, and new solar power panels (Malyshev, 1980).

The fuel system of the Soyuz T was designed so that the main engine and all four attitude control thrusters could utilize a common fuel supply. This meant that the attitude thrusters could serve as a backup to the main engine in an emergency, resulting in higher thrust and ma-

neuvering capabilities. In addition, the orbital module now separated before retrofire instead of after, as with the old Soyuz, saving 10 percent of the fuel (less mass to decelerate). The landing engines also had more thrust, to provide a softer landing.

Soyuz TM

First flown unmanned in May, 1986, the Soyuz TM (an improved version of the Soyuz T) transports crews to and from the Mir Space Station. Improvements include an enhanced onboard computer system and expanded payload capacity, and greater maneuverability and power for rendezvous and docking with the Mir. The new rendezvous system, called "Kurs," precludes the necessity of maneuvering the station in order for the ship to dock (Tarasov, 1987).

SALYUT ORBITAL SPACE STATIONS

Since the beginning of the Salyut program in 1971 to the completion of its mission objectives in 1986, seven Salyut space stations have been placed in orbit (six of them successfully). Powered by solar panels, these spacecraft provided the base for long-term Soviet research missions in Earth orbit and future Soviet plans regarding space manufacturing, materials processing, Earth resources studies, and space research. Although several successive versions were developed, the basic configuration of the station did not vary substantially from one "model" to the next (Figure 4-21).

The Salyut space stations can be grouped in two generations. The first generation (Salyuts 1–5) had only one docking port. The second generation (Salyuts 6–7) had two docking ports, greatly expanding the versatility of the stations, extending mission duration through resupply, and testing expandability concepts through docking of additional modules and vehicles.

First-Generation Space Stations: Salyuts 1–5

Four first-generation Salyut space stations (1971–1976) were launched, while two failed. Design changed with each successive station, both externally (placement of solar panels) and internally (to accommodate different experiments). The single docking port restricted resupply capability and additional crew dockings, limiting the duration and scope of the missions.

Salyut 1

On April 19, 1971, the world's first space station was launched. The station was about 21 meters long, with a 100 cubic meter interior volume. The main habitable portion, or work compartment, was divided into three sections: a small cylinder 3.8 meters long and 2.9 meters in diameter;

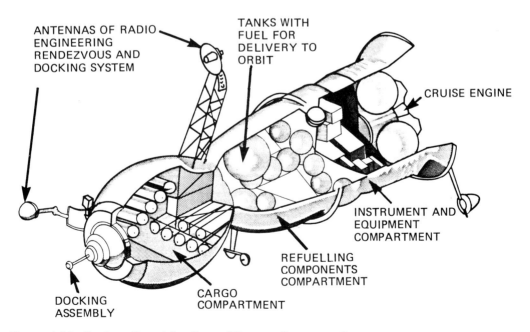

Figure 4-20. Configuration of the Soyuz "Progress" cargo craft.

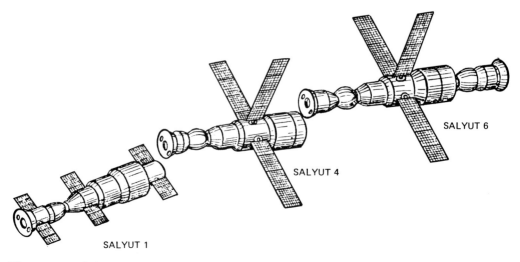

SALYUT 6

SALYUT 4

SALYUT 1

Figure 4-21. Salyut orbital stations of different generations. A Soyuz transport craft is shown docked to each station at the left. Salyut 6 also has a Progress cargo ship docked at the right.

a large cylinder 4.1 meters long and 4.15 meters in diameter; and a cone connecting the two which was 1.2 meters long. The unpressurized assembly module completed the station and was 2.17 meters long and 2.2 meters in diameter (Commit. Comm., Sci., and Transp., 1984).

Two double sets of stationary solar panels were placed at opposite ends of the station's exterior. Heat regulation system radiators, orientation and control devices, and some scientific instruments were also mounted externally.

The interior of Salyut 1 provided the basic configuration for subsequent Salyut stations. Control panels housed navigation instruments, clocks, radio communications monitors and controls, the Globus navigational indicator, and two keyboard command signaling devices. The interior of the Salyut 1 contained 20 portholes for viewing the Earth and stars. Also included was a dining table, with direct feeds for hot and cold water. Farther back was the biomedical area, with a rotatable chair for vestibular studies, and exercise equipment. At the end of the cylinder was the sanitary

hygiene area, which was separated from the rest of the room.

Salyut 3

After two successive space stations failed, the Soviets launched Salyut 3 on June 25, 1974. The station was similar in dimensions to the Salyut 1. Unlike the Salyut 1, however, this station had an aft docking port. Other changes included miniaturized circuitry and more efficient life support and thermal control systems. Three large solar panels (instead of the four small ones on Salyut 1) were capable of rotating 180 degrees so that the station did not have to constantly face the sun.

The interior was designed toward a more "homelike" appearance (Clark, 1981): floors were painted dark, and ceilings were painted a lighter tone. Living quarters included four windows, a special sofa for medical experiments, one fixed-position and one swinging bed (opening from the bulkhead to conserve space), storage space for clothes, linen, and entertainment items (which included a tape recorder, chess set, and small library).

Salyut 4

Salyut 4 was launched December 26, 1974, with the same volume and weight as previous versions. The station walls were thermally insulated with layers of synthetic film sprayed with aluminum, to preclude heat exchange between the station and space. An intricate system of radiators collected solar energy for heating purposes, and radiated surplus thermal energy. Three or more backup systems were available. The interior of the Salyut 4 was dominated by the OST-1 solar telescope, housed in the large conical structure in the cylinder of the spacecraft.

Salyut 5

Launched on June 22, 1976, the Salyut 5 was essentially the same as previous stations. On the recommendation of crews on the previous stations, the entire instrument compartment was covered with blue fabric with a soft inner layer to protect the instruments. In addition, the onboard computer was able to direct the operation of instruments without human interaction (Commit. Comm., Sci., and Transp., 1984).

Second-Generation Space Stations: Salyuts 6–7

Salyut 6

The second-generation Soviet space stations were a significant improvement in that they incorporated two docking ports. This enabled resupply by the Progress cargo ship, and docking capabilities for additional Soyuz vehicles carrying visiting crews. The forward docking port was generally used for Soyuz, while the aft could accommodate either Soyuz or Progress. The first of these space stations, Salyut 6, was launched September 29, 1977.

The basic dimensions were generally the same as for previous Salyut space stations. The three individually rotatable solar panels, spanning 17 meters, had a total area of 60 square meters and produced 4 kilowatts of direct current. AC-DC inverters converted electricity to alternating current.

The interior layout (Figure 4-22) was also much the same as that of previous Salyut versions. The crew entered and egressed through the transfer compartment. Pressure suits and airlock control panels were located in this 8 cubic meter area. The working compartment featured removable walls covered with soft, pastel-colored cloth. Sound insulation was increased 50 percent to soften the noise of onboard equipment (Commit. Comm., Sci., and Transp., 1984).

The scientific equipment area contained a cone which protected the infrared telescope. The shower was located to the right of the equipment compartment on the "ceiling," and nearby were two airlocks for disposal of garbage. One of these was also used for materials processing devices. On the "floor" of this section were cameras and infrared sensors for determining the local vertical positions of the station for navigation purposes. Behind the scientific equipment compartment was the toilet. Beyond this was the intermediate chamber which led to the aft docking hatch.

As dust collected on the 20 portholes in Salyut, problems were encountered with optical quality over a period of time. In a few cases, portholes were apparently scratched by micrometeorites (Commit. Comm., Sci., and Transp., 1984).

Pipes carrying a liquid heat-transfer agent were welded along the inside walls. Heat generated inside the station (by the crew and equipment) was retained by a multilayer thermal material (metalized film). Excess heat was radiated into space with the thermal regulation system. When the station was unoccupied, an electric heater maintained proper temperatures.

Atmospheric regenerators consisting of nonreusable chemical cartridges maintained proper air composition (atmos-

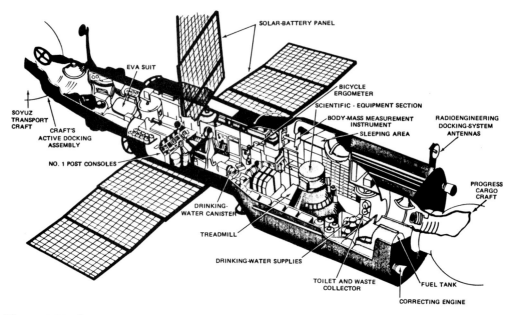

Figure 4-22. Schematic diagram of the Salyut 6 orbital station.

pheric pressure—700–960 mm Hg; partial oxygen pressure—160–240 mm Hg; partial carbon dioxide pressure—7–9 mm Hg). Pressure sensors warned of unplanned drops in pressure. Fans circulated the air, which was replenished by Progress cargo ships (Commit. Comm., Sci., and Transp., 1984).

Salyut 6 contained seven work stations. Work station 1 contained the control panels and posts for the space station systems. Station 2 was used for manual control of the Salyut; station 3 was the control panel for the infrared telescope and its coloring systems; station 4 was used for biomedical equipment (exercise equipment was located nearby); stations 5 and 6 were in the transfer compartment; and station 7 was for the water regeneration systems. The latter removed water vapor from the air (produced by breathing and perspiring) and recycled it for consumption. Additional water was resupplied by Progress cargo ships. There were no provisions for water regeneration from urine (Semenov and Gorshkov, 1981).

Salyut 6 had two main engines (300-kg thrust each) and 32 orientation engines (14-kg thrust each) positioned in four clusters, 90 degrees apart, around the exterior of the aft docking port. Fuel was carried by Progress cargo ships.

The Salyut 6 orientation and motion control system enabled automatic station orientation for scientific observations and experiments, docking maneuvers, and trajectory corrections. An autonomous navigation system forecasted station position 24 hours in advance, and computed times when the station would be within range of tracking sites, automatically activating the communications equipment as appropriate (Commit. Comm., Sci., and Transp., 1984).

Salyut 7

Salyut 7 was launched in April, 1982, and was the final second-generation space station. Like the Salyut 6, it had a second docking unit. Salyut 7 had a combined engine designed for multiple refueling and prolonged fuel storage. Crew comfort was increased through a new ventilation system, new color scheme, new shower, refrigerator, and improved lighting. New scientific equipment included telescopes for studying X-ray sources. Enhanced window protection preserved the clarity of the view for a longer time. A new computer-controlled materials processing furnace could operate automatically when the station was unoccupied. The navigation system was improved, as well as the strength of the forward docking port. The solar panel system was modified to permit attachment of additional arrays.

Experience with the second-generation stations revealed several problems. Expanded scientific investigations led to excessive crowding in the habitation module as equipment was delivered by the numerous Progress resupply ships. This situation affected living conditions and could have threatened crew safety in the event of station evacuation. Because of the inadequate level of automation for onboard operations, the crew was overloaded with numerous housekeeping tasks, with less time available for scientific research activities. Another problem was that the geographic placement of the ground tracking stations forced communication at fixed intervals, rather than continuous communication.

In addition, two docking ports were insufficient when long-term operation modules were docked (e.g., a Soyuz ferry ship and an experimental laboratory module), leaving no room for the Progress resupply ship. It became obvious that a new-generation station was needed, one that was free from the deficiencies of previous stations (Blagov, 1986).

Third-Generation Space Station: Mir

On February 20, 1986, the core of a third-generation space station was launched. This launch marked a significant advancement in Soviet space station design, in particular the inclusion of six docking ports capable of accommodating six spacecraft. Two axial ports for automatic and manual docking can accommodate transport and resupply ships, while four passive lateral ports can accommodate dedicated laboratory modules. A special manipulator arm transfers the modules from the axial to the side ports. The modular principle for the construction of Mir has substantially expanded capabilities for space research, and specialized modules make it possible to conduct research on a regular basis. Such dedicated modules enable specialized studies in astrophysics, environmental studies, materials processing, and biomedical research.

The dimensions of the Mir core module are similar to those of Salyut in length and diameter; however, habitable volume is somewhat greater (130 m^3). The Mir is equipped with seven computers for maximum automation, and the station can be controlled autonomously from the ground.

A special radio has been installed on board with a narrow-beam antenna for communications with the flight control center via the stationary relay transmitter satellite. The period of uninterrupted communications has been extended from 10–25 minutes to 50–60 minutes for each orbit (Blagov, 1986).

The station consists of transfer, working, and equipment modules, a connecting chamber, and two adjacent hermetically sealed airlocks (Pochkayev et al., 1986). The transfer module, spherical in shape with a diameter of 2 meters, has five passive docking ports. The central port is located on the longitudinal axis of the station, while the lateral ports are displaced from it by 90°. The shell of this closed, thermally insulated module contains the ports for the module docking system, the antennas for the approach radio apparatus, video cameras to monitor approach and docking, running lights, and devices for monitoring mutual orientation when the spacecraft is berthed manually.

The transfer module contains the thermal regulation and atmosphere maintenance units, and equipment for inflight measurements, radio and video communication, and lighting.

The working module consists of two cylinders differing in diameter and linked by a cone. To make it easier for cosmonauts to orient themselves within this module, the floor, walls, and ceiling are painted different colors. The smaller cylinder, called the work area, is the principal area where cosmonauts perform their assigned tasks, control the station, and monitor the status of various space flight systems.

The larger living area has been designed and equipped to create comfortable living conditions. There are two private cabins, with sleeping bag, desk, chair, and window. The dining area includes a table with panels for securing food in weightlessness and disposal bags for food wastes. Built into the table is an electrical unit with controls for heating food. Opposite the table is the refrigerator. The dining area can accommodate four crewmembers.

Next to the dining area is a multipurpose physical exercise machine. Behind a screen are the sanitation facility, washroom, waste receptacles and containers. Under the floor of the living area is an airlock for waste disposal.

The connecting chamber at the rear of the core contains a passive docking port. Cosmonauts pass through this port to and from the Soyuz spacecraft to the Mir core module. The connecting chamber contains equipment for docking, water supply, radio communications, personal hygiene, and other systems supporting station functions.

The equipment module contains propellant tanks containing fuel and oxidants, engines, and equipment for heating and docking systems.

The integrated propulsion system includes a low thrust jet system and two high thrust engines. These engines are fuelled with compressed gas, stored in tanks. The cargo ship refuels the station through special hydraulic joints in the docking ports. Cosmonauts operate the propulsion system from consoles located in the living area of the working module.

The power supply system consists of the solar and storage batteries, which provide electricity for core instruments and systems, docked cargo spacecraft, and dedicated modules and their storage batteries. The size of the solar battery panels has been expanded from 51 m^2 in Salyut 7 to 76 m^2 in Mir. Use of gallium arsenide components has also increased efficiency. Solar panels are positioned perpendicular to the sun's rays, by means of special drives controlled by signals from solar position sensors. The station contains several storage batteries connected parallel to the primary power source—the solar batteries. A buffer battery serves as a highly versatile power source during peak demand and creates the stable conditions desirable for equipment operation.

Ventilation is provided within the core station, cargo ship, and dedicated modules. The majority of the hydraulic components of the ventilation system are located on panels outside the station. Heat and moisture are exchanged among the core, dedicated modules, and the cargo ship through air ducts.

The thermal regulation system consists of external and internal heating and cooling loops and maintains a temperature of 18–28°C. A preset temperature regime is maintained on the station automatically, but the crew can also adjust heaters, air conditioners, and fans. Air composition is monitored by gas analyzers.

Mir cosmonauts drink treated water delivered by the Progress cargo ships. The water is processed on Earth with silver ions and stored in 10-liter tanks, remaining potable for up to a year. The core also contains a system for reclaiming water from the spacecraft atmosphere, similar to that on Salyut 7 (Pochkayev et al., 1986).

During the design of Mir, special attention was paid to simplifying repairs. Instruments have been grouped together and installed in the walls, which open inside the habitation module, easing access and replacement. Although the basic repair method is instrument changeout, repairs are necessary at times. Therefore, a special work site in the habitation module has been equipped with a set of various tools.

The Mir space station is expected to operate as the base for Soviet space operations for many years. The multiple docking unit considerably expands the potential for numerous module combinations. As with the Salyut stations, studies onboard Mir will serve to refine and improve research capabilities, reliability of systems, and living and working conditions (Blagov, 1986).

REFERENCES

Blagov, V.D. "Space: Mir—the new generation Soviet orbital station." Zemlya i Vselennaya, 6:2–10, November–December, 1986. (Translated in: JPRS-USP-87-003, U.S.S.R. Report: Space, p. 1, April 22, 1987.)

Clark, P.S. The Design of Salyut Orbital Stations. Spaceflight: 23, 257–258, Oct., 1981.

Committee on Commerce, Science, and Transportation: U.S. Senate Part 2. Soviet Space Programs: 1976–1980 (Supplement 1983). U.S. Government Printing Office, Washington, D.C., 1984.

Grimwood, J.M. Project Mercury: A chronology (NASA SP-4001). National Aeronautics and Space Administration, Washington, D.C., 1963.

Johnston, R.S. Skylab Medical Program Overview. In: Biomedical results from Skylab (NASA SP-377). Edited by R.F. Johnston and L.F. Dietlein. National Aeronautics and Space Administration, Washington, D.C., 1977.

Johnston, R.S., and Hull, W.E. Apollo missions. In: Biomedical results of Apollo (NASA SP-368). Edited by R.S. Johnston, L.F. Dietlein, and C.A. Berry, National Aeronautics and Space Administration, Washington, D.C., 1975.

Lord, D.R. Spacelab: An international success story (NASA SP-487). National Aeronautics and Space Administration, 1987.

Luxenberg, B.A. Space Transportation System. In: United States civilian space programs, 1958–1978. Congressional Research Service, Science Policy Research Division, Washington, D.C., January, 1981.

Malyshev, Yu. Evolution of the Soyuz spacecraft. Aviatsiya i Kosmonavtika, 10:38–39, 1980.

Mueller, G.E. Introduction. In Gemini summary conference (NASA SP-138). National Aeronautics and Space Administration, Washington, D.C., 1967.

NASA. Pocket statistics. National Aeronautics and Space Adminstration, Washington, D.C., March 1973.

Pochkayev, I., Serebrov, A., and Ul'yanov, V. The Mir space station. Aviatsiya i Kosmonavtika, pp. 22–23, November, 1986.

Smith, M.S. Program details of man-related flights. In: Soviet space programs, 1971–1975. Congressional Research Service, Service Policy Research Division, Washington, D.C., August 1976.

Smith, M.S. Manned space flight through 1975. In: United States civilian space programs, 1958–1978. Congressional Research Service, Science Policy Research Division, Washington, D.C., January, 1981.

Tarasov, A. New features of "Soyuz TM-2" spacecraft. Pravda, p. 1 (in Russian), February 7, 1987. Translation in JPRS-USP-87-003, U.S.S.R. Report: Space. Foreign Broadcast Information Service, p. 24, April 22, 1987.

5 Spacecraft Life Support Systems

JAMES M. WALIGORA
RICHARD L. SAUER
JAMES H. BREDT

The essentials of maintaining normal body functions assume new significance on board a spacecraft. The spacecraft environment, principally zero gravity, has specific effects on human physiology and these are treated in other chapters. Equally significant to crew health, however, are problems associated with the need to maintain and control environmental atmospheric conditions, and the logistic problems associated with eating, drinking, personal hygiene, and waste management in a zero-gravity environment.

Spacecraft life support systems have evolved in each of these areas. The general goal has been to achieve systems that are natural and unobtrusive in their impact on the crew, and require a minimum level of crew involvement. In zero gravity, crewmembers should not be expected to expend significantly more effort in life support activities than they would in one gravity.

The elements of each spacecraft life support system will be discussed in this chapter, as well as the evolution of these systems to current Shuttle configurations. Finally, areas of advanced research and development will be discussed.

ATMOSPHERIC CONTROL SYSTEMS

The atmospheric environment that we take for granted on Earth, a certain combination of gas pressure, composition, and temperature, is not present at survivable levels in space. On Earth, atmospheric pressure is 760 torr (14.7 psi) at the surface. The composition of this gaseous medium is 20.9 percent O_2, 78.0 percent N_2, and 0.04 percent CO_2, with trace amounts of other gases. Over much of the Earth's surface average atmospheric temperature ranges from 22°C to 27°C (72–81°F), the ideal temperature range for a lightly clothed man. In contrast, the pressure in space approaches that of a perfect vacuum: there is no question of gas composition, and thermal exchange occurs solely by radiation (from the unshielded sun or to space). For humans to survive in space, there must be living quarters available in which an atmosphere is controlled for proper pressure, gas concentrations, and temperature.

PRESSURE

A minimal atmospheric pressure (about 0.9 psi) is required to keep body fluids in the fluid state, and human tolerance to extremely high pressures is limited. For all practical purposes, however, and particularly in the context of spacecraft, acceptable static pressures for a habitable environment are determined by the required partial pressures of the component gases, their combined ability to support combustion, and the necessity for change in pressure in the course of a mission.

Relative to changes in pressure, several potential physiological problems must be considered in terms of spacecraft atmosphere. The three most significant concerns are barotrauma, explosive decompression syndrome, and altitude decompression sickness.

Barotrauma occurs when gas is temporarily trapped in the middle ear or the sinuses, in teeth if a gas pocket has formed below a tooth restoration or in a decayed tooth, or in the gut. If trapped gas pockets exist, a change in the external pressure will produce pressure differences across the walls of these cavities, resulting in pain and tissue injury. Barotrauma is most likely to occur when (1) swollen mucous membranes associated with a respiratory infection have obstructed passages that normally permit pressure equilibration of the ears and sinuses, (2) poor dental care has resulted in air cavities in teeth, and (3) the diet prior to pressure change has allowed large quantities of gas to form in the gut.

Barotrauma can be avoided by controlling the predisposing factors and operationally limiting the rate of change in pressure. In the Shuttle, for example, cabin pressure is reduced from the normal 14.7 psi to 10.2 psi only prior to extravehicular activity, and later adjusted in the airlock to the level of the pressure suit. For a nominal decompression or recompression, the rate of pressure is limited by specification to 0.1 psi/second and, in practice, to even slower rates. During an emergency recompression, the rate is limited to 1 psi/second.

Explosive decompression syndrome occurs when external pressure drops so rapidly that a transient overpressure develops in the lungs and other air cavities. The lungs may rupture at a pressure differential as low as 80 torr (1.6 psi). Should a tear or rupture of the lungs occur under these conditions, blood vessels would be severed and the positive pressure in the lung would likely force large quantities of gas into the bloodstream, resulting in a fatal air embolism.

The outcome of a rapid decompression or an explosive decompression depends on the following factors:

1. Rate of change of pressure
2. Absolute change in pressure
3. Absolute pressure prior to decompression
4. Ratio of initial pressure to final pressure
5. Ratio of lung volume at the time of decompression to maximum lung capacity
6. Ratio of the cabin orifice over the cabin volume compared to the ratio of airway orifice over the lung volume.

To understand the significance of these factors, it may help to closely examine a scenario of an explosive decompression. Assume that a crewmember is housed in a cabin at 12 psi surrounded by an ambient pressure of 5 psi. A wall of the cabin blows away, so that the area available for gas to leave the cabin is very large relative to the cabin volume. In 0.01 seconds cabin pressure reaches 5 psi. The crewmember's glottis is open at the time of decompression and he has 3 liters of air in his lungs, which have a maximum capacity of 6 liters.

In this example the rate of cabin decompression is extremely high because of the large cabin orifice. The rate of decompression will depend on the area of the orifice, the volume of the cabin, the ratio of the pressure inside and out, and the final absolute pressure.

The rate of cabin pressure change in this example is so high that no appreciable gas volume will be able to escape through the open glottis. The initial pressure in the lungs is 12 psi. During the decompression the lung will expand to its maximal volume, doubling its volume and lowering the pressure by half to 6 psi. At this point, there will be a 1 psi (50-torr) differential pressure across the distended lung. As this pressure is below the 80-torr level at which the lung may rupture, this simple analysis (which does not consider the inertia of the expanding lung) would indicate that the decompression would be survivable. Roth's excellent review of rapid decompression (1968) should be referred to for more rigorous analytical techniques and empirical data.

Explosive decompression was an important consideration for the Shuttle Orbital Flight Test missions. The ejection escape system involved very rapid decompression of the cabin from 14.7 psi to ambient pressure. In certain contingency situations involving a shirtsleeve crewmember with an oxygen supply, the maximum altitude for ejection was limited by considerations of decompression.

Decompression sickness occurs when the pressure of dissolved gases in the tissues exceeds the ambient pressure. Under these conditions, bubbles formed in tissues may be carried by the bloodstream throughout the body. Decompression sickness can manifest itself by subcutaneous bubbles, classic "bends" pain in the joints and muscles, "chokes" or pain in the area of the lungs, neurological manifestations, and circulatory collapse and shock. Normally, decompression is not a problem when the pressure of the diluent gas in the atmosphere does not exceed the final decompression pressure by more than a ratio of 1.3 to 1. When changes in pressure will result in conditions exceeding these limits, it becomes necessary to lower the pressure of dissolved gases in the tissues prior to decompression. Because of the high rate of tissue utilization of oxygen, this gas will not contribute significantly to the formation or growth of bubbles in the tissue. Therefore, an effective means to protect against decompression sickness is to breathe 100 percent O_2 prior to decompression, displacing nitrogen from the tissues, or to lower the concentration of N_2 in the breathing gas, reducing N_2 pressure in the tissue.

In American space missions prior to the Space Shuttle, decompression sickness was a problem primarily on liftoff, when pressure changed from 14.7 psi to 5 psi. To protect against decompression sickness at this time, crewmembers breathed pure oxygen for 3 hours prior to launch. This prebreathing period also protected the crew against cabin decompression early in the mission (which would provide 3.7 psi to the crew in their pressure suits). When extravehicular activities (EVAs) were carried out on subsequent days, decompression from the 5.0-psi cabin pressure to the 3.7-psi suit pressure involved no real hazard of decompression sickness. Because the Shuttle vehicle has a cabin pressure of 14.7 psi, decompression sickness is no longer a concern on liftoff. However, it becomes a concern if crewmembers perform EVA in a pressure suit at a lower pressure.

The method of protection that has been adopted for Shuttle missions involves a 1-hour period breathing oxygen followed by cabin decompression from 14.7 psi to 10.2 psi at least 12 hours prior to EVA (to lower tissue nitrogen), followed by a 40-minute period in the pressure suit at 10.2 psi breathing O_2, then decompression in the airlock to a suit pressure of 4.3 psi (Waligora, 1984).

GAS CONCENTRATIONS

Oxygen

In terms of the well-being of the crew, the most significant gas component of the atmosphere is oxygen. The partial pressure of O_2 at sea level on Earth is 158 torr (3.06 psi). As the atmosphere is breathed, its components are diluted in the lungs by the addition of CO_2 and water vapor so that at the alveoli, where O_2 transfer to the blood takes place, O_2 partial pressure is 104 torr (2.01 psi). This is the physiologically important pressure, which can be calculated for any atmosphere using the following equation:

$$P_A O_2 = F_i O_2 (P_B - 47) - PCO_2$$
$$\times [F_i O_2 + 1 - F_i O_2 / 0.85]$$

where $P_A O_2$ = alveolar partial pressure of oxygen

$F_i O_2$ = oxygen fraction in breathing atmosphere

P_B = barometric pressure of the breathing mixture

0.85 = an assumed respiratory exchange ratio

PCO_2 = partial pressure of CO_2.

On Earth, the total pressure and the O_2 partial pressure vary as a function of altitude. People can live continuously at 3,660 meters (12,000 ft.) with an alveolar

O_2 partial pressure of 54 torr (1.05 psi). However, this requires extensive physiological acclimation, and the acclimation is not complete. Even with acclimation, an individual living at this altitude cannot perform as well as at sea-level. Acclimation can be nearly complete (the exception being maximum oxygen uptake during hard work) at altitudes up to about 1,830 meters (6,000 ft.) with an alveolar O_2 pressure of 77 torr (1.50 psi).

At sea level, humans, without acclimation, show some measurable effects of hypoxia at an alveolar O_2 pressure of 85 torr (1.65 psi). At this level, some aspects of vision (e.g., low-illumination color vision threshold) begin to be affected. At alveolar O_2 pressures between 81 and 69 torr (1.57–1.33 psi), certain discrete types of mental performance (e.g., learning a new task) begin to be affected. As alveolar O_2 drops below this level, the scope and severity of visual, mental, and finally motor impairment increase, until at an alveolar O_2 pressure of about 34 torr (0.67 psi), time of consciousness begins to be affected as shown in Table 5-1.

In the normal Earth environment, man is not exposed to alveolar O_2 levels in excess of 104 torr (2.01 psi). Oxygen at high partial pressures can be toxic. Subjects who breathe 100 percent oxygen at sea level for 6 to 24 hours complain of substernal distress and show a diminution of vital capacity of 500 to 800 milliliters (West, 1974). This loss is probably due to atelectasis, which occurs when all the O_2 in a poorly ventilated alveolus is absorbed by the blood. When this happens, the alveolus collapses. Surface tension tends to prevent reopening of a collapsed alveolus. Astronauts and test subjects exposed to the Apollo spacecraft atmosphere (5.00 psi O_2) for periods of up to 2 weeks showed no acute effects of O_2 toxicity. They did evidence some changes in blood-forming tissue, however (Kimzey et al., 1975). Similar effects on blood-forming tissue have

TABLE 5-1

TIMES OF USEFUL CONSCIOUSNESS AFTER ACUTE EXPOSURE TO REDUCED OXYGEN LEVELS

Altitude, km (ft)	Alveolar O_2 Partial Pressure (torr)	Time of useful consciousness, sec	
		(moderate activity)	(sitting quietly)
6.7 (22000)	32.8	300	600
7.6 (25000)	30.4	120	180
8.5 (28000)	<30	60	90
9.1 (30000)	<30	45	75
10.7 (35000)	<30	30	45
12.2 (40000)	<30	18	30
19.8 (65000)	<30	12	12

Adapted from Horrigan, 1979.

been reported after 8 hours/day exposure to 8.00 psi O_2 (Hendler, 1974).

The Shuttle environmental control system (ECS) maintains O_2 at 3.2 ± 0.25 psi (165 ± 12.9 torr), or essentially Earth-normal O_2 pressure. Mission rules require that O_2 masks be donned should O_2 pressure fall below 2.34 psi (121 torr). Hyperoxia is not a concern; but it can be a consideration in altitude chamber training where N_2 elimination is accomplished by breathing 100 percent O_2 at 14.7 psi. If a test is delayed once prebreathe has begun, the prebreathe is not to be extended beyond 6 hours, the threshold time after which some symptoms of oxygen toxicity may begin to appear.

Carbon Dioxide

On Earth, carbon dioxide (CO_2) is normally present outdoors at a concentration of 0.04 percent. CO_2 is a product of respiration, so its concentration increases in indoor environments that are crowded or poorly ventilated. Its production by the crewmember presents a problem in the closed-loop environmental control systems of the spacecraft cabin and pressure suit.

Effects of increased CO_2 in the atmosphere depend on the concentration and duration of exposure. Acute responses to increased CO_2 are increases in heart rate, respiration rate, and minute volume (Figure 5-1). Chronic exposure to CO_2 disturbs the acid-base balance of the body.

The PCO_2 limit for nominal Shuttle operations is 7.6 torr (0.15 psi). Exceeding this limit constitutes a mission contingency and every effort is taken to correct the situation. Breathing masks are donned if PCO_2 exceeds 15 torr (0.30 psi). In the pressure suit, PCO_2 is limited to 7.6 torr for metabolic rates up to 1,600 Btu/hr., and to 15 torr (0.20 psi) for higher work rates.

WATER VAPOR (HUMIDITY)

Water vapor is a normal constituent of Earth's atmosphere. The partial pressure of water in the atmosphere is a function of (1) exposure of the atmosphere to free water and (2) temperature, which may limit water vapor pressure. Percent relative humidity is a measure of the water vapor pressure relative to the maximum water vapor pressure that the atmosphere will hold at a given temperature. High relative humidity is sometimes associated with condensation and can be conducive to microbial and fungal growth. Absolute humidity, the actual partial pressure of water vapor, is the more important physiological measure of humidity. Low humidity, encompassing levels that are common in winter, causes drying of the eyes and skin and the mucous membranes of the nose and throat, as well as chapping of the lips. Inactivation of cilia protecting the respiratory tract leads to an increased incidence of respiratory infections under these conditions (Carleton, 1971). In addition to its direct physiological effects, humidity also significantly influences heat loss and heat balance. Water vapor pressure of 10 torr (0.19 psi) is optimum for habitability. The Shuttle ECS controls water vapor pressure between 6 torr and 14 torr (0.12–0.27 psi).

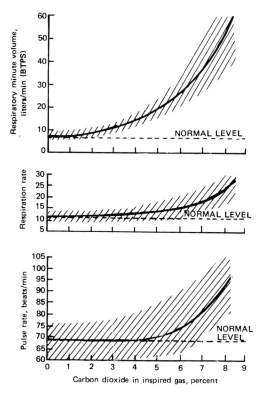

Figure 5-1. Immediate effects of increased CO_2 on pulse rate, respiration rate, and respiratory minute volume (BTPS = body temperature and pressure, saturated with water) for subjects at rest. Hatched areas represent one standard deviation on each side of the mean. To convert percentage of CO_2 to partial pressure, multiply percent value by 1.013 for kilonewtons per square meter or by 7.6 for torr. (Horrigan, 1979).

TEMPERATURE

The temperature of the atmosphere is an important aspect of the heat balance that must be maintained in the bodies of spacecraft crewmembers. Body temperature is closely guarded by physiological responses and sensory behavioral responses. In addition, the thermal mass of the body resists change in temperature due to temporary imbalances in heat gain and heat loss. Physiological thermoregulatory control responses include shivering and vasoconstriction in the cold, and sweating and vasodilation in the heat. The element of behavioral control in temperature regulation is dependent on a compelling sense of discomfort when the environment is too hot or too cold. This discomfort has a deleterious effect on performance. Thermal comfort is, then, a critical factor if optimum performance is to be maintained. The observation has been made that at least 5 percent of a large group will find any given temperature uncomfortable (Fanger, 1970). An inclusive and practical approach to achieving comfort is to provide thermostatic temperature control around an optimum point, and to provide some means for individuals to modify their heat balance, either by clothing selection or by individual air motion control.

The Shuttle ECS provides temperature control within a range of 18°C to 27°C (64°–

81°F). Under conditions in which a comfortable heat balance is maintained, variations in humidity do not have a strong effect on comfort. However, when heat balance can only be maintained at the upper limit of a comfort band or outside a comfort band, humidity becomes very significant. To preserve a strong and effective thermoregulation response to overheating, particularly during exercise, an upper value of 14 torr (0.27 psi) PH_2O is a component of the Space Shuttle Orbiter specification.

EVOLUTION OF THE SPACECRAFT ATMOSPHERIC CONTROL SYSTEMS

A number of options are available in providing a viable spacecraft atmosphere; the choice of options has a major impact on crew comfort and safety, as well as on vehicle cost, weight, complexity, and reliability. Spacecraft atmosphere control systems have evolved as space missions have increased in complexity.

The Mercury spacecraft had a 5.0 psi O_2 atmosphere supplied from a store of pressurized oxygen. CO_2 was controlled by a lithium hydroxide absorber in the environmental control loop. Temperature was controlled through cooling provided by a sublimator heat exchanger, which was supplied by a tank of cooling water augmented by condensate water from the ECS water separator. The sublimator vented water vapor overboard and cooling resulted from the change of state. The crew stayed in their pressure suits and the ECS system controlled both the pressure suit and the cabin environment (Mercury Project Summary, 1963).

The Gemini spacecraft retained the 5.0 psi O_2 atmosphere used in Mercury; however, the primary source of oxygen was a liquid O_2 tank, with secondary O_2 supplies stored as high-pressure O_2. CO_2 was again controlled by the use of lithium hydroxide absorber. The primary means of heat rejection in the Gemini vehicle was a spacecraft radiator which radiated the heat to space. Heat loss was controlled by the flow of coolant to the radiator and ECS heat exchangers. A secondary system permitted sublimation of water to the space vacuum if required for additional cooling. In later Gemini flights, extensive periods were spent outside the pressure suit. Gemini was, incidentally, the first American spacecraft to support a pressure suit in space. Its ECS system supplied the pressure suit through an umbilical connection (Gemini Midprogram Conference, 1966).

The Apollo atmosphere control systems were similar to the Gemini systems, but improved and more elaborate. The Apollo system involved three separate environmental control systems: a Command Module ECS system, a Lunar Landing Module ECS system, and one within the Service Module which carried consumables to support the Command Module system. The atmosphere was 5.0 psi O_2, supplied from a cryogenic O_2 supply in the Service Module. Lithium hydroxide was used to absorb CO_2. Cabin temperature was maintained at 24°C ± 2.8° (75°F ± 5°), with relative humidity limited to the range of 40–70 percent. The primary system for heat rejection was again a space radiator. Use of the radiators was facilitated by a slow, controlled roll of the Command and Service Modules called the passive thermal control flight mode. An evaporator was installed to provide additional cooling, but was not used after Apollo 11 except for launch, Earth orbit, and reentry (Brady et al., 1975).

The Skylab atmosphere control system incorporated some significant changes. Cabin pressure was 5.0 psi, but a two-gas environment was used to avoid minor chronic effects of hyperoxia over a long mission and possible interference of such effects with medical experiments. The atmospheric composition was 70 percent O_2 and 30 percent N_2, to provide an O_2 partial pressure just slightly higher than Earth-normal. There was automatic control of the two gases, but in practice much of the control was done manually to provide constant O_2 pressure during certain medical experiments. CO_2 absorption was accomplished with a regenerable molecular sieve system. This system allowed CO_2 to be flushed out of one bed by vacuum and heat and vented from the spacecraft while a second bed was absorbing CO_2. This regenerable system has obvious advantages for a long mission. However, a characteristic of this system was that it operated at a nominal CO_2 level of about 5 torr, so that although it met the same 7.6-torr CO_2 limit as earlier lithium hydroxide systems, the average CO_2 level was higher than on earlier spacecraft. Earlier systems had kept CO_2 near 1 torr most of the time. The thermal control system for Skylab was primarily a passive system. The vehicle was carefully coated with paints of varying emissivity in specific patterns, so that very little active control with radiators or evaporators was necessary. Several large exterior surface panels were lost during Skylab's launch, and later two separate types of shades were used to cover this exposed area (Belew, 1977).

As noted earlier, the Shuttle is the first American spacecraft to use a 14.7-psi atmospheric pressure. Gas composition is 80 percent N_2 and 20 percent O_2, as on Earth. CO_2 is absorbed with disposable lithium hydroxide cartridges, as in pre-Skylab flights, and thermal control is accomplished using radiators on the insides of the cargo bay doors.

FACTORS IMPACTING PRESSURE AND GAS CONTROL

A number of competing requirements influence the selection of cabin pressure and gas composition. Some of these factors are listed below:

- An O_2 partial pressure that is neither hyperoxic nor hypoxic
- An O_2 concentration that minimizes flammability of materials
- A gas density that will provide adequate cooling to gas-cooled electronics
- A total cabin/pressure suit pressure differential that is not conducive to dysbarism
- Structural strength sufficient to contain the cabin pressure
- Compensation for gas leakage.

To demonstrate how these factors interact, and the tradeoffs involved in emphasizing certain system parameters at the expense of others, let us examine a current pressure/gas control system. The Shuttle cabin atmosphere (14.7 psi with 20 percent O_2 and 80 percent N_2) incorporates most of these factors; however, it does present a dysbarism problem when considered in combination with a 4.3-psi pressure suit. This pressure differential requires 3 to 4 hours prebreathing with O_2 prior to decompression in the suit. This lengthy prebreathing requirement reduces the time available for EVA during a reasonable workday. To arrive at a more acceptable combination of cabin and suit pressures, either suit pressure must be increased or cabin pressure must be reduced. If cabin pressure is reduced and O_2 pressure is held constant, the percentage concentration of O_2 increases, and flammability is increased. If cabin pressure is reduced and O_2 concentration is held constant, then O_2 partial pressure is reduced and hypoxia becomes a problem. If suit pressure is increased, then suit mobility becomes a problem. The ideal solution to this dilemma may ultimately be provided by the development of a high-pressure suit (8.0–10.0 psi) with good mobility. In the meantime, the compromise solution for the Shuttle is to use a 10.2-psi decompression stop for 12 hours, breathe O_2 for 40 minutes, and then decompress to a 4.3-psi pressure suit. This protocol involves an acceptable degree of reduction in gas cooling, an acceptable increase in flammability, some reduction in O_2 pressure (to 1.830 meters equivalent) that will not result in clinical hypoxia, a prebreathing requirement that reduces EVA time, and some increase in suit pressure.

ADVANCED ATMOSPHERIC CONTROL SYSTEMS

When permanent stations are established in space, it will become desirable to reduce the weight of consumable life support supplies that must be launched to maintain operations. Since a significant fraction of oxygen breathed by the crew will be incorporated in water vapor, the air and water cycles will interact in a regenerative life support system.

In the Space Shuttle, CO_2 is removed from the atmosphere by absorption in lithium hydroxide, excess water vapor is condensed and sent to flash evaporation units within the temperature control system, and losses of O_2 and N_2 are replenished from supplies of liquefied gas. A regenerative life support system would still need a source of N_2 to compensate for leakage from the spacecraft into the ambient vacuum.

However, a makeup supply of O_2 might not be necessary, because O_2 could be regenerated by electrolyzing water, and substantial amounts of water would be present in the onboard food supply. It is expected that a Space Station life support system would not be permitted to vent water because of its effects on sensitive optical instruments outside. Therefore, water brought onboard in food would be retained in the system and its oxygen con-

tent could more than compensate for leakage losses if the cabin were tightly sealed.

On Skylab, which used consumable oxygen supplies, CO_2 was adsorbed on molecular sieve material and periodically desorbed to the space vacuum by heating the adsorbent. This could be done on a Space Station without requiring an oxygen supply if the leak rate were low enough. More advanced solid amine adsorbents and electrochemical CO_2 removal systems can deliver CO_2 at atmospheric pressure; catalytic reaction with H provides water, which is then electrolyzed to give O_2, and methane, which can be broken down further to recover its H_2 content or disposed of without chemical transformation.

The cabin pressure to be used on a Space Station is a major question that remains unresolved. Most considerations in pressure favor the selection of a 14.7-psi cabin pressure. However, early planning for the Space Station Freedom, based on projected Space Station missions at the turn of the century, anticipates a very heavy requirement for and involvement in extravehicular activity (EVA). Consideration of this frequent, perhaps daily, requirement for EVA lends attractiveness to environmental control systems utilizing a cabin pressure lower than 14.7. Such a cabin pressure would allow a lower suit pressure and perhaps greater mobility.

Operational tests conducted to verify acceptability of the 10 psi protocol (Waligora, 1984) have shown that particular types of exercise performed during EVA result in higher incidences of decompression sickness symptoms than have been reported in other studies in the aviation medicine literature. EVAs are of long duration, 4–8 hours, and involve fairly continuous low to moderate levels of activity. In altitude chamber studies involving this type of exercise, both a conventional 4-hour prebreathe and the 10.2 psi staged decompression protocol led to a high incidence of venous bubbles, detected by a precordial Doppler bubble detector, and a substantial incidence of very mild symptoms of decompression sickness. In view of the very mild and transient nature of the altitude decompression sickness symptoms encountered, it was determined that the denitrogenation procedures were acceptable for Shuttle operations. As a result of these findings, procedures were developed to provide treatment for altitude decompression sickness in flight, should this be required.

In view of the heavy emphasis on EVA in Space Station operations and the likelihood of daily or near-daily EVA, the cabin pressure-suit pressure combination selected should preclude symptoms of decompression sickness and preclude or minimize its presymptomatic expressions. One assumption that has been the basis for high suit pressure research and development testing for a number of years is that a zero prebreathe decompression could be made from 14.7 psi to 8.00 psi without fear of decompression sickness. After the unexpected incidence of decompression sickness during protocol verification tests at the L. B. Johnson Space Center (JSC), a series of tests were sponsored at the School of Aerospace Medicine to verify that decompressions from 14.7 psi to 8.00 psi

could be made without symptoms or bubbles. These tests utilized the same 6-hour exercise protocol as the tests at JSC. Preliminary findings indicate that a pressure of 9.00 psi or higher would have to be used to preclude symptoms and to minimize venous bubbles (Adams, 1984). Subsequent to and using results from the tests conducted at JSC, a table of zero prebreathe options of suit and cabin pressures was prepared, referenced to, and equivalent to an 8.00-psi suit and a 14.7-psi cabin (Waligora, 1984). The table (Table 5-2) has been updated in view of the Adams data with sets of cabin and suit pressure equivalent to a 9.00-psi suit and a 14.7-psi cabin.

The above combinations of cabin and suit pressures are values based on current information that will not require pre-EVA oxygen breathing, will not limit decompressions per day, nor require a minimum interval between EVAs. They will preclude symptom and presymptomatic expressions of decompression sickness. Probably 11.0 psi is the lowest cabin pressure that is compatible with automatic cabin and oxygen pressure control, 30 percent maximum oxygen concentration, and a 2.8 psi or higher nominal oxygen pressure.

TABLE 5-2

ZERO PREBREATHE OPTIONS OF SUIT AND CABIN PRESSURES

Cabin Pressure (psi)	Suit Pressure (psi)	Nominal O_2 Pressure (psi)	Constraints Prior to EVA
14.7	9.0	3.1–2.8	None
11.0	6.5	3.1–2.8	1 hr prebreathe prior to depress to 11.0 + 24 hrs at 11.0 psi.
10.2	6.0	3.1–2.8	1 hr prebreathe prior to depress to 10.2 + 24 hrs at 10.2 psi.
8.0	4.1	3.2–2.9	4 hrs prebreathe prior to depress to 8.0 + 24 hrs at 8.0 psi.

Tests at JSC and the School of Aerospace Medicine are continuing and will lead to more definitive pressure options for Space Station Freedom.

The problems and progress associated with zero prebreathe "hard" suit development are covered in Chapter 6, Extravehicular Systems.

CREW SUPPORT SYSTEMS

WATER SUPPLY

Introduction

As space missions lengthen, the need to recycle water for personal hygiene, housekeeping, and drinking becomes more critical. This is evident when one considers the penalty of storing the amounts of water required for these functions. Estimates for the amounts of water required per person are in the range of 2.6 kg/day for food and beverage reconstitution, 5.5 kg/day for personal hygiene activities, and up to 50 kg/day for housekeeping, clothes laundering, and dishwashing. In terms of a 90-day mission for 6 persons, this volume of water equals some 31,400 kg (9,400 gallons) or 31.4 m^3 of water. The prohibitive penalty to launch and store water quantities of this size in flight will force varying degrees of water reclamation on future missions of longer duration. Associated with water recycling will be the requirement to establish and monitor water quality parameters.

History

The initial manned space flights, Mercury and Gemini, used only launch-stowed water. This was feasible because the requirement for water was minimal and mostly limited to drinking water. The Apollo Command Module incorporated fuel cells for electrical power. Water was a by-product of the fuel cells, and this water was of sufficient quality and quantity to serve as potable water for food rehydration and drinking (Sauer and Calley, 1975). Mission lengths and vehicle constraints were such that personal hygiene activities requiring water were minimal. The Skylab missions were of a length that fuel cells were not practical for power production. As a result, all inflight water requirements were provided by launch-stored water (Sauer and Westover, 1975). The Shuttle vehicle, designed for relatively brief flights, has fuel cells that produce water for food reconstitution, drinking, and personal hygiene.

Inflight potable water that has been provided to date by either launch-storing or production from fuel cells has met potability standards similar to those for terrestrial potable water. The potable water specification for the shuttle is shown in Table 5-3.

Future Systems

Planned future manned missions such as Space Station Freedom will incorporate a system to recycle water for metabolic, personal hygiene, housekeeping, and other purposes. Sources for this water are humidity condensate, spent wash water, urine, and water contained in feces. Because of the small amount of water in feces and the relative difficulty in reclaiming it, however, feces are not normally considered a source of water for the Space Station (Sauer and Bustamante, 1971).

Unlike terrestrial application, where all water brought into the home must meet potable water requirements, quality requirements for inflight uses may vary. Only the relatively small amount of water designated for metabolic purposes will be required to meet the more stringent potable water requirement. In general, per-

TABLE 5-3

SHUTTLE POTABLE WATER SPECIFICATION

Characteristic	Requirement
Prior to biocide addition:	
Electrical conductivity	3.3 $\times$ 10-6 OHM-1 CM-1 (max) @ 25°C
pH	6.0 $-$ 8.0 @ 25°C
Total solids	2 mg / liter (max)
Total organic carbon	1 mg / liter (max)
Taste and odor	None at threshold odor No. of 3
Turbidity	11 units (max)
Color, true	15 units (max)
Ionic species	
Cadmium	0.01 mg / liter (max)
Chromium	0.05 mg / liter (max)
Copper	1.0 mg / liter (max)
Iron	0.3 mg / liter (max)
Lead	0.05 mg / liter (max)
Manganese	0.05 mg / liter (max)
Mercury	0.005 mg / liter (max)
Nickel	0.05 mg / liter (max)
Selenium	0.01 mg / liter (max)
Silver	0.05 mg / liter (max)
Zinc	5.0 mg / liter (max)
Sterility	Determine viable organism count for reference only
Dissolved gas	No free gas when subjected to one (1) atmosphere pressure at 37°C
After biocide addition:	
Sterility	Free of viable microorganisms
Electrical conductivity	Measure for reference only
Iodine	10 ppm by weight (max)
pH	Measure for reference only
Space Shuttle Program Specification	Space Shuttle Fluid Procurement and Use Control, Change 30

sonal hygiene and housekeeping water requirements can be less demanding relative to inorganic and organic constituents. Microbiological requirements, however, will be equal for all water uses: essential sterility or no detectable organisms when a specific analytical procedure is used, e.g., Millipore Filter using 150 ml of sample. Because of the nature of the sources of recycled potable water, the organic constituents of water intended for metabolic support will be critical.

Various methods of water reclamation adaptable to flight constraints are being investigated and developed. Specific processes include filtration, hyperfiltration, chemical coagulation, reverse osmosis, membrane evaporation, distillation (phase change), and sorption by ion exchange and activated carbon. Microbiological control through the use of a residual bactericide will be required. Iodine has been successfully used in the Skylab and Shuttle programs for this purpose.

Developmental Needs

Reclamation and System Hardware. Further work is required in the development of reliable and efficient systems to recycle water for inflight uses, and to better define the housekeeping and personal hygiene water quantity requirements for long-term space missions. The latter requirement cannot be met completely until inflight data is developed using prototype hardware supportive of long-term flight requirements. These data, along with the more fully developed reclamation hardware, will permit definition and design of the integrated water recycling and supply system for long-term use.

Water Quality Requirements. Quality criteria for recycled water need to be established. These criteria, particularly the organic content, cannot be totally defined until the constituents of reclaimed water are characterized through development and testing of treatment hardware and procedures. It is expected that quality criteria will vary for different uses, with the most constraining being those for recycled water for metabolic needs.

Water Quality Monitoring Hardware. Following definition of the constituents and potential contaminants of reclaimed water, inflight monitoring capabilities will be developed to provided continuing verification that maximum allowable concentrations are not exceeded. It is projected that this capability will serve not only as a final check on the acceptability of the water, but also as a backup capability to water reclamation process control instrumentation.

WASTE MANAGEMENT

Introduction

Waste management activities include collection and disposal of biologically active or potentially active materials, such as metabolic wastes, urine and feces, and food residues. Other than eventual disposal requirements for food residue, this waste does not present any particular physiological challenge and will not be discussed in detail.

History

One of the greatest challenges to crew life support has been providing effective and acceptable methods of inflight collection of urine and feces under microgravity conditions. The first systems provided for this purpose were intimate contact devices. In-suit urine collection was accomplished with a roll-on cuff and bag system. Feces management, if required, was provided by absorbent diaper-type underwear and a tape- or stick-on colostomy-type bag for feces collection. While functional, those systems were difficult to use, time consuming, and tended to be messy (Sauer and Jorgensen, 1975).

In an attempt to develop a more acceptable system, the Skylab systems for urine and feces collection were designed to incorporate air flow for pneumatic collection and transport of wastes. This air flow served as an artificial gravity causing separation and transportation of wastes from the body into waste processing equipment. Intimate contact with the collection system was not required. (A similar method of urine and feces collection and transport is used on the Space Shuttle.) The Skylab system was also designed to provide volume and mass measurement and samples of wastes in support of biomedical experimentation. Disposal of urine, with the exception of very early space flight missions, has been accomplished by dumping to the space vacuum. Feces disposal in early missions was accomplished by chemical disinfection and eventual return to Earth in bags. Feces were freeze-dried on Skylab to support biomedical sample preservation requirements and returned to Earth for clinical analysis (NASA TM X64813, 1974). On the Shuttle, feces are collected in a single container, vacuum dried, and returned to Earth for final disposal. The Shuttle waste management system has been designed to support both male and female use.

Future Systems

Urine and feces management systems for future long-duration space flight programs must be at least as effective and efficient as the one-gravity systems used on Earth. In addition to collection, flight systems will provide for stabilization of wastes and total control of odors. The eventual disposal of urine will be an integral part of the water reclamation process, as discussed previously. Eventual disposal of solid or semi-solid wastes resulting from the water reclamation process and the feces will be provided. In the event that biomedical experimental or operational requirements dictate a need, volume and mass measurement and sampling of metabolic wastes will be required. This will most likely include inflight analysis of specific metabolic waste constituents.

Development Needs

Collection. It is anticipated that the development work being undertaken in support of Shuttle waste collection will be directly applicable to comparable systems designed for use on long-term space missions. One exception is the development of a means to ensure positive separation of feces from the anal area—a continuing flight problem.

Disposal. Again, developmental efforts in support of Shuttle flights should provide technical solutions for long-term disposal of solid wastes. The waste reclamation system, if it uses urine for re-

cycling of water, will result in eventual disposal of urine. If this system does not recycle urine, then either onboard storage for eventual return to Earth or controlled overboard dumping will be required.

Measurement, Sampling and Analysis. Skylab techniques for measurement and sampling of urine and feces are, for the most part, inappropriate for future use because of the crew time and large amount of expendable bags and equipment required. The technology being developed to provide the urine monitoring system for Shuttle will be directly applicable to future needs. However, there is nothing comparable being developed for feces monitoring. Technology is needed for feces sampling and measurement and real-time analysis of waste constituents in support of operational and experimental requirements.

PERSONAL HYGIENE

Introduction

For general crew well-being it is projected that the personal hygiene requirements for long on-orbit stays will approximate those required in a normal (Earth) environment. These will include requirements for hand and face washing, bathing, hair washing, grooming, shaving, and oral hygiene.

History

Means for personal hygiene, while not a major impetus in previous space flights, have been provided on a continuing if not complete basis. Concepts and systems currently used for many personal hygiene needs such as shaving and tooth brushing are directly applicable to future needs. However, in general, systems to support major requirements are inadequate or nonexistent. A shower developed for Skylab involved such a significant amount of crew time to set up and operate that it was judged to be ineffectual. The hand washer as provided in Shuttle does not provide adequate fluid handling and control to be useful in long-term space flight.

Future Systems

As noted, future long-duration space flight will require devices and levels of personal hygiene similar to those to which civilized man has become accustomed. This includes the convenience of an onboard shower and lavatory. The greatest challenges to developing workable systems for space flight are the effects of microgravity on water management. The relatively large volumes of water required for bathing drive the need for wash-water recycling. Soap will be selected according to compatibility with the crew as well as the water recycling system.

Development Needs

Development requirements for personal hygiene systems primarily involve inflight showering or bathing and hand or face washing capabilities. The systems provided in Skylab and Shuttle are inadequate for long-duration space flight. The development of these capabilities to support future needs is considered a major effort.

EMERGENCY SURVIVAL SYSTEMS

The atmospheric control systems and crew support systems described in this chapter are critical to the health and well-being of the crew. Because failures of atmospheric control can quickly result in acute prob-

lems, there is a basic requirement for emergency survival systems. However, in emergency situations in which crew retrieval may take many days, survival systems must provide backups for all environmental control functions.

Launch Escape Systems. Possible failure of the booster rocket during launch is one of the contingencies that must be addressed. The emergency system must rapidly separate crewmembers from the booster and return them safely to the ground. Approaches that have been utilized are: (1) ejection seats combined with pressure suits and seat-contained life support systems and parachute system, and (2) separable crew module systems incorporating a high-G rocket motor to pull the capsule away after explosive bolts free it from its connection to the booster.

Emergency Pressure Systems. In the event of a failure of the pressure envelope, an emergency system is required to provide O_2 at levels that will support life. Some of the approaches that have been used include a pressure suit as a pressure refuge, an emergency gas makeup system to maintain pressure in the event of a leak, and systems involving a pressure refuge in a portion of the spacecraft or in a second spacecraft.

Emergency O_2 System and Breathing Systems. An O_2 breathing system must be available in the event of contamination of the cabin breathing environment with toxic materials or smoke, or in the case of loss of O_2 pressure. Such a system may also serve as an O_2 prebreathe system as part of a pre-EVA denitrogenation system. These systems are frequently incorporated in suits and worn on launch and entry to protect against low altitude loss of pressure and aftereffects of a survivable crash landing in which release of toxic gases from reaction motors would be very likely.

Emergency Transfer Pressure Envelopes. Should it be necessary to transfer crewmembers from a disabled vehicle to a rescue vehicle, a pressure suit or similar pressure envelope may be utilized.

HISTORY

The Mercury spacecraft's escape system employed a rocket motor mounted above the cabin, capable of separating the cabin from the booster in the event of a booster failure. Emergency pressure was provided by a pressure suit worn throughout flight. Each suit incorporated a urine collection device, described earlier in this chapter. The ventilation system in the suit provided emergency O_2 in the event of smoke or other contamination of the cabin atmosphere.

The Gemini spacecraft utilized ejection seats as the escape system in the event of a booster failure up to an altitude of 15,000 ft. Above 15,000 ft. the retro rockets could separate the cabin from the booster, with ejection retained as a backup mode after separation. Pressure suits provided a pressure refuge and were worn during launch, rendezvous, and reentry. The O_2 supply system was backed with two emergency O_2 bottles that would have supplied enough O_2 for an emergency deorbit abort and sufficient time for redonning pressure suits in the event of a cabin leak.

The Apollo spacecraft incorporated an escape system similar to the Mercury system, with a high impulse rocket motor mounted above the cabin to pull the cabin away from the booster in the event of a booster failure. Apollo pressure suits were designed specifically for EVA and, although they could be used as a pressure refuge, the primary emergency pressure system for orbital flights was an emergency gas supply that would sustain cabin pressure with a leak of a given size, and

sustain this pressure for sufficient time to allow an emergency return to Earth. In lunar Apollo flights, the Lunar Module (LM) served as a potential pressure refuge. During the Apollo 13 incident, after the Service Module cryogenic oxygen supply was lost and the Command Module was left without its main source of supply for oxygen, water, and electrical power, the LM's ECS sustained the crew. The LM was not utilized as an exclusive pressure refuge during this incident, because it was able to maintain normal cabin pressure in the Command Module as well as the LM. In Apollo, a separate smoke mask system was provided to handle a low O_2 or smoke in case of a cabin emergency.

The Skylab complex incorporated features of the Apollo Program. In addition, Skylab contained several pressure-tight compartments that could have been used as pressure refuges. Early in the Skylab Program a "lifeboat" system was contemplated that included a retro rocket to allow reentry. This concept was not pursued, however, and the Apollo capsule with reentry capability always remained docked to Skylab.

Shuttle approach and landing tests and orbital flight tests utilized ejection seats as an emergency escape system. These tests did not exceed an altitude of 22,000 ft. The crew wore flight suits and O_2 masks to provide life support after ejection. During orbital flight tests an escape and ejection pressure suit was worn, which allowed for ejection up to about 100,000 ft.

The configuration of the operational Shuttle vehicle through 51-L did not include an ejection escape system, and the Shuttle vehicle was not designed to be capable of separation from the boosters and fuel tank while the rocket motors were thrusting. The pressure suits on board the Shuttle vehicle are for EVA and do not provide a pressure refuge. Shuttle avionics require at least an 8.00-psi atmosphere for cooling. The emergency pressure system consists of a gas supply that will maintain cabin pressure at an emergency level of 8.00 psi with a 0.45-inch hole in the cabin for 165 minutes, sufficient time for a forced abort landing at a contingency landing site. As a result of the 51-L accident investigation, consideration is being given to additional emergency systems.

REFERENCES

Adams, J.D. Preliminary results of 8.00 psi zero prebreathe study. NASA/Defense PRT 82170, 1984.

Belew, L.F. (Ed.). Skylab, our first Space Station (NASA SP-400). U.S. Government Printing Office, Washington, D.C., 1977.

Brady, J.C., Hughes, D.F., Samonski, F.H., Jr., Young, R.W., and Browne, D.M. Apollo command and service module and lunar module environmental control systems. In: Biomedical results of Apollo (NASA SP-368). Edited by R.S. Johnston, L.F. Dietlein, and C.A. Berry. U.S. Government Printing Office, Washington, D.C., 1975.

Carleton, W.M. and Welch, B.E. Fluid balance in artificial environments: Role of environmental variables. Final Report (NASA/Defense PRT 74393-G) April, 1971.

Fanger, P.O. Thermal comfort. Copenhagen, Danish Technical Press, 1970.

Gemini Midprogram Conference (NASA SP-121). U.S. Government Printing Office, Washington, D.C., 1966.

Hendler, E. Physiological responses to intermittent oxygen and exercise exposures (NADC-74 241-40; AD BOOO 348L). November, 1974.

Horrigan, D.J., Jr. Atmosphere. In: The physiological basis for spacecraft environmental limits. NASA Reference Publication 1045, 1979.

Kimzey, S.L., Fisher, C.L., Johnson, P.C., Ritzman, S.E., and Mengel, C.E. Hematology and Immunology Studies. In: Biomedical Results of Apollo, (NASA SP-368), Edited by R.S. Johnston, L.F. Dietlein, and C.A. Berry, U.S. Government Printing Office, Washington, D.C., 1975.

Mercury Project Summary (NASA SP-45), National Aeronautics and Space Administration, 1963.

NASA Technical Memorandum X-64813. MSFC Skylab Orbital Workshop, Vol. III, May 1974.

Roth, E.M. Rapid explosive decompression emergencies in pressure-suited subjects (NASA CR-1223), 1968.

Sauer, R.L. and Calley, D.J. Potable Water Supply. In: Biomedical Results of Apollo (NASA SP-368). Edited by R.S. Johnston, L.F. Dietlein, and C.A. Berry. U.S. Government Printing Office, Washington, D.C., 1975.

Sauer, R.L. and Jorgensen, G.K. Waste Management System. In: Biomedical Results of Apollo (NASA SP-368). Edited by R.S. Johnston, L.F. Dietlein, and C.A. Berry. U.S. Government Printing Office, Washington, D.C., 1975.

Sauer, R.L. and Westover, J.B. The Potable Water System in Skylab. 74-ENAs-17, ASME Intersociety Conference on Environmental Systems, 1975.

Sauer, R.L. and Bustamante, R.B. Water Supply in Spacecraft—Past, Present and Future. Paper presented at 26th Purdue Industrial Waste Conference, Lafayette, Indiana, May 4–6, 1971.

Space Shuttle Program Specification: Space Shuttle Fluid Procurement and Use Control Change #30 dated 5/8/84.

Waligora, J.M., Horrigan, D., Jr., Conkin, J. and Hadley, A.T., III. Verification of an altitude decompression sickness prevention protocol for Shuttle operations utilizing a 10.2 psi pressure stage. NASA Technical Memorandum 58259, June, 1984.

Waligora, J.M. "Extravehicular Activities" and Appendix C "Physiologically Acceptable Space Station and Pressure Suit Pressures." In: Space Station Medical Sciences Concepts. NASA Technical Memorandum 58255, February, 1984.

West, J.B. Respiratory Physiology. Baltimore, MD, The Williams and Wilkins Co., 1974.

6 Extravehicular Activities

DAVID J. HORRIGAN, JR.
JAMES M. WALIGORA
JAMES H. BREDT

Since the time of the Gemini missions, extravehicular activity (EVA) has been one of the most dramatic challenges of space flight. Although various problems were encountered in the five Gemini EVAs, those early missions demonstrated the feasibility of placing a human into free space, outside the protective confines of the space vehicle. The practicality of EVA was firmly established in subsequent manned missions; lunar surface activities during the Apollo Program were highly successful in the deployment and conduct of numerous experiments, and a series of EVAs in Skylab permitted the completion of repairs crucial to successful station operation. In the Shuttle era, crewmembers have demonstrated abilities to retrieve and service satellites and to fly untethered using the Manned Maneuvering Unit (MMU).

During the Apollo Program, 12 crewmembers spent a total of 160 hours on the one-sixth gravity lunar surface. Apollo crews also spent a total of almost 8 hours in zero-gravity EVAs (Waligora and Horrigan, 1975). The EVAs planned for Skylab originally required a total of 18 to 20 hours, including the replacement of film used in Apollo Telescope Mount (ATM) cameras. These plans were changed, however, when the Orbital Workshop was damaged during the launch of Skylab 1. An initial set of EVAs was conducted to deploy the solar power panel. After it was demonstrated that a considerable amount of work could be performed successfully in zero gravity, the number and duration of EVAs were extended, and additional EVAs were carried out to erect a solar canopy, repair an Earth Resources antenna, replace a gyro power pack, and perform other vehicle and experiment repairs (Waligora and Horrigan, 1977).

Paramount among the planning considerations relative to EVA is the need to meet essential physiological requirements. The pressurized suit must supply oxygen and

121

remove carbon dioxide, while protecting the body from temperature extremes and micrometeoroids. But physiology is not the only factor involved. Operational and engineering considerations create separate sets of requirements that must be effectively integrated with physiological considerations in planning EVA operations. One example, encountered during preparations for a contingency EVA in the initial flight tests of the Shuttle, involved the use of enriched onboard oxygen concentrations (Horrigan and Waligora, 1980). Increased flammability is an operational consideration which sets an upper limit to the O_2 concentration used, while the danger of hypoxia and the need for nitrogen elimination prior to decompression are physiological considerations which set a lower limit on O_2 and an upper limit on nitrogen. If the Shuttle suit pressure is raised to decrease the extent of the decompression and thereby reduce the time required for preoxygenation, then mobility within the suit is compromised. These factors must be balanced to find the ideal "window" for O_2 concentration on the spacecraft. Cumulative experience through the years of various manned space programs has enhanced our ability to understand and integrate the matrix of spacecraft life support, operational, and engineering requirements. However, features introduced by future EVAs in conjunction with the Space Shuttle and Space Station Freedom present a number of new requirements. Thus, it is necessary to examine the current status of EVA technology and the basic problems that drive its development.

SPACE SUITS

Pressure garments were utilized in lieu of total cabin pressurization as early as 1935 by Wiley Post, and developed into more sophisticated full-pressure suits by the military for jet aircraft flights exceeding altitudes of 50,000 feet. The pressurized suit was retained as a backup for cabin pressure through the Mercury Program. However, for Gemini, Apollo, and Skylab, suits were required for EVA as well. EVA required that the suits be compatible with Command Module and Lunar Module pressures, and capable of independent interaction with the portable life support system (PLSS) (Correale, 1979).

The Shuttle Extravehicular Mobility Unit (EMU) consists of the space suit and an integrated life support system. It differs from previous suits in that it is not custommade for each astronaut. Instead, it consists of ten separate components such as the hard upper torso, arm and lower torso assemblies. These component items can be combined and integrated to form a suit appropriate to individual anthropometric proportions. The Shuttle EMU is designed to provide a 4.3 psi nominal pressure, higher than that provided for earlier suits such as the Skylab suit (3.85 psia). The suit is purged to a minimum O_2 concentration of 95 percent prior to EVA and all makeup gas is O_2. CO_2 is absorbed by a lithium hydroxide canister which maintains CO_2 at 0.15 psi or less at metabolic rates up to 1,600 BTU/hr., and below 0.29 psi at higher metabolic rates. A liquid-cooling garment removes body heat by a combination of conduction, convection, and evaporation. Coolant is pumped through the garment to a heat exchanger in contact with a sublimator which dissipates heat to the vacuum of space through controlled sublimation of a water supply.

Future suits may have a pressure as high as 9.5 psia. Although joint mobility has been shown to be independent of total pressure in these ranges (Vykukal, 1984), a system permitting adequate hand mobility at higher pressures remains to be developed (Flugel and Kosmo, 1984) (Horrigan, Waligora and Dierlam, 1983).

Development of a suit in the 8 to 10 psia range would eliminate the lengthy pre-breathing period prior to EVA (required to eliminate nitrogen gas from the body to reduce the risk of decompression sickness), since the decompression would be only the equivalent of sea level to about 12,000 feet.

LIFE SUPPORT SYSTEMS

The EMU is actually a small, self-contained spacecraft that can supply all the essentials of life support for as long as 7 or 8 hours. It must provide adequate pressure, suitable O_2 partial pressure, and a means of removing the CO_2 generated by the crewmember. In addition, sufficient cooling must be available to remove the metabolic heat generated by the crewmember, the heat generated in absorbing CO_2, and that generated by pumps and fans.

Given these requirements, the greatest concern in terms of the space suit's life support capability is that of workload. Before the pressurized suit was developed for the first Gemini EVAs, planners had to make educated guesses as to the metabolic cost of work in zero gravity and the one-sixth gravity on the lunar surface. As it happened, although the Gemini life support system was generally adequate for average metabolic rates during EVA, it was not able to handle short-term increases in the work and metabolic rates. Although metabolic rates were not measured directly, it was obvious on several occasions that they exceeded the thermal control and carbon dioxide washout capabilities of the life support system.

LIQUID-COOLED GARMENT

The answer to these problems was the development, in the Apollo Program, of a liquid-cooled garment (LCG). This system suppressed perspiration at work rates up to 400 kcal/hr, and allowed sustained operations at work rates as high as 500 kcal/hr without thermal stress. By comparison, the heat removal capacity of the improved gas cooling system used on the later Gemini missions was limited to about 250 kcal/hr. The Apollo LCG was able to handle without difficulty all of the peak workloads encountered on the lunar surface during tasks involving heavy lifting, lengthy walking, and vigorous calisthenic-like exercise (Waligora and Horrigan, 1975). Later, the suit also proved adequate for all the EVAs on Skylab.

The average metabolic rate of crewmembers performing Shuttle EVAs is lower than both the Apollo and Skylab values (significance at .01 level, Table 6-1). This was expected with the addition of specialized tools, foot restraints, and devices such as the Manned Maneuvering Unit (MMU). These devices, along with careful training of the crewmembers in the Water Environment Test Facility at the Lyndon B. Johnson Space Center and ease of joint mobility in the Shuttle space suit, explain the reduction in required human energy expenditure.

DECOMPRESSION SICKNESS

Apart from the problems of cooling and oxygen supply, another important concern relative to EVA is the danger of decompression sickness. Because of limitations on mobility of the limbs and hands as suit pressure increases, an astronaut is subjected to lower pressures in the suit than in the spacecraft cabin. The difference between these two pressures is, generally speaking, proportional to the risk of developing decompression sickness.

TABLE 6–1

METABOLIC RATES DURING EVAS

Mission	Kcal/Hr	Crewmember-Hrs EVA
Apollo ⅙ G	234	162
0 G	151	9
Skylab	238	83
Shuttle	197	137

ETIOLOGY

Decompression sickness may occur when the partial pressure of dissolved gases in bodily tissues exceeds the ambient atmospheric pressure. Typically this is the result of rapid decompression, as when a diver ascends quickly to the surface or an astronaut dons a space suit which is then rapidly decompressed. Under these conditions, bubbles may form in tissues and blood and be carried in the venous blood to the heart and lungs. Decompression sickness can manifest itself by bubbles underneath the skin, by classic "bends" pain around the joints and muscles, by "chokes" or pain in the area of the lungs, by neurological manifestations such as a skin rash or numbness, and, in extreme cases, by paralysis, circulatory collapse, and shock. Most commonly, decompression sickness symptoms are divided into two main categories: Type I and Type II (Kidd and Elliott, 1969). Type I includes those cases in which pain is the only symptom, or in which cutaneous and lymphatic involvement are seen either alone or with joint pain. Type II symptoms include cases of a more serious nature, with nervous system and respiratory involvement. Other authors further subdivide these categories. Table 6-2 presents a detailed listing of symptoms, drawing on the paradigm of Hills (1982). Type I bends are the main concern in space flight. The expectation is that preventing Type I bends will also pre-

vent the more severe symptoms. However, evidence described by Hills (1982) suggests that spinal, cerebral, and vestibular symptoms can be elicited by choice of conditions and may have different and independent etiologies. Thus, there is not necessarily a progression from Type I to Type II. They may occur in parallel, or Type II may appear without Type I, depending on the site of bubble formation. Since intra-arterial bubbles appear to be a cause of Type II, one concern has been the possibility of transpulmonary passage of venous emboli. Work by Butler and Hills (1979) has shown that the lung is an efficient bubble filter; and unless there is a pathological condition such as a patent foramen ovale, transmission of bubbles from the venous to arterial side would not be expected under levels of decompression found in normal space operations. Another factor that could impair the bubble-trapping action of the lungs is excessive oxygen toxicity (Butler and Hills, 1981), which may interfere with the functioning of pulmonary surfactant. Moreover, changes in pulmonary surfactant have also been reported to be involved in the pathophysiology of transpulmonary passage of venous gas emboli (Hills and Butler, 1981). Neither of these conditions is associated with atmospheres designed for use in space.

PREVENTION

Decompression is not normally a problem when the original partial pressure of the diluent gas (usually nitrogen) in the atmosphere, and thus in the tissues, does not exceed the final decompression pressure by more than a ratio of 1.3 to 1. The actual rate varies from individual to individual and from tissue to tissue (for example, muscle absorbs and expels nitrogen much more quickly than does fatty tissue). But when changes in pressure result in con-

TABLE 6–2

DECOMPRESSION SICKNESS MANIFESTATIONS FOR THE SIX TYPES OF DYSBARISM

| Organs Involved | Symptoms | | | | | |
	I	II	III	IV	V	VI
Bends						
Skin	Rash Urticaria Pruritus					
Extremities	Localized joint pains					
Central Nervous System		Unconsciousness, Visual disturbances				
Cerebral		Convulsions Headache Collapse Paresthesia				
Spinal cord			Hemiplegia Paresthesia Abdominal pain Muscular weakness			
Vestibular/ Cochlear				Vertigo Nausea/Vomiting Nystagmus Incoordination Deafness Tinnitus		
Lungs					"Chokes" Cough Irritation	
Bones						Type A Osteonecrosis (juxta-articular) Type B Osteonecrosis (head, neck, shaft) Pain Neurologic manifestations

Based on the paradigm developed by Hills, 1982.

ditions exceeding these limits, it is necessary to lower the pressure of dissolved gases in the tissues prior to decompression. There are at least two basic ways of accomplishing this denitrogenation of tissues.

Preoxygenation. Because of the high rate of tissue utilization of oxygen, this gas does not contribute significantly to the formation or growth of bubbles in tissue. Therefore, an effective method to protect against decompression sickness is to breathe 100 percent O_2 prior to decompression, displacing nitrogen from the tissues, or to lower the concentration of N_2 in the breathing gas, thus reducing N_2 pressure in the tissue to a point at which the ratio is within the "safe" zone.

In Gemini and Apollo missions, the potential for decompression sickness was greatest at liftoff, when pressure changed from 14.7 psi to 5 psi. To protect against decompression sickness, crews breathed pure oxygen for 3 hours prior to launch, flushing nitrogen from their tissues. This procedure is known as "whole-body washout." It decreased the ratio of tissue nitrogen pressure to cabin pressure at launch to about 1.6, which was considered acceptable (Figure 6-1). Preoxygenation also protected the crew against both sudden cabin decompression and the need for an immediate ("contingency") EVA, which would have exposed crewmembers to 3.7 psi in their space suits. In either event, the N_2/suit pressure ratio would have been considerably higher—about 2.1 (Figure 6-1). However, in the case of the lunar EVAs, N_2 tension in the tissues had been lowered sufficiently so that the 3.7-psi suit presented little danger of bends by the time crews embarked on their planned EVAs several days later.

The situation in Skylab was similar, except that the Skylab cabin contained a two-gas atmosphere (70 percent O_2, 30 percent N_2, at 5 psi). However, delivery

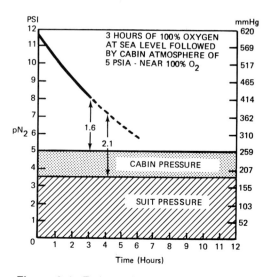

Figure 6-1. Estimated relationships of N_2 tension to cabin and suit pressures in early U.S. space flights. The curve is for N_2 tension in a 360-minute tissue—that is, a tissue with an N_2-elimination half-time of 360 minutes.

to Skylab was accomplished via the 100 percent O_2 Apollo vehicle, so that an additional period of nitrogen washout was undergone. No cases of decompression sickness were reported. The Apollo-Soyuz Test Project presented an interesting variation, in that there were repetitive transfers of personnel between the 5-psi Apollo spacecraft and the 10-psi Soyuz vehicle. The scenario was tested on the ground beforehand (Cooke et al., 1975a) and, as expected, proved safe. Again, no cases of bends were reported.

Space Shuttle: N_2 Equilibration. The Space Shuttle presents a very different set of concerns in the prevention of decompression sickness during EVA. In contrast to all preceding U.S. spacecraft, the Shuttle cabin has an "Earth-normal" atmosphere of 14.7 psi, with 21 percent O_2 and 79 percent N_2. Consequently, decompression sickness is a possibility not at liftoff but during preparation for EVA. Initially, a 3-hour denitrogenation using 100 percent O_2 was contemplated. The assumption was that this would be adequate for individuals with a low fat-to-lean body mass ratio who were also bends-free during the space suit certification trials, and assuming EVA work rates similar to or less than those experienced on Apollo EVAs. However, when planners examined the results of O_2-prebreathing studies in which similar final decompression pressures were obtained, they were disturbed by some of the findings (Table 6-3).

Although some researchers achieved total protection from bends on a 3-hour preoxygenation regimen, other results ranged as low as 58 percent protection. Four hours of prebreathing appeared to offer consistently good protection.

Another problem with onboard prebreathing was a physical, or technical, one. When the crewmember dons the EVA suit, he must not break the prebreathing regimen. As shown in Figure 6-2, this presents considerable difficulty. A nose clip and mouthpiece would be provided to permit hands-free manipulation, but to get completely into the suit the crewmember would have had to remove the mouthpiece and hold his breath, then resume prebreathing once in the suit. When the helmet is attached, the crewmember must hold his breath for another 30 seconds before the helmet is flushed of nitrogen. Considering these two operations, it is difficult to verify that some of the 80 percent nitrogen cabin air has not been inhaled.

This is an important concern because of the rate at which tissues become resaturated with nitrogen during washout (Figure 6-3). Air Force studies (Cooke, 1975b) showed an increased incidence of decompression sickness in subjects who interrupted their prebreathing with selected periods of air breathing for 5 or 10 minutes as compared with those who did not in-

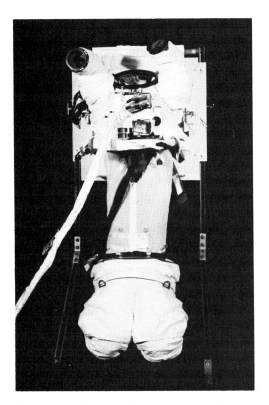

Figure 6-2. Donning the space suit while prebreathing was difficult and could have compromised the prebreathing process.

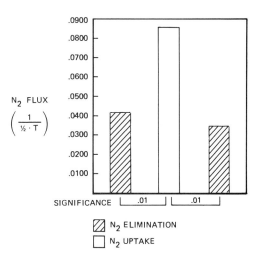

Figure 6-3. Uptake of nitrogen in muscle during an air break in nitrogen washout (Horrigan, 1979a).

TABLE 6–3

PERCENT PROTECTION FROM BENDS PROVIDED BY SELECTED PERIODS OF O_2 PREBREATHING

Final Pressure (psi)	Duration of Prebreathing at Sea Level (hours)						
	0.5	1.0	1.5	2.0	3.0	3.5	4.0
2.8	24	–	–	–	–	–	96
3.5	26	45	–	70	83	–	91
3.5	–	–	50	–	60	77	93
3.7	–	–	–	–	100	–	–
3.8	–	–	–	–	58	–	–
3.0	–	30.4	–	–	–	–	–
4.4	–	4.2	–	–	–	–	–
3.8	–	–	–	–	100[a]	–	–

[a]This represents space suit training conducted at Johnson Space Center. The policy was to provide at least 3 hours prebreathing; some individuals may have had substantially more than this.
Studies from different laboratories; data compiled by NASA.

terrupt the oxygen breathing. Further studies (Adams et al., 1977) indicated that a 1-minute interruption, or "air break," would require 34 minutes of additional prebreathing to compensate for the renitrogenation of tissues. A human study conducted at the Shrine Burn Hospital in Galveston (Horrigan et al., 1979a, 1979b), using 80 percent argon and 20 percent oxygen for a normoxic denitrogenation, revealed a sharp slope of renitrogenation in quadriceps muscle tissue (Figure 6-4). The relatively rapid, subsequent denitrogenation upon exposure to 30 minutes of 100 percent O_2 prebreathing is probably due to the high rate of N_2 elimination in muscle tissue.

The various problems encountered with onboard preoxygenation led planners to search for alternative means of proper decompression prior to EVA in the Space Shuttle. The search centered on a diving physiology technique, the Haldane method of using N_2 tissue/total pressure ratios (Boycott, Damant, and Haldane, 1908) to determine optimum pressure combinations. Initially, "equilibration" to 11-psi and 12-psi cabin pressure for 12

hours was considered. But in order to achieve final ratios comparable to those obtained with sea-level oxygenation, suit pressure would have to be raised from 4 psi to 5 psi (Figure 6-5). As this was not feasible due to suit engineering, the procedure selected for the operational flight tests (OFT) of the Shuttle was to decompress the cabin to 9 psi at 28 percent O_2 for 12 hours, then don the suit for 30-45 minutes of 100 percent oxygen breathing at that pressure before decompressing the suit to 4 psi for EVA. Tests showed an approximately 6 percent incidence of Type I bends with this procedure (Adams et al., 1981), which was deemed a satisfactory risk in the event of contingency EVA during the OFTs. Since no EVAs were required during these missions, the procedure was not put to the test in space.

On the basis of decompression parameters alone, the Haldane method compared favorably with preoxygenation while allowing freedom of movement and activity. At the end of 12 hours of equilibration to this atmosphere, the pressure ratio would be 1.9—comparable to about 3 hours of preoxygenation. The final 30-40 minutes

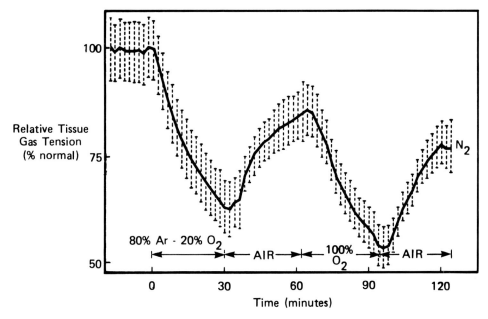

Figure 6-4. Nitrogen tension measured in the quadriceps muscle of human subjects exposed to selected atmospheres. (Horrigan, 1979b).

on oxygen reduces the ratio to a still lower and safer level. Comparing these figures to the previous results of decompression studies (Figure 6-6), it is clear that as the ratio drops below 2.0 into the 1.6-1.8 range, the incidence of bends decreases.

However, one potential problem emerged with the 9-psi equilibration. To minimize flammability, which is a consideration when using certain spacecraft cabin materials, a limitation of 30 percent was placed on oxygen concentration. At 9 psi, when fluctuations of the gas pressure controller are taken into account, the worst-case oxygen level during the 12-hour equilibration period would approach the pO_2 level found at 2,500 meters. Normally (on Earth) this is a safe altitude. But considering that the effects of pulmonary function changes and fluid redistribution in zero gravity are not completely known, the problem of potential hypoxia had to be faced. Although bed rest studies suggest that oxygenation of the blood is not impaired at that pO_2 level in zero gravity

(Waligora et al., 1982), definitive assurance of the procedure's safety was not possible until pulmonary function data were obtained from Shuttle and Spacelab

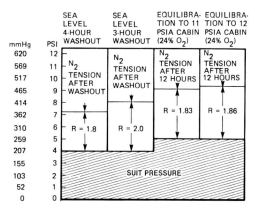

Figure 6-5. Comparison of sea level nitrogen washout with suit/cabin pressure combinations which permit equilibrium to lower N_2 tension without oxygen breathing by mask. R = ratio of N_2 partial pressure before decompression to suit pressure after decompression.

NASA AND USAF ALTITUDE EXPERIENCE (1980-1984)

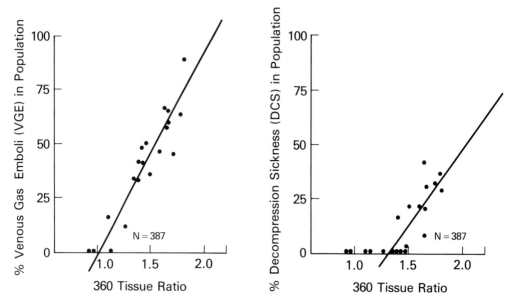

Figure 6-6. Linear plots of DCS and VGE incidence using 360 tissue ratios.

flights. Nevertheless, the 9-psi cabin pressure was adopted for the Shuttle OFT flights, in the event that an EVA was required. However, the decompression ratio was useful only in determining general guidelines. The complexity of decompression physiology required empirical testing of candidate procedures.

For the "mature" Shuttle runs (STS-5 and beyond), a compromise equilibration procedure was developed which alleviates the problem of potential hypoxia. This procedure involves reducing cabin pressure to 10.2 psi at 26.5 percent O_2. Although this is a slightly lower concentration of oxygen, the pO_2 is higher (now equivalent to about 1,200 meters, well below hypoxic limits). With this procedure, suit pressure is increased to 4.3 psi. Equilibration still requires 12 hours, and 100 percent O_2 is still breathed for 60 minutes prior to initial depressurization, and for 40 minutes in the suit before final depressurization. Rapid EVA would still re-

quire 4 hours prebreathing of O_2 at sea-level pressure, in the suit, followed by depressurization of the airlock. The above procedures require further validation in both ground and flight tests. In any event, emergency EVAs in early operational Shuttle flights could have been conducted with minimal risk of bends by prebreathing O_2 at 14.7 psi in the suit prior to EVA.

An extensive series of ground tests was performed at the Johnson Space Center to verify the acceptability of utilizing the 10.2 psi pressure stage in pre-EVA procedures (Waligora, Horrigan, Conkin, and Hadley, 1984). The tests involved 173 man-runs to evaluate the procedure in terms of eliciting venous bubbles and symptoms of altitude decompression sickness. The tests also addressed the safety, in terms of incidence of decompression sickness, of conducting EVAs on consecutive rather than on alternate days. The testing involved up to 6 hours of exercise at 4.3 psia using anticipated EVA work rates (Figure 6-7). The incidence of venous bubbles (55 percent) and symptoms (26 percent) were higher than anticipated. This is thought to be due to the type and duration of exercise, as well as the sensitivity of the reporting technique to minor symptoms. The procedure was modified to include an hour of oxygen breathing prior to the first decompression as well as 40 minutes in the suit prior to the final depressurization to 4.3 psia (Figure 6-8).

The procedure shown in Figure 6-8 was accepted for flight and has been used successfully (no signs or reports of bends symptoms) on 12 EVAs (129 crewmember hours) as of this writing (Horrigan et al., 1985, 1987). This procedure, nevertheless, retains about a 20 percent risk of mild limb bends symptoms. Inflight occurrence of such symptoms would be treated by repressurization to cabin pressure, and the use of the suit for additional pressure, if required. Most cases of altitude bends are relieved by return to sea-level pressure. Procedures, equipment, and techniques are

being developed to eliminate the need for any prebreathing prior to EVA and eliminate any symptoms, regardless of type or level, of decompression sickness. Table 5-2 in Chapter 5 provides examples of selected cabin and suit pressures designed to eliminate symptoms of decompression sickness.

SHUTTLE EVA HARDWARE

The Extravehicular Mobility Unit (EMU) described above includes an in-suit drink bag which holds drinking water during a 7-hour EVA, and a urine collection device. It has a communication system to allow voice contact with the spacecraft and the ground, and a display and control module which allows the crewmember to control cooling temperature and select one of several operational modes. This module pro-

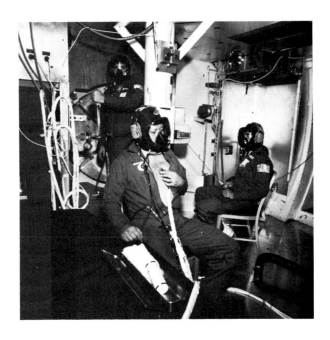

Figure 6-7. Doppler technician monitors himself for intravenous bubbles during NASA JSC bends prevention test as test crewmembers perform selected exercise. Conditions are 4.3 psia, ambient pressure and pure oxygen in the breathing masks.

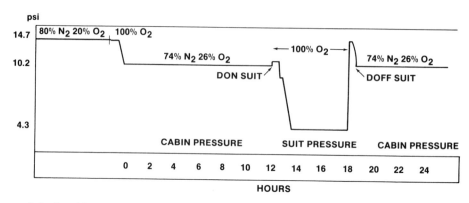

Figure 6-8. Combination of straight oxygen prebreathing and staged decompression.

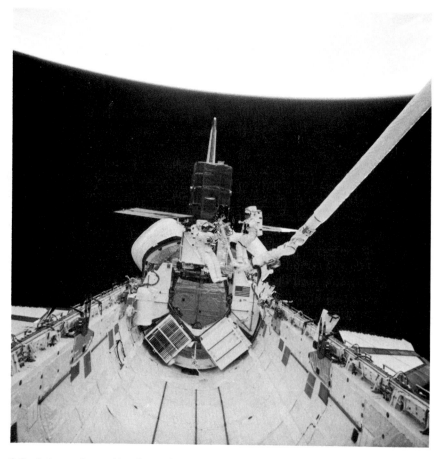

Figure 6-9. Astronauts working in payload bay.

vides the crewmember with status of consumables through a visual display, as well as warning of possible system failures. The multiple visors of the Extravehicular Visor Assembly allow the crewmember to select the appropriate degree of protection from glare and ultraviolet radiation. Finally, a secondary oxygen pack provides emergency pressure, O_2, CO_2 washout, and cooling for a 30-minute period by controlled release of a high-pressure O_2 supply in an open loop mode (not recirculated).

Many new devices to expand the capability and efficiency of the crewmember during EVA have been tested. Among these are the Manned Maneuvering Unit (MMU), the Manipulator Foot Restraint (MFR), the MMU docking device, and hand tools such as a power screwdriver. Moreover, the EMU itself permits easier joint flexing than its earlier counterparts. Figure 6-9 shows two EVA crewmembers working in the Shuttle payload bay, and Figure 6-10 shows a crewmember operating the MMU.

OUTLOOK FOR EVA OPERATIONS

SHUTTLE EVAS

Shuttle EVAs are carried out primarily in the Orbiter's payload bay. Crewmembers use a slide wire to translate between the forward and aft portions of the bay. On the starboard side, next to the forward bulkhead, a Task Simulation Device (TSD) was used in early missions as a test bed for representative tasks. TSD simulations included tasks typical for satellite servicing, such as cutting a thermal blanket, removing screws, disconnecting and reconnecting electrical contacts, and cutting grounding wires. Foot restraints and handholds have been developed for Shuttle EVA operations using experience gained in earlier missions. Experience with these procedures was helpful in preparing for later Shuttle EVAs, in which crewmembers successfully repaired satellites. The two EVAs of Shuttle flight

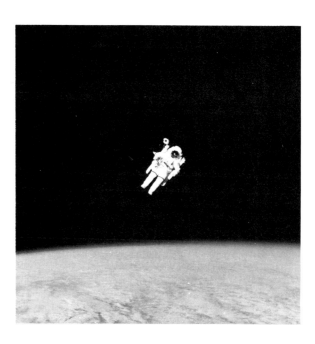

Figure 6-10. Astronaut operating MMU.

61-B in November and December of 1985 demonstrated the capabilities of crewmembers to effectively build large structures in space and provided useful data for future space construction.

FUTURE EVA REQUIREMENTS

The feasibility and utility of EVA has been amply demonstrated. While allowing useful work to be performed, the space suit life support system has protected astronauts against the space vacuum, temperature extremes of $-118°$ to $+136°C$ ($-180°$ to $+277°F$), and the impact of micrometeoroids. A wider variety of tasks and increasingly diverse crew populations require continuous reevaluation of the physiological limits, procedures, and hardware systems that have been established for EVA.

Long-term space operations, such as those planned for Space Station Freedom, are expected to require quantum improvements in the flexibility, durability, and reliability of EVA hardware. One such improvement could be the development of a suit at a higher pressure, which would make EVA operations much more efficient (Vykukal and Webbon, 1984; Flugel et al., 1984). Another would be the combination of an increased suit pressure with a decreased cabin pressure. If engineering difficulties can be successfully overcome, this may in fact be the next step forward in the direction of simplifying and "normalizing" man's activity in space.

REFERENCES

Adams, J.D., Theis, C.F. and Stevens, K.W. Denitrogenation/renitrogenation profiles: Interruption of oxygen prebreathing. Proceedings of the Aerospace Medical Association Meeting, Las Vegas, NV, May 1977.

Adams, J.D., Dixon, G.A., Olson, R.M., Bassett, B.E., and Fitzpatrick, E.L. Prevention of bends during Space Shuttle EVAs using stage decompression. Proceedings of the Aerospace Medical Association Meeting, San Antonio, TX, 1981.

Boycott, A.E., Damant, G.C.C. and Haldane, J.S. The prevention of compressed air illness. Journal of Hygiene, 1908, 8:342-443.

Butler, B.D. and Hills, B.A. The lung as a filter for microbubbles. Journal of Applied Physiology, 47:537-543, 1979.

Butler, B.D. and Hills, B.A. Effect of excessive oxygen upon the capability of the lungs to filter gas emboli. In: Underwater Physiology VII, Edited by A.J. Bachrach and M.M. Matzen, Bethesda, MD, Undersea Medical Society, 1981.

Cooke, J.P., Bollinger, R.R. and Richardson, B. Prevention of decompression sickness during a simulated space docking mission. Aviat., Space, and Envir. Med., p. 930, July 1975.

Cooke, J.P. Interruption of denitrogenation by air breathing, summary report NASA contract T-82170, USAF School of Aerospace Medicine, Brooks AFB, TX, 1975.

Correale, J.V. Evolution of the Shuttle Extravehicular Mobility Unit, ASME Publication No. 79-ENAs-24. Presented at ICES meeting July, 1979.

Flugel, C.W., Kosmo, J.J. and Rayfield, J.R. Development of a Zero-Prebreathe Space Suit; SAE No. 840981, Warrendale, PA. Presented at the 14th Intersociety Conference on Environmental Systems, San Diego, CA, July 16–19, 1984.

Hills, B.A. Basic issues in prescribing preventive decompression (letter to the Editor). Undersea Biomedical Research, September, 1982.

Hills, B.A. and Butler, B.D. Migration of lung surfactant to pulmonary air emboli. In: Underwater Physiology VII, Edited by A.J. Bachrach and M.M. Matzen. Bethesda, MD, Undersea Medical Society, 1981.

Horrigan, D.J., Wells, C.H., Guest, M.M., Hart, G.B. and Goodpasture, J.E. Tissue gas and blood analyses of human subjects breathing 80% argon and 20% oxygen. Aviat., Space, and Envir. Med. 50(4): 357–362, 1979a.

Horrigan, D.J., Wells, C.H., Hart, G.B. and Goodpasture, J.E. Elimination and uptake of inert gases in muscle and subcutaneous tissue of human subjects. Proceedings of the 50th Scientific Meeting of the Aerospace Medical Association, Washington, D.C., May 13–17, 1979b.

Horrigan, D.J. and Waligora, J.M. The development of effective procedures for the protection of Space Shuttle crewmembers against decompression sickness during extravehicular activities. Proceedings of the Aerospace Medical Association Meeting, Anaheim, CA, May 1980.

Horrigan, D.J., Waligora, J.M. and Dierlam, J. Hypobaric hand exposure test report. NASA JSC Internal Report, December 12, 1983.

Horrigan, D.J., Waligora, J.M. and Stanford, J. A physiological evaluation of Space Shuttle extravehicular activities. Abstract No. 18, 1985 Scientific Program Aerospace Medical Association, Aviat., Space, and Envir. Med. 56:484, 1985.

Horrigan, D.J., Waligora, J.M., Gilbert, J.H., Edwards, B.F., and Stanford, J. Results of metabolic rate assessment during Shuttle extravehicular activities. Abstract No. 3, 1987 Scientific Program Aerospace Medical Association, Aviat., Space, and Envir. Med. 58(5):483, 1987.

Kidd, D.J. and Elliott, D.H. Clinical manifestations and treatment of decompression sickness in divers. In: The physiology and medicine of diving and compressed air work. Edited by P.B. Bennett and D.H. Elliott, Baltimore, MD, Williams and Wilkins Company, 1969.

Vykukal, H.C. and Webbon, B. A comparison of space suit joint flex forces as a function of suit pressure. SAE Technical Paper series No. 840980, presented at the 14th Intersociety Conference on Environmental Systems, San Diego, CA, July, 1984.

Waligora, J.M. and Horrigan, D.J. Metabolism and heat dissipation during Apollo EVA periods. In: Biomedical results of Apollo (NASA SP-368). Edited by R.S. Johnston, L.F. Dietlein, and C.A. Berry, U.S. Government Printing Office, Washington, D.C.: NASA, 1975.

Waligora, J.M. and Horrigan, D.J. Metabolic cost of extravehicular activities. In: Biomedical results from Skylab (NASA SP-377). Edited by R.S. Johnston and L.F. Dietlein, U.S. Government Printing Office, Washington, D.C., 1977.

Waligora, J.M., Horrigan, D.J., Jr., Bungo, M.W. and Conkin, J. Investigation of the combined effects of bed rest and mild hypoxia. Aviat., Space, and Envir. Med., 53(7):643–646, 1982.

Waligora, J.M., Horrigan, D.J., Jr., Conkin, J. and Hadley, A.T., III. Verification of an altitude decompression sickness prevention protocol for Shuttle operations utilizing a 10.2-psi pressure stage, NASA Technical Memorandum 58259, June, 1984.

PHYSIOLOGICAL ADAPTATION TO SPACE FLIGHT

7 Overall Physiological Response to Space Flight

ARNAULD E. NICOGOSSIAN

Understanding the physiology of the human response to extreme environments requires that the sequence of underlying mechanisms be identified. Knowledge of these mechanisms is of great importance to the development of rational and appropriate prophylactic or therapeutic treatments. In obtaining this knowledge, it is advantageous to observe the process of change in its entirety, without intervention. However, it has been difficult to avoid intervention in studies of human response to space stresses (principally weightlessness), since medical personnel are also responsible for ensuring the health, well-being, and optimum performance of the crews under observation. This invariably requires some type of intervention during the period of exposure, further complicating and slowing the study of physiological processes.

There are a number of additional factors that complicate attempts to clearly delineate the time course of response to weight-lessness and the overall acclimation process in space. These include:

- Sample Size. To date, only a small number of individuals have flown in space. This small sample size makes it difficult to generalize to a larger population (Table 7-1).
- Limited Capabilities for Scientific Observations. Biomedical observations have been restricted by the operational constraints imposed on most space missions, and also by time, since the longest mission flown so far has not exceeded 1 year.
- Extensive Use of Countermeasures. Prophylactic and therapeutic use of countermeasures, such as those for neurovestibular symptoms, cardiovascular deconditioning, and loss of lean body mass, has masked some of the direct effects attributable to weightlessness alone.
- Different Mission Types. More individ-

139

TABLE 7-1

NUMBER OF ASTRONAUTS FLOWN IN SPACE[a]

Mission	Flights < 2 wk	Flights > 2 wk	Repeated Flights
U.S.	133 (including 8 non-U.S. astronauts)	9	57
U.S.S.R.	80 (including 14 non-U.S.S.R. astronauts)	36	38

[a] April, 1961 to December, 1988.

uals have flown on short-duration missions and mission profiles have markedly changed with time and number of crewmembers involved.

Despite these limitations, Skylab and Salyut missions have generated a wealth of biomedical data that points toward definite trends and lends itself to the formulation of hypotheses concerning acute responses in zero gravity and subsequent adjustments. Table 7-2 presents these trends for short missions (up to 14 days) and for longer missions (in excess of 2 weeks).

TIME COURSE OF INFLIGHT ACCLIMATION

Figure 7-1 presents a graphic summary of the time course of physiological shifts associated with space acclimation. It presupposes that all biological systems are in a state of homeostasis in the one-gravity environment at the beginning of the flight (one-gravity set point). Soon after orbital insertion, changes are exhibited by more susceptible physiological systems, although not necessarily simultaneously. For example, neurovestibular adjustments, with associated initial symptomatology, are likely to occur during the first few days

on orbit, while decrease in red blood cell (RBC) mass is detected only after a period of subclinical latency and peak at 60 days in flight. Other physiological functions do not exhibit detectable shifts early in flight, but are later shown to have undergone gradual and progressive changes. In particular, calcium loss, loss of lean body mass, and possible effects from cumulative radiation appear to increase continually, regardless of flight duration or level of acclimation achieved by other body systems.

Most physiological systems appear to reach a new steady state compatible with "normal" function in the space environment within 4 to 6 weeks. This acclimation process may not be complete for any physiological system, however, without a very long period of exposure to weightlessness.

READAPTATION TO EARTH'S ENVIRONMENT

The biomedical data collected on returning crews indicate that a compensatory period of physiological readaptation to one gravity is required after each space flight. The amount of time necessary for readaptation and the characteristic features of the process exhibit large individual differences.

TABLE 7-2

PHYSIOLOGICAL CHANGES ASSOCIATED WITH SHORT-TERM AND LONG-TERM SPACE FLIGHT

Physiological Parameter	Short-Term Space Flights[a] (1–14 days)	Long-Term Space Flights (more than 2 weeks)[b]	
		Pre- vs. Inflight	Pre- vs. Postflight
Cardiopulmonary System			
Heart rate (resting)	Slight increase inflight. Increased postflight; peaks during launch and reentry, normal or slightly increased during mission. RPB[c]: up to one week.	Normal or slightly increased.	Increased. RPB[c]: 3 weeks.
Blood pressure (resting)	Normal; decreased postflight.	Diastolic blood pressure reduced.	Decreased mean arterial pressure.
Orthostatic tolerance	Decreased after flights longer than 5 hours. Exaggerated cardiovascular responses to tilt test, stand test, and LBNP postflight. RPB[c]: 3–14 days.	Highly exaggerated cardiovascular responses to inflight LBNP (especially during first 2 weeks), sometimes resulting in presyncope. Last inflight test comparable to R + O[d] (recovery day) test.	Exaggerated cardiovascular responses to LBNP. RPB[c]: up to 3 weeks.
Cardiac size	Normal or slightly decreased cardio / thoracic ratio (C/T) postflight.		C/T ratio decreased postflight.
Stroke volume	Increased the first 24 hours inflight, then decreased by 15%.	Same as short duration missions.	12% decrease on average.
Left end diastolic volume	Same as stroke volume.	Same as short duration missions.	16% decrease on average.
Cardiac output	Unchanged.	Unchanged.	Variable RPB[c]: 3–4 weeks.
Central venous pressure (indirect measurement)	Gradual decrease over 7 days inflight.	Not measured.	Not measured.
Left cardiac muscle mass thickness	Unchanged.	Unchanged.	11% decrease, return to normal after 3 weeks.
Cardiac electrical activity (ECG/VCG)	Moderate rightward shift in QRS and T postflight.	Increased PR interval, QT_c interval, and QRS vector magnitude.	Slight increase in QRS duration and magnitude; increase in PR interval duration.
Arrhythmias	Usually premature atrial and ventricular beats (PABs, PVBs). Isolated cases of nodal tachycardia, ectopic beats, and supraventricular bigeminy inflight.	PVBs and occasional PABs; sinus or nodal arrhythmia at release of LBNP inflight.	Occasional unifocal PABs and PVBs.

141

TABLE 7-2 (Continued)

PHYSIOLOGICAL CHANGES ASSOCIATED WITH SHORT-TERM AND LONG-TERM SPACE FLIGHT

Physiological Parameter	Short-Term Space Flights[a] (1–14 days)	Long-Term Space Flights (more than 2 weeks)[b]	
		Pre- vs. Inflight	Pre- vs. Postflight
Systolic time intervals	Not measured.	Not measured.	Increase in resting and LBNP-stressed PEP/ET Ratio. RPB[c]: 2 weeks.
Exercise capacity	No change or decreased postflight; increased HR for same O_2 consumption; no change in efficiency. RPB[c]: 3–8 days.	Submaximal exercise capacity unchanged.	Decreased postflight, recovery time inversely related to amount of inflight exercise, rather than mission duration.
Lung volume	Not measured.	Vital capacity decreased 10%.	No change.
Leg volume	Decreased up to 3% postflight. Inflight, leg volume decreases exponentially during first 24 hours, and plateaus within 3 to 5 days.	Same as short missions.	15% decrease in calf circumference.
Leg blood flow	Not measured.	Marked increase.	Normal or slightly increased.
Venous compliance in legs	Not measured.	Increased: continues to increase for 10 days or more; slow decrease later inflight.	Normal or slightly increased.
Body Fluids			
Total body water	3% decrease inflight.		Decreased postflight.
Plasma volume	Decreased postflight (except Gemini 7 and 8).		Markedly decreased postflight. RPB: 2 weeks increased at R + 0; decreased R + 2 (hydration effect).
Hematocrit	Slightly increased postflight.		
Hemoglobin	Normal or slightly increased postflight.	Increased first inflight sample; slowly declines later inflight.	Decreased postflight RPB: 1–2 months.
Red blood cell (RBC) mass	Decreased postflight; RPB: at least 2 weeks.	Decreased ~15% during first 2–3 weeks inflight; begins to recover after about 60 days; recovery of RBC mass is independent of the stay time in space.	Decreased postflight RPB: 2 weeks to 3 months following landing.
Red cell half-life (^{51}Cr)	No change.		No change.

Measurement			
Iron turnover			No change.
Mean corpuscular volume (MCV)	Increased postflight; RPB: at least 2 weeks.		Variable, but within normal limits.
Mean corpuscular hemoglobin (MCH)	Increased postflight; RPB: 2 weeks.		Variable, but within normal limits.
Mean corpuscular hemoglobin concentration (MCHC)	Increased postflight; RPB: at least 2 weeks.		Variable, but within normal limits.
Reticulocytes	Decreased postflight; RPB: 1 week.		Decreased postflight. In Skylab, RPB: 2–3 weeks for 28-day mission, 1 week for 59-day mission, and 1 day for 84-day mission.
White blood cells	Increased postflight, especially neutrophils; lymphocytes decreased; RPB: 1–2 days. No significant changes in the T/B lymphocyte ratios.		Increased, especially neutrophils; postflight reduction in number of T-cells and reduced T-cell function as measured by PHA^e responsiveness; RPB: 3–7 days; transient postflight elevation in B-cells; RPB: 3 days.
Red blood cell morphology	No significant changes observed postflight.	Increase in percentage of echinocytes; decrease in discocytes.	Rapid reversal of inflight changes in distribution of red cell shapes; significantly increased potassium influx; RPB: 3 days.
Plasma proteins	Occasional postflight elevations in $\alpha2$-Globulin, due to increases of haptoglobin, ceruloplasmin, and $\alpha2$-Macroglobulin; elevated IgA and C_3 factor.		No significant changes.
Red cell enzymes	No consistent postflight changes.	Decrease in phosphofructokinase; no evidence of lipid peroxidation and red blood cell damage.	No consistent postflight changes.
Serum/plasma electrolytes	Decreased K and Mg postflight.	Decreased Na, Cl, and osmolality; slight increase in K and PO_4.	Postflight decreases in Na, K, Cl, Mg; increase in PO_4 and osmolality.
Serum/plasma hormones	Inflight increases in ADH, ANF, and decreases in ACTH, aldosterone and cortisol. Inflight decrease in glucose.	Increases in cortisol. Decreases in ACTH, insulin.	Postflight increases in angiotensin, aldosterone, thyroxine, TSH and GH; decrease in ACTH.

TABLE 7-2 (Continued)

PHYSIOLOGICAL CHANGES ASSOCIATED WITH SHORT-TERM AND LONG-TERM SPACE FLIGHT

Physiological Parameter	Short-Term Space Flights[a] (1–14 days)	Long-Term Space Flights (more than 2 weeks)[b] Pre- vs. Inflight	Pre- vs. Postflight
Serum/plasma metabolites & enzymes	Postflight increases in blood urea nitrogen, creatinine, and glucose; decreases in lactic acid dehydrogenase, creatinine phosphokinase, creatinine phosphokinase, creatinine phosphokinase, albumin, triglycerides, cholesterol, and uric acid.		Postflight decrease in cholesterol, uric acid.
Urine volume	Decreased postflight.	Decreased early inflight.	Decreased postflight.
Urine electrolytes	Postflight increases in Ca, creatinine, PO₄, and osmolality. Decreases in Na, K, Cl, Mg.	Increased osmolality, Na, K, Cl, Mg, Ca, PO₄. Decrease in uric acid excretion.	Increase in Ca excretion; initial postflight decreases in Na, K, Cl, Mg, PO₄, uric acid; Na and Cl excretion increased in 2nd and 3rd week postflight.
Urinary hormones	Inflight decreases in 17-OH-corticosteroids, increase in aldosterone; postflight increases in cortisol, aldosterone, ADH, and pregnanediol; decreases in epinephrine, 17-OH-corticosteroids, androsterone, and etiocholanolone.	Inflight increases in cortisol, aldosterone, and total 17-ketosteroids; decrease in ADH.	Increase in cortisol, aldosterone, norepinephrine; decrease in total 17-OH-corticosteroids, ADH.
Urinary amino acids	Postflight increases in taurine and β-alanine; decreases in glycine, alanine, and tyrosine.	Increased inflight.	Increased postflight.
Sensory Systems			
Audition	No change in thresholds postflight.		No change in thresholds postflight.
Gustation & olfaction	Subjective and varied human experience. No impairments noted.	Same as shorter missions.	Same as shorter missions.
Somatosensory	Subjective and varied human experience. No impairments noted.	Subjective experiences (e.g., tingling of feet).	

144

Vision	Transitory postflight decrease in intra-ocular tension; postflight decreases in visual field; constriction of blood vessels in retina observed postflight; dark adapted crews reported light flashes with eyes open or closed; possible postflight changes in color vision. Decrease in visual motor task performance and contrast discrimination. No change in inflight contrast discrimination, or distant and near visual acuity.	Light flashes reported by dark adapted subjects frequency related to latitude (highest in South Atlantic Anomaly, lowest over poles).	No significant changes except for transient decreases in intraocular pressures.
Vestibular system	40–50% of astronauts / cosmonauts exhibit inflight neurovestibular effects including immediate reflex motor responses (postural illusions, sensations of tumbling or rotation, nystagmus, dizziness, vertigo) and space motion sickness (pallor, cold sweating, nausea, vomiting). Motion sickness symptoms appear early inflight, and subside or disappear in 2–7 days. Postflight difficulties in postural equilibrium with eyes closed, or other vestibular disturbances.	Inflight vestibular disturbances are same as for shorter missions; markedly decreased susceptibility to provocative motion stimuli (cross-coupled angular acceleration) after 2–7 days adaptation period. Cosmonauts have reported occasional reappearance of illusions during long-duration missions.	Immunity to provocative motion continues for several days postflight. Marked postflight disturbances in postural equilibrium with eyes closed. Some cosmonauts exhibited additional vestibular disturbances postflight, including dizziness, nausea, and vomiting.
Musculoskeletal system			
Height	Slight increase during first week inflight (~1.3 cm). RPB: 1 day.	Increased during first 2 weeks inflight (maximum 3–6 cm); stabilizes thereafter.	Height returns to normal on R + 0.
Mass	Postflight weight losses, average about 3.4%; about 2/3 of the loss is due to water loss, the remainder due to loss of lean body mass and fat.	Inflight weight losses average 3–4% during first 5 days; thereafter, weight gradually declines for the remainder of the mission. Early inflight losses are probably mainly due to loss of fluids; later losses are metabolic.	Rapid weight gain during first 5 days postflight, mainly due to replenishment of fluids. Slower weight gain from R + 5** to R + 2 or 3 weeks. Amount of postflight weight loss is inversely related to inflight caloric intake.

TABLE 7-2 (Continued)

PHYSIOLOGICAL CHANGES ASSOCIATED WITH SHORT-TERM AND LONG-TERM SPACE FLIGHT

Physiological Parameter	Short-Term Space Flights[a] (1–14 days)	Long-Term Space Flights (more than 2 weeks)[b]	
		Pre- vs. Inflight	Pre- vs. Postflight
Body composition		Fat is probably replacing muscle tissue. Muscle mass, depending on exercise regimens, is partially preserved.	
Total body volume	Decreased postflight.	Center of mass shifts headward.	Decreased postflight.
Limb volume	Inflight leg volume decreases exponentially during first mission day; thereafter, rate of decrease declines until reaching a plateau within 3–5 days. Postflight decrements in leg volume up to 3%; rapid increase immediately postflight, followed by slower RPB.	Early inflight period same as short missions. Leg volume may continue to decrease slightly throughout mission. Arm volume decreases slightly.	Rapid increase in leg volume immediately postflight, followed by slower RPB.
Muscle strength	Decreased inflight and postflight; RPB: 1–2 weeks.		Postflight decrease in leg muscle strength, particularly extensors. Increased use of inflight exercise appears to reduce postflight strength losses, regardless of mission duration. Arm strength is normal or slightly decreased postflight.
EMG analysis	Postflight EMGs from gastrocnemius suggest increased susceptibility to fatigue and reduced muscular efficiency. EMGs from arm muscles show no change.		Postflight EMGs from gastrocnemius show shift to higher frequencies, suggesting deterioration of muscle tissue; EMGs indicate increased susceptibility to fatigue. RPB: about 4 days.
Reflexes (Achilles tendon)	Reflex duration decreased postflight.		Reflex duration decreased postflight (by 30% or more). Reflex magnitude increased. Compensatory increase in reflex duration about 2 weeks postflight; RPB: about 1 month.

Nitrogen & phosphorus balance		Negative balances early inflight; less negative or slightly positive balances later inflight.	Rapid return to markedly positive balances postflight.
Bone density	Os calcis density decreased postflight. Radius and ulna show variable changes, depending upon method used to measure density.		Os calcis density decreased postflight; amount of loss is correlated with mission duration. Little or no loss from non-weightbearing bones. RPB is gradual; recovery time is about the same as mission duration.
Calcium balance	Increasing negative calcium balance inflight.	Excretion of Ca in urine increases during 1st month inflight, then plateaus. Fecal Ca excretion declines until day 10, then increases continually throughout flight. Ca balance is positive preflight, becoming increasingly negative throughout flight.	Urine Ca content drops below preflight baselines by day 10; fecal Ca content declines, but does not reach preflight baseline by day 20. Markedly negative Ca balance postflight, becoming much less negative by day 10. Ca balance still slightly negative on day 20. RPB: at least several weeks.

a Compiled from biomedical data collected during the following space programs: Mercury, Gemini, Apollo, ASTP, Vostok, Voskhod, Soyuz and Shuttle Spacelab.
b Compiled from biomedical data collected during Skylab and Salyut missions.
c RPB: Return to preflight baseline.

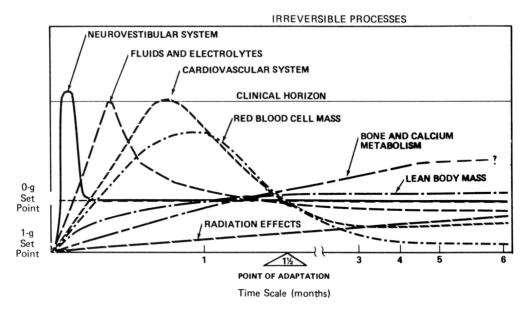

Figure 7-1. Time course of physiological shifts associated with acclimation to weightlessness. 1-g set point represents physiological status on Earth. 0-g set point denotes a complete physiological adaptation level in space, which probably can only be achieved by individuals born in space. Point of adaptation is the average time of 6 weeks required for a visitor to space to exhibit partial adaptation to the environment.

Some differences may be attributed to variations in mission profile and duration, sample size, or the use of countermeasures. Furthermore, different physiological systems appear to readapt at varying rates. Nevertheless, it is possible to draw tentative conclusions concerning the time course of readaptation, especially for those systems that are minimally affected by mission duration. Figure 7-2 illustrates these trends.

The return to Earth's environment is invariably characterized by the reappearance of shifts in several physiological systems, sometimes leading to overt symptomatology. For example, astronauts and cosmonauts have consistently demonstrated postflight orthostatic intolerance, associated with major physiological realignments due to body fluid shifts and associated reflex responses of the cardiopulmonary neuroreceptors. The post-

flight readaptation process in the neurovestibular system is usually heralded by difficulties in postural equilibrium; an array of symptoms ranging from mild to frank sickness has been observed in some individuals. However, most of the measured parameters return to preflight baselines within 1 to 3 months postflight. Longer space missions usually require more time for readaptation, although the reverse has been observed for some parameters (e.g., RBC mass). Again, concern remains regarding the recovery of bone mineral mass and tissue damaged by radiation. Another unknown involves the effects of weightlessness on lean body mass, which raises the possibility of focal atrophy in the antigravity muscles even when countermeasures, such as vigorous exercise, are employed. Recent studies performed after Shuttle and Spacelab missions suggest that readaptation is not a linear process, but that significant fluctuations and oscillatory-type manifestations occur before return to preflight baseline levels.

Despite these numerous shifts, humans appear to acclimate adequately to environmental effects of space flight and return to Earth, particularly with the help of empiric countermeasures and the application of principles of preventive medicine. So far, astronauts have not demonstrated overt, progressive, or documented residual pathology upon return to Earth. Nevertheless, there is probably wide variability in individual tolerance and ability to acclimate to weightlessness and to readapt to Earth's gravity.

This leads to the hypothesis that there may be two major groups of individuals who respond differently to the space environment. The first group makes the transition from Earth to space and back with

no apparent difficulty and no significant deterioration in performance or health. The second group responds with significant early physiological shifts associated with symptomatic responses during the first week of exposure; this group reaches a reasonably steady state later in flight. It is possible that there is a small third group of individuals who do not reach equilibrium in the space environment, and who will continue to show progressive pathophysiological deterioration despite extensive use of countermeasures. So far, there have been many conjectures regarding the full restoration to the preflight norms of muscle and bone morphology and function after flights in excess of 6 months' duration. Hard scientific data regarding the recovery process are lacking and need to be obtained before more ambitious undertakings such as manned solar system explorations are executed.

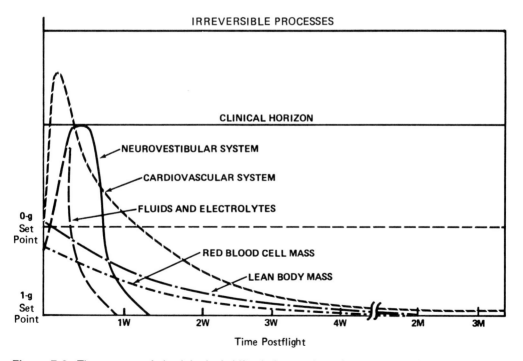

Figure 7-2. Time course of physiological shifts during readaptation to one gravity in body systems in which the characteristics of readaptation are minimally dependent on flight duration. Calcium recovery curve is missing because adequate postflight data have not been collected at this time.

SUPERIMPOSED EFFECTS OF COMBINED STRESSES

Although space flight is associated with numerous environmental changes that influence biological systems, the most remarkable and consistent feature is the relative absence of gravity. The continuous gravitational pull has been a major factor in shaping the evolutionary process of all biological systems on Earth. Growth, development, structure, function, orientation, and motion have all evolved features to cope with and take advantage of gravity.

Gross structural changes have been observed in space. For example, astronauts typically demonstrate increases in height (Thornton, Hoffler, and Rummel, 1977). The weightless environment is also associated with a tendency to assume a fetal position, as shown in Figure 7-3. The well-documented fluid shifts provide additional substantiation for the profound effects of weightlessness (Gazenko, Grigor'yev, 1980; Hoffler, Bergman, and Nicogossian, 1977) and, by inference, for the reliance of structural architecture and functional dynamics on gravity.

These changes in elastic forces in body tissues may be accompanied by changes at the cellular level. Presumably, some of the endocrine and metabolic alterations observed in flight are related to the mechanical effects of weightlessness.

Although weightlessness is the primary contributing factor to the observed physiological changes, it is probably not the sole operant factor. Launch and reentry into Earth's atmosphere entail exposure to increased G forces and vibration which may have distinct physiological impacts

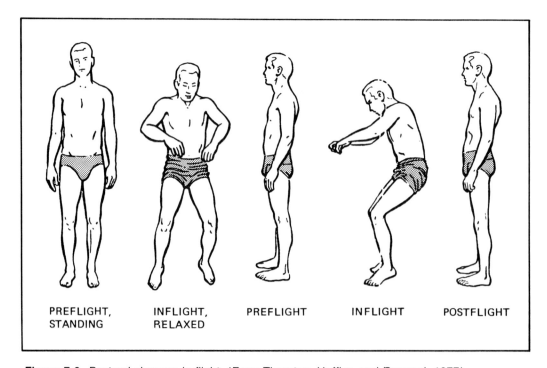

PREFLIGHT, STANDING   INFLIGHT, RELAXED   PREFLIGHT   INFLIGHT   POSTFLIGHT

Figure 7-3. Postural changes in flight. (From Thornton, Hoffler, and Rummel, 1977)

(Hordinsky et al., 1981). Once in space, it is impossible for humans to live without the protection and life support provided by spacecraft. This kind of self-contained and confined habitat, rarely encountered on Earth, is an additional environmental stressor.

On a physiological level, the spacecraft must supply life support systems, such as atmospheric control and food and waste management, in the relative absence of gravity. On a psychological level, the crew must contend with reliance on these life support systems, as well as with sustained workloads, altered work/rest cycles, isolation, confinement, and restricted quarters. The environment outside Earth's atmosphere also exposes humans to more intense radiation and altered geomagnetic and electrical fields. More research is required to determine the physiological changes for which these conditions are responsible and, especially, how they interact with the influence of weightlessness.

It is worth restating that there is still a poor understanding of the mechanisms governing the physiological changes in space flight, despite impressive recent breakthroughs in delineating the time course of adaptation in short- and long-duration space missions. The prevailing hypothesis is that the removal of gravitational force triggers a series of changes as a result of cephalic fluid shifts, thus increasing intravascular pressures. In addition, the gravity receptors of the peripheral and central nervous systems are also directly affected. While the role of the vestibular system as a gravity receptor is well documented, other receptor sites have yet to be demonstrated. The sensory system in the absence of gravity produces the so-called "sensory conflict" with the resultant motion sickness (described fully in Chapter 8). The translocation of fluids from the lower to the upper part of the body, on the other hand, has the net effect

of reducing the total body water content, and represents a hypovolemic state by Earth's standards. On Earth, true hypovolemia triggers several systemic responses in order to maintain critical organ (e.g., brain) perfusion. This leads to the activation of the adrenergic system, renal splanchnic hypoperfusion, secretion of vasoactive hormones, fluid shifts to extravascular compartments, and metabolic acidosis. In contrast, in space flight hypovolemia is secondary to the initial fluid shifts, which start while crewmembers are awaiting launch in a supine, legs-up position. The fluid shifts are complete following insertion into Earth orbit.

Physiological adjustments which follow probably consist of a transient metabolic alkalosis, increased secretions of adrenergic and mineralocorticoid hormones, and enhanced sympathetic responses, both central and peripheral, including activation of the renin-angiotensin system (Figure 7-4). These changes may partially explain the symptoms of motion sickness, transient changes in sleep pattern, as well as fatigue observed after 6 months' stay time in space. Such findings as increases in resting heart rates, intermittent benign arrhythmias, increased total peripheral vascular resistance, and decreased cardiac stroke volume may be related to the action of hormones and neurotransmitters at the receptor sites. Still unknown is the role of the baroreceptors, and their moderating effect on the activation of adrenergic responses. Baroreceptor adjustments may provide the necessary clues to the rapid reestablishment of normal function of certain organs under space flight conditions, such as the splanchnic and renal circulation, which is affected by hypovolemia under Earth's conditions, thus allowing astronauts to perform strenuous tasks in space without overt symptoms of cardiovascular or metabolic dysfunction. It is also unknown at this time whether hemato-

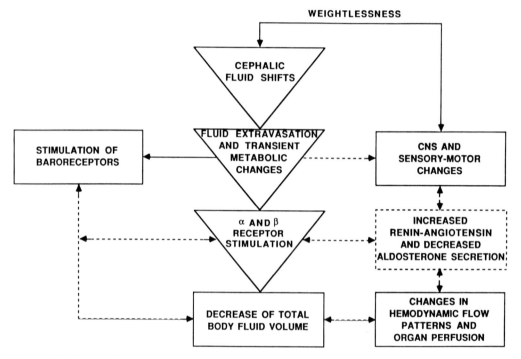

Figure 7-4. A hypothesis for space flight-induced metabolic changes.

logical and musculoskeletal function is directly or indirectly affected in some way by autonomic nervous system responses. Most of these issues await resolution in the early 1990's, when data obtained from Spacelab life sciences missions will serve as a basis for developing the next generation of countermeasures.

REFERENCES

Gazenko, O.G., Genin, A.M., and Yegorov, A.D. Major Medical Results of the Salyut-6/Soyuz 185-Day Space Flight. NASA NDB 2747. Paper presented at the XXXII Congress of the International Astronautical Federation, Rome, Italy, September 6–12, 1981.

Gazenko, O.G., Grigor'yev, A.I., and Natochin, Uy.V. Fluid-Electrolyte Homeostasis and Weightlessness. In: JPRS, USSR Report: Space Biology and Aerospace Medicine, October 30, 1980, 14(5):1–11.

Hoffler, G.W., Bergman, S.A., and Nicogossian, A.E. In-flight Lower Limb Volume Measurement. In: The Apollo-Soyuz Test Project: Medical Report (NASA SP-411). Edited by A.E. Nicogossian. National Aeronautics and Space Administration, Washington, D.C., 1977.

Hordinsky, J.R., Gebhardt, U., Wegmann, H.M., and Schafer, G. Cardiovascular and biochemical response to simulated space flight entry. Aviation, Space, and Environmental Medicine, 52(1):16–18, 1981.

Thornton, W.E., Hoffler, G.W., and Rummel, J.A. Anthropometric Changes and Fluid Shifts. In: Biomedical Results from Skylab (NASA SP-377). Edited by R.S. Johnston and L.F. Dietlein. National Aeronautics and Space Administration, Washington, D.C., 1977.

References Used in Compiling Table 7-2

Akulinichev, I.T., et al. Results of physiological investigations on the space ships Vostok 3 and Vostok 4. In: Aviation and Space Medicine (NASA TT F-228). Edited by V.V. Parin. National Aeronautics and Space Administration, Washington, D.C.

Biomedical Results of Apollo (NASA SP-368). Edited by R.S. Johnston, L.F. Dietlein, and C.A. Berry. National Aeronautics and Space Administration, Washington, D.C., 1975.

Biomedical Results from Skylab (NASA SP-377). Edited by R.S. Johnston and L.F. Dietlein. National Aeronautics and Space Administration, 1977.

Bungo, M.W., Bagian, T.M., Bowman, M.A., and Levitan, B.M. Results of Life Sciences Detailed Supplementary Objectives (DSOs) Conducted Aboard the Space Shuttle from 1981 to 1986. NASA TM 58280, 1987.

Foundations of Space Biology and Medicine. Edited by M. Calvin and O.G. Gazenko. NASA SP-374, Washington, D.C., 1975.

Gazenko, O.G., Kakurin, L.I., Kuznetsova, A.G. Biomedical Investigations on Soyuz Spacecraft. Nauka Press, Moscow, 1976.

Gemini Midprogram Conference (NASA SP-121). National Aeronautics and Space Administration, Washington, D.C., 1967.

Gemini Summary Conference (NASA SP-138). National Aeronautics and Space Administration, Washington, D.C., 1967.

Mercury Project Summary Including Results of the Fourth Manned Orbital Flight (NASA SP-45). U.S. Government Printing Office, Washington, D.C., 1963.

Physiologic Adaptation of Man in Space. Edited by A.W. Holland. Aviation, Space, and Environmental Medicine, 58(9):A1–A148, September, 1987.

Results of Medical Evaluations Performed on the Orbital Station "Salyut-6"-"Soyuz." Edited by O.G. Gazenko and N.N. Gurovskii. Moscow, Nauka Press, 1986.

Space Life Sciences, Acta Astronautica. Special Issue, Edited by H.M. Wegmann and R.J. White. Pergamon Press, 17(2), February, 1988.

The Apollo-Soyuz Test Project: Medical Report (NASA SP-411). Edited by A.E. Nicogossian. National Aeronautics and Space Administration, 1977.

Volynkin, Yu.M., and Vasil'yev, P.F. Some results of medical studies conducted during the flight of the Voskhod. In: The Problems of Space Biology. Vol. VI (NASA TT F-528). Edited by N.M. Sisakyan. National Aeronautics and Space Administration, Washington, D.C., 1969.

Vorob'yev, Ye.I., et al. Some results of medical investigations made during flights of the Soyuz 2-6, Soyuz 7, and Soyuz 8 space ships. Space Biology of Medicine, 4(2):65–73, 1970.

Vorob'yev, Ye.I., Gazenko, O.G., Gurovskiy, N.N., Nefedov, Yu.G., Yegorov, B.B., Bayevsky, R.M., Bryanov, I.I., Genin, A.M., Degtyarev, V.A., Yegorov, A.D., Yeremin, A.V., and Pestov, I.D. Preliminary results of medical investigations carried out during the second mission of the Salyut-4 orbital station. Space Biology and Aerospace Medicine, 10(5):3–18, September–October, 1976.

Yorob'yev, Ye.I., Gazenko, O.G., Shulzhenko, E.B., et al. Preliminary medical results of investigations conducted during the five month spaceflight on the "Salyut 7"-"Soyuz T" orbital complex. Space Biology and Aerospace Medicine 2:27–33, Medical Press, Moscow, 1986.

8 The Neurovestibular System

JERRY L. HOMICK

JAMES M. VANDERPLOEG

The neurovestibular system provides information concerning the direction and magnitude of the net gravito-inertial forces acting on the information necessary to maintain equilibrium and spatial orientation of the body. On Earth, the gravitational component is an important part of this total force. During space flight, when the gravitational force is neutralized, significant adaptive processes occur in the components of this sensory system, in particular in vestibular interactions with other sensory systems. Disturbances in spatial orientation and an array of clinical symptoms may appear during the initial phase of adaptation to weightlessness. The most important disturbance associated with space flight is so-called "space motion sickness," or SMS, a condition that has affected 40 to 50 percent of individuals flying in space.

VESTIBULAR SYSTEM STRUCTURE

The principal components of the peripheral vestibular system are the otolith organ and the semicircular canals. The otolith organ includes the saccule and utricule, which provide information about gravity and linear acceleration. The receptor cells of the otolith are embedded in a gelatinous mass containing otoconia (crystals of calcium carbonate). The weight of the crystals causes the gelatinous mass to shift position during changes in head orientation in one gravity, and during linear acceleration in both one and zero gravity. This produces a shearing force on sensory hair cells (cilia) and results in the transmission of neural impulses to the central nervous system.

The three semicircular canals provide information about angular accelerations of the head. Each canal consists of a membranous tube filled with endolymph, floating within a bony canal filled with perilymph. At the end of each membranous canal is an enlargement called the ampulla, which contains the sensory receptors. The orientation of each canal roughly corresponds to one of the three anatomical planes of the head; each canal responds maximally to angular acceleration in its plane.

The two components of the vestibular system deal with independent aspects of orientation, but do not function entirely independently of each other or of certain other body systems. According to Guedry (1978), the semicircular canals localize the angular acceleration vector relative to the head during head movement and contribute to sensory inputs for (1) appropriate reflex action relative to an anatomical axis and (2) perception of angular velocity about that axis. Perception of orientation relative to the Earth depends upon sensory inputs from the otolith and somatosensory systems. The otoliths provide both static and dynamic orientation information (relative to gravity) and contribute to perception of tilt.

A complex network of nerve pathways connects the peripheral vestibular receptors with the brain and spinal cord. Although these pathways are not fully understood, physiological and anatomical studies indicate that the vestibular afferent fibers terminate either in the brain stem vestibular nuclei or the cerebellum (Correia and Guedry, 1978). Interactions in these areas involve nerve fibers that subserve the extraocular muscles of the eye; fibers that subserve neck, limb, and body skeletal muscles; and the reticular formation that regulates a variety of vegetative responses of the organism.

SPACE MOTION SICKNESS

Graybiel et al. (1977) distinguish between two categories of vestibular side effects associated with space flight: (1) immediate reflex motor responses, which include postural illusions, sensations of rotation, nystagmus, dizziness, and vertigo; and (2) space motion sickness, or SMS.

SYMPTOMS

Table 8-1 presents the clinical symptoms and biochemical changes variably recorded with motion sickness in Earth environments, as compared to those in space environments. In general, the progressive cardinal symptoms of most terrestrial forms of motion sickness consist of pallor, increased body warmth, cold sweating, nausea, and vomiting. Although symptoms of SMS appear to be similar to those experienced on Earth, there are some significant differences. Data obtained from Space Shuttle crewmembers indicate that anorexia, lethargy, malaise, and headache are predominant symptoms of SMS. Also, there have been a number of instances in which vomiting occurred suddenly in space, without prodromal symptoms (Homick et al., 1984). Diagnostic criteria commonly used to evaluate motion sickness in the laboratory as well as in space flight are shown in Table 8-2 (Graybiel et al., 1977). In Skylab, as subjects made experimental head movements while rotating in a chair, an observer estimated the severity of each predesignated symptom and recorded this data for postflight analysis. This and similar techniques have been used to systematically document symptoms of SMS during Space Shuttle missions (Homick et al., 1984; Oman et al., 1984).

INCIDENCE

Table 8-3 lists the reported incidence of SMS in U.S. and U.S.S.R. space missions. About one-half of all astronauts and cosmonauts have experienced at least some symptoms, ranging from mild dizziness and stomach awareness to nausea and vomiting. Since many space crews took anti-motion sickness drugs prophylactically, it is possible that the severity of vestibular symptoms would otherwise have been greater.

It is interesting to note that of the 12 Apollo astronauts who walked on the moon, only three reported mild symptoms, such as stomach awareness or loss of appetite, prior to their moon walk. None reported symptoms while in the one-sixth gravity of the lunar surface, and no symptoms were noted upon return to weightlessness (Homick and Miller, 1975). Likewise, symptoms have never occurred during extravehicular activity (EVA).

SUSCEPTIBILITY TO SPACE MOTION SICKNESS

A number of different research techniques have been used over the years to elicit motion sickness symptomatology in susceptible subjects. Examples of these include:

- Vertical oscillators
- Swings
- Caloric irrigation
- Roll and pitch rockers
- Visual inversion or reversal techniques
- Off-vertical rotation
- Optokinetic stimulation
- Z-axis recumbent rotation
- Cross-coupling accelerations produced by head movements
- Parabolic flights.

Although some of these tests (particularly those that involve exposure to cross-coupled stimulation) have been useful in predicting susceptibility in one-gravity motion environments, they have not successfully predicted SMS susceptibility (Homick et al., 1984). Nor do personal motion sickness histories, which document previous incidences of motion sickness in provocative one-gravity environments, predict susceptibility to SMS. There are several probable reasons for the failure of these tests to predict motion sickness susceptibility in space. First, individual susceptibility to different motion environments in one gravity often varies widely, and it is common for individuals to be susceptible under certain motion conditions without transfer to other motion environments. Second, an astronaut's susceptibility to SMS probably involves three major components:

1. Initial "susceptibility" to the provocative motion environment
2. Rate of adaptation
3. Degree of adaptation.

Most of the tests that have been used to predict susceptibility to SMS measure only the first component. However, an individual's capacity to adapt to a new motion environment may be more important than his initial susceptibility to an acute motion stimulus. Other variables that may have interfered with the predictive accuracy of these tests include the prophylactic and therapeutic use of anti-motion sickness remedies, and the lack of reliable quantitative methods for measuring symptoms.

TIME COURSE OF ADAPTATION

Susceptibility to SMS varies not only among individuals, but within the same individual over time. On any particular flight, symptoms usually appear in susceptible individuals early after insertion into orbit, and are aggravated by head and

TABLE 8–1

MOTION SICKNESS MANIFESTATIONS

Physiological System	Terrestrial Manifestations	Space Flight Findings
Cardiovascular	Changes in pulse rate and/or blood pressure	Reported
	Increased tone of arterial portion of capillaries in the fingernail bed	Not measured
	Decreased diameter of retinal vessels	Not measured
	Decreased peripheral circulation	Not measured
	Increased muscle blood flow	Not measured
Respiratory	Alterations in respiration rate	Not measured
	Sighing or yawning	Reported
Gastrointestinal	Inhibition of gastric intestinal tone and motility	Reported
	Salivation	Reported
	Gas or belching	Reported
	Epigastric discomfort or awareness	Reported
	Sudden relief from symptoms after vomiting	Reported
Body fluids, blood[a]	Changes in LDH concentrations	
	Changes in glucose utilization	
	Decreased concentration of eosinophils	
	Increased 17-hydroxycorticosteroids	
	Increased plasma proteins	
Urine[a]	Increased 17-hydroxycorticosteroids	
	Increased catecholamines	
Temperature	Decreased body temperature	Variable
	Coldness of extremities	Variable
Visual system	Ocular imbalance	Not present
	Dilated pupils during emesis	Not present
	Small pupils	Not present
Behavioral	Apathy, lethargy, sleepiness, fatigue, and weakness	Reported
	Depression and/or anxiety	Reported
	Mental confusion, spatial disorientation, dizziness, and giddiness	Variable
	Anorexia	Reported
	Headache, especially frontal headache	Reported
	Decreased muscular coordination and psychomotor performance	Reported
	Decreased time estimation	Reported
	Decreased motivation	Reported

[a]Measured inflight, but presently not correlated with space motion sickness.
Adapted from Money, 1970; Reason and Brand, 1975.

body movement, especially when the eyes are open. In most cases, symptoms disappear within 2 to 4 days, and do not recur. According to Yakovleva et al. (1980), adaptation follows one of three patterns: (1) very little or no sensory discomfort, (2) intense discomfort for a short period, or (3) prolonged adaptation without severe symptoms.

To determine changes in thresholds for vestibular response on the Skylab missions, Graybiel et al. (1977) measured susceptibility to provocative motion stimuli preflight, inflight (beginning on or after mission day 5), and postflight. A stressful motion environment was produced by rotating subjects in a chair and requiring them to execute head movements with eyes covered. Symptoms were scored using the criteria in Table 8-2. In general, once acclimatized, astronauts demonstrated a marked increase in the threshold of susceptibility to motion sickness during the inflight provocative tests. This "immunity" to cross-coupled angular acceleration stimuli continued in these subjects for a week or more postflight. Limited postflight data obtained on Space Shuttle

TABLE 8-2

DIAGNOSTIC CATEGORIZATION OF DIFFERENT LEVELS OF SEVERITY OF ACUTE MOTION SICKNESS

Category	Pathognomonic (16 points)	Major (8 points)	Minor (8 points)	Minimal (2 points)	AQS[a] (1 point)
Nausea syndrome	Nausea III[b] Vomiting or retching	Nausea II	Nausea I	Epigastric discomfort	Epigastric awareness
Skin		Pallor III	Pallor II	Pallor I	Flushing / subjective warmth > II
Cold sweating		III	II	I	
Increased salivation		III	II	I	
Drowsiness		III	II	I	
Pain					Headache (persistent) > II
Central nervous system					Dizziness (persistent) Eyes closed > II Eyes open > III

LEVELS OF SEVERITY IDENTIFIED BY TOTAL POINTS SCORED

Frank Sickness (FS)	Severe Malaise (M III)	Moderate Malaise A (M IIIA)	Moderate Malaise B (M IIB)	Slight Malaise (M I)
> 16 points	8–15 points	5–7 points	3–4 points	1–2 points

[a] AQS = Additional qualifying symptoms.
[b] III, severe or marked; II, moderate; I, slight.
From Graybiel et al., 1977.

crewmembers, particularly the crew of the Spacelab 1 mission (Oman et al., 1984), confirm that motion sickness susceptibility thresholds remain elevated for some time postflight.

Most experiments and observations indicate that readaptation to one gravity involves a reappearance of vestibular side effects, particularly after longer missions. Tests of postural equilibrium with eyes closed revealed marked postflight deficits in one Apollo crewmember and all Skylab crews (Homick and Miller, 1975; Homick and Reschke, 1977). In the Skylab crewmembers, postural stability appeared to return to normal within 10 days. Using more refined measurement techniques, similar postflight postural instability, and especially significant changes in postural sensory motor reflexes were observed in the Spacelab 1 crewmembers (Reschke et al., 1984; Young et al., 1984). The Spacelab 1 data suggest that postural reflex readaptation occurred in 1 to 7 days, depending upon the specific response under investigation. Several of the returning astronauts from Skylab and Apollo reported a variety of additional postflight disturbances, which appear to be vestibular in origin and included dizziness and lightheadedness, vertigo during rapid head movements, and difficulty in turning corners. Similar responses, but of a lesser magnitude, have been reported postflight by several Space Shuttle crewmembers. With the exception of one episode experienced by a Skylab crewmember, naturally occurring motion sickness has not been experienced by U.S. astronauts during the first few days following return from space flight.

Soviet cosmonauts have experienced more pronounced postflight vestibular disturbances, including persisting postural instability, sweating while walking, dizziness, nausea, and vomiting, particularly during head movements (Gazenko, 1979). One of the crewmembers of the 175-day Salyut mission had, in addition to most of the foregoing, pronounced illusory reactions (autokinetic illusions during fixation) postflight (Matsnev, in press). Some Soviet investigators (Kornilova et al., 1979), comparing postflight measures of

measures of otolith reflex and statokinetic disorders in several Salyut crews, concluded that the degree and duration of symptoms were proportional to mission length.

MECHANISMS UNDERLYING SPACE MOTION SICKNESS

Two major theories that have been advanced to account for SMS are the sensory conflict (or "sensory rearrangement") theory and the fluid shift hypothesis. A third hypothesis suggests that slight functional differences between the left and right otolith receptors may cause disturbances due to increased bilateral differential sensitivity of the peripheral vestibular apparatus and its central connections, or erroneous compensation of bilateral asymmetries of the otolith system in microgravity.

TABLE 8-3

INCIDENCE OF SPACE MOTION SICKNESS IN U.S. AND U.S.S.R. SPACE MISSIONS[a]

United States (as of October 1984)

Program	Number of Crewmen[b]	Incidence of Motion Sickness
Mercury	6	0
Gemini	20	0
Apollo	33	11
Skylab	9	5
ASTP	3	0
Shuttle	48	25

Soviet Union (as of 1981)

Program	Number of Crewmen[b]	Incidence of Motion Sickness
Vostok	6	1
Voskhod	5	3
Soyuz	38	21
ASTP	2	2
Salyut 5	6	2
Salyut 6	27	12

[a] Reports of one or more symptoms of space motion sickness are included. No attempt was made to categorize by severity of symptoms.
[b] Includes some crewmen who flew more than once.

Sensory Conflict Theory

The most probable theory to explain the onset of SMS, and motion sickness in general, is the sensory conflict or "sensory rearrangement" theory. Under one-gravity conditions, human orientation in three-dimensional space is based on four sensory inputs. These are (1) otolith information on gravity vector and linear accelerations, (2) angular acceleration data provided by the semicircular canals, (3) visual information concerning body orientation, and (4) touch pressure and kinesthetic information. In normal environments, information from these systems is compatible and complementary, and matches that expected on the basis of previous experience. When the motion environment is altered in such a way that information from body sensory systems is not compatible and/or does not match previously stored neural patterns, motion sickness may result. Reason and Brand (1975) distinguish between two different kinds of sensory rearrangements that can induce motion sickness:

1. Visual-inertial rearrangement, in which the sensory conflict arises between input from the visual system and vestibular apparatus
2. Canal-otolith rearrangement, in which the conflict is between the input from the semicircular canals and the otolith organ.

Fluid Shift Hypothesis

According to this hypothesis, the cephalad fluid shifts accompanying weightlessness produce concomitant changes in intracranial pressure, thereby altering the response properties of vestibular receptors. For example, engorgement of the blood vessels surrounding the endolymphatic duct might restrict the flow of endolymph from the cochlea to the endolymphatic sac, resulting in hydrops.

Parker and Money (1978) point out that most evidence does not favor this hypothesis. Graybiel and Lackner (1977) did not find an increased susceptibility to provocative motion stimulation during head-down tilt. Anecdotal reports from Space Shuttle astronauts and limited inflight measurements of responses (e.g., auditory evoked potentials and intraocular pressure), presumably sensitive to increased intracranial fluid pressure, do not favor the fluid shift hypothesis (Thornton, personal communication).

Although in recent years Soviet investigators have begun to place greater emphasis on sensory motor conflict as the primary cause of SMS, they continue to investigate the possible role of cephalad fluid shifts as an etiological factor (Matsnev and Bodo, 1984). It is interesting to note, however, that in the past Soviet scientists have not been able to predict in-

dividual susceptibility to SMS using this hypothesis (Homick, 1978).

Otolith Asymmetry

Von Baumgarten and Thumler (1979) have proposed a mechanism which complements the sensory conflict theory to explain adaptation to weightlessness and readaptation to one gravity, and individual differences in SMS susceptibility. They suggest that some individuals possess slight functional imbalances (for example, weight differences) between the right and left otolith receptors that are compensated for by the central nervous system in one gravity. This compensation is inappropriate in zero gravity, however, since the weight differential is nullified. The result is a temporary asymmetry producing rotary vertigo, eye movements, and posture changes until the central "compensating centers" adjust to the new situation. A similar imbalance would be produced upon return to one gravity, resulting in postflight vestibular disturbances. Individuals with a greater degree of asymmetry in otolith morphology would thus be more susceptible to SMS. Von Baumgarten et al. (1981) have stated that this hypothesis is difficult to evaluate, because no practical test procedures for otolith bilateral asymmetries in humans exist.

PREVENTION AND TREATMENT OF SPACE MOTION SICKNESS

The disruptive nature of SMS, occurring as it does during the early, critical stages of a mission, has led to a variety of approaches to prevention or control of this malady. Only limited success has been achieved to date. Research directed toward prevention has proceeded along four broad lines of inquiry. Each of these research areas is described below in terms of its potential for control and problems associated with its use.

Training

Training procedures for the control of SMS are based on the general physiological principle that increasing the levels of a stress agent will lead to a heightened level of adaptation. The problem is that training for SMS prior to a mission cannot be conducted in a zero-gravity environment, but must be conducted in a one-gravity situation on Earth, recognizing that transfer of the training effect to the space situation may be limited or even nonexistent.

It is difficult to assess the training effectiveness of any of these procedures inasmuch as control groups are not used. Therefore, there is no baseline against which to measure the amount of protection afforded. However, there is at least a basis in theory for each of these procedures.

Aerobatic maneuvers in high performance aircraft may produce the stimulation known to cause motion sickness in susceptible individuals. Astronauts frequently have participated in flights of this type prior to missions. Based on anecdotal reports, one can assume that some protection is afforded. However, results from space missions in which astronauts have suffered SMS make it clear that this protection is not total.

A procedure for adaptation training places the subject in a rotating environment, such as a rotating chair or a slow-rotation room. Work by Graybiel and his colleagues has shown that it is possible to lower an individual's susceptibility to motion sickness in a particular environment by exposing him to gradually increasing levels of stress intensity. In one study (Graybiel and Knepton, 1978), it was found that over-adaptation in one motion environment appears to provide protection in other motion environments. Using the slow-rotation room, subjects executed standardized head and body movements leftward or rightward until either the motion sickness end point was reached or 1200 head movements were executed. Next, subjects executed head movements in the three unpracticed quadrants. A marked adaptation effect was measured under these conditions. This training effect now needs to be evaluated for possible transfer to weightless conditions.

A sensory-motor training approach, which has yet to be fully developed and evaluated, is derived in part from self-motion perception and eye movement changes measured in Space Shuttle crewmembers. Using these data and other applicable ground-based and space flight data, Parker et al. (1985) have proposed preflight adaptation training procedures and apparatus based upon an otolith tilt-translation reinterpretation hypothesis. The preflight adaptation trainer is intended to produce preflight recalibration in the brain of relationships between vestibular and visual neural signals. The result would be self-motion reports, eye movements, and postural orientation reflexes corresponding to those exhibited by astronauts after they have adapted to zero gravity.

Pharmacological Countermeasures

It has long been known that drug therapy offers some relief from motion sickness in aircraft or in any moving vehicle. Logically, therefore, as soon as a motion sickness problem was identified in space flight, a search for effective pharmacological control began. Selection of drugs for evaluation began with those known to offer some relief from motion sickness in one gravity.

Graybiel et al. (1975) reported on a series of evaluations using drugs of known effectiveness, administered singly and in combinations. The authors concluded that a fixed-dose combination of promethazine hydrochloride plus ephedrine sulfate (25 mg each) administered orally proved outstanding, as this combination exhibited a supra-summation effect. An oral combination of scopolamine hydrobromide (0.3 mg) plus d-amphetamine (5.0 mg) was also highly efficacious. Substantial individual differences in response to the drugs also were noted, implying that individual assessments must be made for best protection. Finally, based on a few tests conducted using larger than usual doses, it was concluded that individuals may vary both with regard to choice of drug and amount administered. More recent studies continue to indicate that scopolamine plus dexedrine and promethazine plus ephedrine are among the most effective anti-motion sickness drugs.

Operational experience has shown that orally administered anti-motion sickness drugs lose much of their effectiveness when taken after symptoms have appeared. Therefore, alternative methods of administration which bypass the gastrointestinal system have been investigated.

Wurster et al. (1981) compared the transdermal application of scopolamine with other drug combinations administered orally. Because of the great intra- and inter-individual variations, the responses to the drugs were not statistically significant. However, they revealed strong tendencies for a promethazine-ephedrine combination and scopolamine, both administered orally, to reduce motion sickness. Scopolamine administered transdermally could not be distinguished from the placebo.

A more recent evaluation of transdermally administered scopolamine (Homick et al., 1983) reached many of the same conclusions as earlier studies. Here, the particular interest was in a form of administration which would allow a drug such as scopolamine to be effective for a longer period than the 4 to 6 hours achieved with oral administration. Results of this study showed average improvements of 45, 32, 53, and 54 percent, relative to placebo, when measured at 16-, 24-, 48-, and 72-hour intervals. Although there was a consistent beneficial effect, it was not statistically significant since individual differences were large. The authors feel that one causal factor may be variations in rates of scopolamine absorption or metabolism. On the basis of a number of side effects noted, particularly drowsiness and blurred vision, and the large individual variations, it was concluded that operational use of transdermal scopolamine should be contingent upon careful screening and further efficacy testing.

Graybiel and his colleagues (unpublished data) have demonstrated that scopolamine or promethazine administered by intramuscular injection is highly effective in alleviating severe nausea and vomiting in subjects exposed to parabolic flight. A major drawback with this approach is the pronounced sedation typically induced by the injected drug. Investigators at the NASA Johnson Space Center have evaluated scopolamine administered by sublingual and buccal capsules. The amount and time course of plasma levels of the drug were no different from those measured with orally administered scopolamine.

Regardless of the route of administration, all the studies cited above evaluated the prophylactic or therapeutic effect of drugs which act on the central nervous system. Recently, NASA has begun to investigate the utility of drugs which act primarily on the gastrointestinal tract to promote normal motility and gastric emptying. Metachlopramide, for example, has been used by astronauts with varying success to alleviate nausea and vomiting. Additional research with centrally-acting and peripherally-acting pharmacological countermeasures is indicated.

Biofeedback Procedures

Autogenic biofeedback techniques are being considered for use in training subjects to control the symptoms of SMS, especially in light of a U.S. Air Force program for rehabilitating crewmembers grounded with supposedly disqualifying air sickness. The premise of the Air Force work was that air sickness (pallor, cold sweating, stomach awareness, nausea, etc.) is an autonomic nervous system response. Interruption of this response through voluntary control of the autonomic nervous system should therefore lead to prevention of air sickness. In the U.S. Air Force program (Levy, 1980), selected air crews were given relaxation training and biofeedback training in a two-axis motion chair with the individual connected to physiological monitoring equipment. As rotation increased, the subject was required to recognize physiological responses prior to actual motion sickness symptoms, and bring these responses under control. According to a recent review (Jones and Hartman, 1984), this program was about 75 percent successful in returning air crewmembers to flying status. Similar psychological intervention techniques are being used successfully by the German Air Force (Kemmler, 1984) to prevent air sickness.

Additional support for the feasibility of biofeedback techniques comes from research at the NASA Ames Research Center. Cowings and Toscano (1982) used biofeedback techniques with one group highly susceptible to motion sickness and another identified as moderately susceptible. These were compared with two control groups of matched susceptibility. Both treatment groups showed significantly improved performance on the Coriolis Sickness Susceptibility Index.

Although biofeedback procedures are promising, investigators have identified potential problems with their use. Lackner (1978) notes substantial individual differences in the extent to which subjects are able to gain control over the variable being "reinforced." He further states that laboratory training may not transfer to situations where the subject's active participation in other tasks is required. The effectiveness of biofeedback techniques in preventing motion sickness under operational conditions remains to be determined.

Mechanical Devices

Astronauts and cosmonauts have reported that SMS is aggravated by movement of the body, especially the head and neck. Soviet scientists, operating on the principle that reducing movement should decrease the severity of symptoms of SMS, have developed a head restraint system termed "Neck Pneumatic Shock-Absorber" (Matsnev et al., 1983). The device supplies a controlled load of known force to the cervical vertebrae and neck anti-gravitational muscles and restricts head movements during adaptation to weightlessness. The device consists of a soft cap with loop holes for rubber cords. With the cap on, a crewmember must exert considerable force with the neck muscles in order to move his head from its natural erect position. The device includes straps attached to the right and left shoulders, which restrict head tilt and turn. Flight test results from the Salyut missions indicate that the head restraint cap was of benefit in controlling the development of SMS symptomatology. Matsnev concludes that the benefit of this head restraint system may be a result of its control of the vestibulo-cervical reflex, known to involve the labyrinth (semicircular canals and otolith organs) as a receptor and neck muscles as effectors. Reports from U.S. astronauts, however, indicate that such mechanical devices seem unnecessary, because crewmembers quickly learn to voluntarily restrict head movements to prevent symptoms.

SUMMARY

The weightless environment of space produces disturbances in the functioning of the vestibular apparatus that result in a number of side effects, the most important of which is space motion sickness, or SMS. The major symptoms of this disorder, which occurs in susceptible individuals soon after insertion into orbit, include anorexia, lethargy, malaise, nausea, and vomiting. These symptoms typically subside or disappear within 2 to 4 days. Almost one-half of the astronaut and cosmonaut population has shown at least some symptoms of SMS in flight. However, tests designed to measure vestibular function or susceptibility to motion sickness in one gravity have not successfully predicted which individuals will be susceptible in flight. Likewise, totally effective and operationally acceptable countermeasures have yet to be validated.

Dietlein and Johnston (1981) state that SMS "represents the greatest research challenge facing life scientists in contemporary space medicine and physiology." Solutions will not come easily. Progress in all likelihood will extend principally from experiments carried out in space. Indeed, significant new data have already been obtained from the Spacelab 1 mission and other recent Space Shuttle flights. Further investigations to be conducted in the Spacelab missions and the Shuttle middeck will examine the function of the vestibular apparatus in humans and the morphology of the otolith in animals. Through these programs, new knowledge may be acquired concerning the functioning of the vestibular system, its interaction with other neurosensory components, its rate of adaptation, and the effectiveness of procedural and pharmacological preventive measures.

REFERENCES

Armstrong, H.S. Air sickness. In: Aerospace Medicine. Edited by H.G. Armstrong, Baltimore, MD, Williams and Wilkins Co., 1961.

Barrett, S.V., and Thornton, C.L. Relationship between perceptual style and simulator sickness. Journal of Applied Psychology, 52:304–308, 1968.

Chinn, H.I. Motion sickness in the military service. Military Surgeon, 198:20–29, 1951.

Chinn, H.I. Evaluation of drugs for protection against motion sickness aboard transport ships. Journal of the American Medical Association, 106:755–760, 1956.

Corria, M.V. and Guedry, F.E. The vestibular system: Basic biophysical and psychological mechanisms. In: Handbook of Behavioral Neurobiology, Vol 1, Sensory Integration. Edited by R.B. Masterton, New York, Plenum Press, 1978, 311–351.

Cowings, P.S., and Toscano, W.B. The relationship of motion sickness susceptibility to learned autonomic control for symptom suppression. Aviat., Space, and Envir. Med., 53(6):570–575, 1982.

Dietlein, L.F., and Johnston, R.S. U.S. manned space flight: The first twenty years. A biomedical status report. Acta Astronautica, 8(9–10):893–906, 1981.

Gazenko, O.G. (Ed.) Summaries of reports of the 6th All-Soviet Union Conference on Space Biology and Medicine (Vol. 1 and 11). Kaluga, U.S.S.R., June 5–7, 1979.

Graybiel, A. Measurement of otolith function in men. In: Vestibular system—Part 2: Psychophysics, applied aspects and general interpretations. Edited by H.H. Kornhuber, Berlin, Springer-Verlag, 1974.

Graybiel, A. Prevention and treatment of space sickness in Shuttle-Orbiter missions. Aviat., Space, and Envir. Med., 50(2):171–176, 1979.

Graybiel, A., and Knepton, J. Bidirectional overadaptation achieved by executing leftward or rightward head movements during unidirectional rotation. Aviat., Space, and Envir. Med., 49(1):1–4, 1978.

Graybiel, A., and Lackner, J.R. Comparison of susceptibility to motion sickness during rotation at 30 rpm in the Earth-horizontal, 10° head-down positions. Aviat., Space, and Envir. Med., 48(1):7–11, 1977.

Graybiel, A., Miller, E.F., and Homick, J.L. Experiment M131: Human vestibular function. In: Biomedical results from Skylab (NASA SP-377). Edited by R.S. Johnston and L.F. Dietlein, U.S. Government Printing Office, Washington, D.C., 1977.

Graybiel, A., Wood, C.D., Knepton, J., Hoche, J.P., and Perkins, G.F. Human assay of antimotion sickness drugs. Aviat., Space, and Envir. Med., 46(9):1107–1118, 1975.

Graybiel, A., Wood, C.D., Miller, E.F., II, and Cramer, D.B. Diagnostic criteria for grading the severity of acute motion sickness. Aerospace Medicine, 39:453–455, 1968.

Guedry, F.E., Jr. Vestibular function. In: U.S. Naval Flight Surgeon's Manual (2nd ed.). Prepared under Office of Naval Research Contract N00014-76-C-1010 by the Naval Aerospace Medical Institute and BioTechnology, Inc., U.S. Government Printing Office, Washington, D.C., 1978.

Hemingway, A. Airsickness during early flying training. Journal of Aviation Medicine, 16:409–416, 1945.

Hill, J. The care of the sea-sick. British Medical Journal, Oct.–Dec.: 802–807, 1936.

Homick, J.L. Special note: Space motion sickness in the Soviet manned space flight program. In: Space motion sickness symposium proceedings. Edited by J.L. Homick, Lyndon B. Johnson Space Center, Houston, TX, 15–17 November, 1978. (Prepared by General Electric Company under Purchase Order T-1830G).

Homick, J.L., Kohl, R.L., Reschke, M.F., Degioanni, J., and Cintron-Trevino, N. Transdermal scopolamine in the prevention of motion sickness: Evaluation of the time course of efficacy. Aviat., Space, and Envir. Med. 54(11):994–1000, 1983.

Homick, J.L., and Miller, E.F., II. Apollo flight crew vestibular assessment. In: Biomedical results of Apollo (NASA SP-368). Edited by R.S. Johnston, L.F. Dietlein, and C.A. Berry, U.S. Government Printing Office, Washington, D.C., 1975.

Homick, J.L. and Reschke, M.F. Postural equilibrium following exposure to weightless space flight. Acta Otolaryngol. 83:455–454, 1977.

Homick, J.L., Reschke, M.F. and Vanderploeg, J.M. Space adaptation syndrome. Incidence and operational implications for the Space Transportation System Program. In: AGARD Conference Proceedings (CP-372) on Motion Sickness: Mecha-

nisms, Prediction, Prevention and Treatment. Williamsburg, VA, 1984.

Jones, D.R. and Hartman, B.O. Biofeedback treatment of airsickness: A review, In: AGARD Conference Proceedings (CP-372) on Motion Sickness: Mechanisms, Prediction, Prevention and Treatment. Williamsburg, VA, 1984.

Kaplan, I. Motion sickness on railroads. Industrial Medicine and Surgery, 33:648–651, 1964.

Kemmler, R.W. Psychological components in the development and prevention of airsickness. In: AGARD Conference Proceedings (CP-372) on Motion Sickness: Mechanisms, Prediction, Prevention, and Treatment. Williamsburg, VA, 1984.

Kornilova, L.N., Syrykh, G.D., Tarasov, I.K., and Yakovleva, I.Ya. Results of the investigation of the otolith function in manned space flights (NASA TM-76103). Translated from Vestnik Otorinolaringologii, 6:21–24, 1979.

Lackner, J.R. Training countermeasures. In: Space motion sickness symposium proceedings. Edited by J.L. Homick, Lyndon B. Johnson Space Center, Houston, TX, 15–17 November 1978. (Prepared by General Electric Company Purchase Order T-1830G).

Levy, R.A. Biofeedback rehabilitation of airsick aircrew. Preprints of the 1980 Annual Scientific Meeting of the Aerospace Medical Association, Anaheim, CA, 1980.

Matsnev, E.I. Space motion sickness: Phenomenology, countermeasures, mechanisms. Moscow, U.S.S.R., Institute of Biomedical Problems, U.S.S.R. Ministry of Health, (in press).

Matsnev, E.T. and Bodo, D. Experimental assessment of selected anti-motion sickness drugs. Aviat., Space, and Envir. Med., 55(4):281–286, 1984.

Matsnev, E.I., I.Y. Yakovleva, I.K. Tarasov, V.N. Alekseyev, L.N. Kornilova, A.D. Matveev and G.I. Gorgiladze. Space motion sickness: Phenomenology, countermeasures, and mechanisms. Aviat., Space, and Envir. Med., 54(4):312–317, 1983.

McDonough, F.E. NRC Committee on Aviation Medicine, Report No. 181, 1943.

Miller, E.F., II. Evaluation of otolith organ function by means of ocular counter-rolling. In: Vestibular function on Earth and in Space. Edited by J. Stahle, Oxford, Pergamon Press, 1970.

Money, K.E. Motion sickness. Physiology Review, 50:1–39, 1970.

Oman, C.M., Lichtenberg, B.R. and Money, K.E. Space motion sickness monitoring experiment: Spacelab 1. In: AGARD Conference Proceedings (CP-372) on Motion Sickness: Mechanisms, Prediction, Prevention and Treatment. Williamsburg, VA, 1984.

Parker, D.E., and Money, K.E. Vestibular/motion sickness mechanism. In: Space motion sickness symposium proceedings. Edited by J.L. Homick, Lyndon B. Johnson Space Center, Houston, TX, 15017 November, 1978. (Prepared by General Electric Company under Purchase Order T-1830G).

Parker, D.E., Reschke, M.F., Arrott, A.P., Homick, J.L. and Lichtenberg, B.K. Otolith tilt-translation reinterpretation following prolonged weightlessness: Implications for preflight training. Aviat., Space, and Envir. Med., 56:601–606 1985.

Reason, J.T. Relations between motion sickness susceptibility, the spiral after-effect and loudness estimation. British Journal of Psychology, 59:385–393, 1968.

Reason, J.T., and Brand, J.J. Motion sickness. London, Academic Press, 1975.

Reason, J.T., and Graybiel, A. An attempt to measure the degree of adaptation produced by differing amounts of Coriolis vestibular stimulation in the Slow Rotation Room (NAMI–1084, NASA Order R–93). Naval Aerospace Medical Institute, Pensacola, FL, 1969.

Reschke, M.F., Anderson, D.V., and Homick, J.L. Vestibulospinal reflexes as a function of microgravity. Science, 225:212–214, 1984.

von Baumgarten, R.J., and Thumler, R.R. A model for vestibular function in altered gravitational states. In: Life sciences and space research (Vol. XVII). Edited by R. Holmquist, Oxford, Pergamon Press, 1979.

von Baumgarten, R.J., Vogel, H., and Kass, J.R. Nausogenic properties of various dynamic and static force environments. Acta Astronautica, 8(9–10):1005–1013, 1981.

Whittingham, H.E. Medical aspects of air travel. I. Environment and immunization requirements. British Medical Journal, 1:556–558, 1953.

Wilding, J.M., and Meddis, R. Personality correlates of motion sickness. British Journal of Psychology, 63:619–620, 1972.

Wurster, W.H. Burchard, E.C. and von Restorff, W. Comparison of oral and TTS-scopolamine with respect to anti-motion sickness potency and psychomotor performance. Preprints of the 1981 Annual Scientific Meeting of the Aerospace Medical Association (ISSN 0065-3764), San Antonio, TX, 1981.

Yakovleva, I. Ya., Kornilova, L.N., Tarasov, I.K., and Alekseyev, V.N. Results of the study of the vestibular apparatus and the functions of the perception of space in cosmonauts (pre- and postflight observations) (NASA TM-76485). Translated into English from Report to the XI Joint Soviet-American Working Group on Space Biology and Medicine, Moscow, October, 1980.

Yegorov, A.D. Results of medical research during the 175-day flight of the third prime crew on the Salyut 6-Soyuz orbital complex (NASA TM-76450). Moscow, U.S.S.R.: Academy of Sciences U.S.S.R., Ministry of Health, 1980.

Young, L.R., Oman, C.M. Watt, D.G.D., Money, K.E., and Lichtenberg. Spatial orientation in weightlessness and readaptation to Earth's gravity. Science, 225:205–208, 1984.

9 Performance

DONALD E. PARKER
MILLARD F. RESCHKE
NANCY G. ALDRICH

Since the beginning of the U.S. Mercury Program and the Soviet Vostok flights, many investigators have examined variables of task performance associated with exposure to the space environment. This chapter reviews observed and reported changes in sensory and motor systems, illusions, and sleep disturbances, with the goal of comprehending or predicting their possible impact on astronaut performance during and immediately after weightless space flight.

Prior to the actual undertaking of manned space flight, concerns were expressed that sensory disturbances in weightlessness would be so great that astronauts would be unable to perform even simple tasks. With the possible exception of deficits due to space motion sickness (discussed in a separate chapter), these initial concerns proved unfounded. During brief missions under nominal conditions, performance disturbance associated with changes in sensory and motor systems, illusions, or altered sleep patterns do not appear to have significant operational impact. However, questions remain concerning possible deficits after prolonged

exposure to weightlessness over the course of long-term missions such as a tour of duty on a space station, or an interplanetary flight.

Volumes of new data have been gathered by international teams of scientists affiliated with the American and Soviet space programs. Partial summaries of these efforts may be found in special issues of *Science* (13 July 1984, Volume 225, Number 4658), and *Experimental Brain Research* (Volume 64, 1986), devoted to Spacelab 1 findings, and in the "Proceedings of the 7th International Academy of Astronautics Man in Space Symposium: Physiologic Adaptation of Man in Space," published in *Aviation, Space and Environmental Medicine* (Vol. 58, Number 9, September Supplement, 1987).

SENSORY-MOTOR DISTURBANCE

Task performance requires both adequate sensory information and appropriate motor capability. This section summarizes major findings concerning the effects of weightlessness on vision, proprioception, mass perception, motor performance, and posture.

VISION

Because accurate perception of the environment is critical for orientation and adaptation to the space environment, vision has received particular attention. Initially, it was expected that exposure to the space environment would induce changes in visual performance. These changes could result from several factors, including altered light conditions, modified receptor physiology, and disturbances of the eye-movement control system as a secondary effect of vestibular changes.

The visual environment in space is altered in several ways. First, objects are brighter under solar illumination. Earth's atmosphere absorbs at least 15 percent of the incoming solar radiation. Water vapor, smog, and clouds can make this absorption considerably higher. In general, this means that the level of illumination in which astronauts work during daylight is about one-fourth higher than on Earth. Second, on surfaces such as the moon, there is no atmospheric scattering of light (Figure 9-1). This causes areas not under direct solar illumination to appear much darker and results in a transformation of normal visual intensity relationships.

Improved visual acuity was suggested by astronauts' reports that, while in orbit, they were able to see objects such as trucks and cars moving along highways. However, extensive testing of Gemini 5 astronauts indicated that visual performance was neither degraded nor improved during the 8-day mission: performance was within limits predicted by preflight measures of visual acuity (Duntley et al., 1966). The astronauts' reported ability to detect cars was probably due to dust clouds or shadows associated with traffic, which could significantly enlarge visual images.

Studies of visual system physiology were undertaken during the Apollo program. Photographic studies of the retinal vasculature showed a significant decrease in the size of veins for one crewmember after 4 hours, and of both veins and arteries about $3\frac{1}{2}$ hours after flight for another crewmember. The degree of constriction of retinal vasculature postflight in this crew was greater and more persistent than could be accounted for by the vasoconstrictive effect of oxygen alone (Hawkins and Zieglschmid, 1975). Such constriction may also be associated with an incompletely understood decrease in central venous pressure in the upper part of the body (Kirsch et al., 1986), coupled with an increase in intraocular pressure.

Intraocular pressure rises during flight and drops below preflight level after landing, as was shown during the Spacelab D-1 mission. Three crewmembers measured intraocular pressure using a hand-applanation tonometer; the mean pressure rise was 20–25 percent (Draeger et al., 1986). These intraocular tension changes are probably associated with the headward shift of body fluids following orbital insertion and the subsequent pooling of fluid in the trunk and lower extremities after return to Earth.

Space Shuttle flights have offered several opportunities for more refined visual testing. A specially-designed visual test apparatus was used to assess contrast sensitivity, phoria, eye dominance, flicker fusion frequency, stereopsis, and acuity. An investigation undertaken by Task and Genco (1986) employed 16 crewmembers from three Shuttle missions. With the exception of slightly improved stereopsis, no significant changes due to weightlessness were found. A second study (Ginsburg and Vanderploeg, 1986), which examined near visual acuity and contrast sensitivity

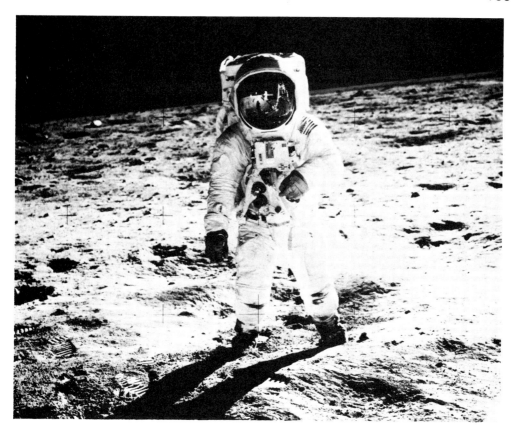

Figure 9-1. Dark shadows from astronaut and rocks illustrate lack of light scattering in the lunar environment.

in 23 crewmembers (four flights), reported evidence of reduced contrast sensitivity with little or no change in visual acuity. The spatial frequencies at which the contrast sensitivity changes were noted varied for crewmembers. The changes were smaller than a factor of two, too insignificant to impact operational performance. However, if contrast sensitivity changes continued to develop during protracted exposure to weightlessness, as suggested by the work of Lazarev et al. (1981), the decrement could become operationally significant.

The effects of weightlessness on vision, noted above, may be attributable to intravascular fluid shifts and associated changes in the physical characteristics of the eye. Microgravity is known to produce a headward shift of 700–1400 ml of fluid. Linder and Trick (1986) noted that head-down tilt on Earth produces fluid shifts similar to those observed during space flight. This suggests that the contrast sensitivity changes could result from physiological changes that are a direct consequence of the intraocular pressure changes.

Possible changes during weightlessness in the ability to maintain visual fixation on targets while moving the head, and the ability to track moving targets, have not been fully examined. However, results of several experiments on eye-movement control suggest that performance of these tasks might be diminished during the initial period of exposure to weightlessness and immediately after landing. The vestibular nuclei located in the brain stem are part of a system that allows one to fix the gaze on a stationary target during voluntary head motions as well as to track moving targets. This system appears to be disturbed during flight, perhaps as a consequence of altered vestibular receptor function due to the absence of gravity. Vieville et al. (1986) reported that the amplitudes (eye movement "gain") of vertical eye movements were diminished during the first 3 days of weightlessness, both when astronauts moved their heads voluntarily and when they attempted to track a moving visual target. After 4 days in orbit, the gains returned to the preflight level, perhaps as a consequence of substitution of neck receptor cues for vestibular receptor cues. Grigoriev et al. (1986) reported that after 237 days of space flight the pattern of movements was significantly altered when cosmonauts moved their heads and eyes to fixate a laterally displaced target. The authors reported that similar disturbances have been observed in patients suffering from cerebellar disorders.

Perceived light flashes in the absence of normal visual stimulation were studied by Hoffman et al. (1977) during the Skylab 4 mission. These flashes are caused by heavy ionized cosmic particles passing through retinal cells. During this study, consisting of two observation sessions of 70 and 55 minutes, respectively, a total of 168 flashes were reported. Although no performance disturbance has been associated with these light flashes, it is likely that the flashes mask transient visual stimuli.

PROPRIOCEPTION

Disturbance of proprioception, particularly with respect to perceived limb ori-

entation, has been reported anecdotally (Schmitt and Reid, 1985). Watt and his colleagues examined crewmembers' ability to distinguish joint angles following passive bending (Watt et al., 1985). Although the crewmembers rarely made errors when performing this task on the ground, they made a significant number of errors in estimating elbow and knee angles during the initial 3 days of weightlessness. A similar proprioceptive deficit was noted during an active pointing task. Crewmember subjects were blindfolded after viewing the locations of several targets. After 5 minutes they were asked to point several times to each target. While this task was accomplished easily both before and after flight, two crewmembers exhibited very poor performance in weightlessness. One showed improvement during the flight, but the other did not. These observations suggest that task performance may be disturbed when visual cues are unavailable.

ILLUSIONS

Various visual, orientational, proprioceptive, and self-motion illusions have been reported both during and after flight. Oscillopsia refers to an apparent displacement of visual targets during passive or voluntary head movement. Apparent oscillation of visual targets was reported by some Skylab astronauts (Graybiel et al., 1977), but was attributed to drowsiness. Young and his colleagues (1984) systematically investigated oscillopsia on the Spacelab 1 mission. Their subjects reported instability of visual targets during head movement immediately after landing.

During reentry and immediately after landing, astronauts frequently report that voluntary head motions produce illusions of self-motion or motion of the visual surroundings (oscillopsia) (Reschke and Parker, 1987). It is likely that these illusions are related to disturbances of the gaze control system.

Oscillopsia is readily understood in terms of miscalibrated compensatory eye movements (inappropriate vestibular-ocular reflex gain) during head movement in an unusual force environment. The appearance of oscillopsia postflight indicates that the compensatory eye movements had adjusted to the microgravity condition and were no longer appropriate to normal gravity. This suggests that a carefully designed experiment would reveal oscillopsia during the period immediately following orbital insertion, before astronauts have adapted to weightlessness.

Anecdotal reports from the Soviet and American space programs include illusions of orientation. Yakovleva and her colleagues (1982) reported that cosmonauts often described illusions of inversion ("hanging upside down"). These reactions usually occurred immediately after onset of weightlessness and persisted for periods ranging from minutes to hours. Mittelstaedt (1986) has proposed that the inversion illusion may be understood using a model that includes an internal ("ideotropic") orientation vector.

Proprioceptive illusions have been noted during and after extended space flight. Watt and his associates (1985) asked subjects on Space Shuttle Mission 41-G to perform knee and arm bends. The two types of illusions reported are illustrated in Figure 9-2. During arm flexions, subjects felt as though the wall moved toward them. During leg bends, subjects felt as though the floor were moving up and down (like a trampoline). Similar illusions were reported by Spacelab 1 astronauts (Reschke et al., 1986) and during the two-gravity phase of parabolic flight (Lackner and Graybiel, 1981). These data are consistent with the view that altered force environments disturb the system that compares motor commands with associated sensory consequences.

Illusions of self-motion or unusual surround motion have been addressed in several studies. Perceived translational self-motion was reported during roll stimulation in darkness 1–3 hours after Shuttle landing (Parker et al., 1985). Unexpected illusory translation of either the subject or the visual surround was reported by two astronauts who performed voluntary pitch or roll head movements during reentry and after the orbiter had stopped on the runway (Reschke and Parker, 1987). These observations, as well as similar ones reported by Young et al. (1984), support the hypothesis that signals from receptors that respond to linear acceleration are reinterpreted during adaptation to weightlessness (Parker et al., 1985).

MASS PERCEPTION

Ross and her associates (1986) demonstrated that the ability to discriminate between the masses of small objects was poorer in weightlessness. It is reasonable that this should be so, because mass information was detectable by the astronauts only during periods of positive and negative acceleration as they shook the objects, whereas on Earth that information is also available through skin pressure receptors that allow detection of an object's weight. In addition to the loss of weight information, incomplete adaptation to the altered force environment could contribute to performance decline.

POSTURE

Normal locomotion and postural stability are consequences of evolution in one gravity. The structural and anatomical features that allow upright movement on Earth are not appropriate for orientation in microgravity. Disturbances in postural equilib-

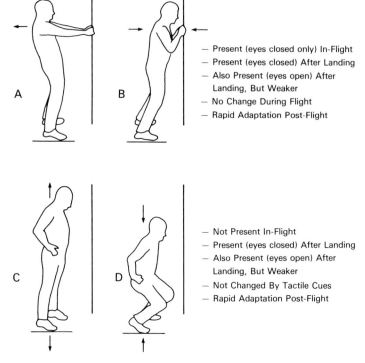

— Present (eyes closed only) In-Flight
— Present (eyes closed) After Landing
— Also Present (eyes open) After
   Landing, But Weaker
— No Change During Flight
— Rapid Adaptation Post-Flight

— Not Present In-Flight
— Present (eyes closed) After Landing
— Also Present (eyes open) After
   Landing, But Weaker
— Not Changed By Tactile Cues
— Rapid Adaptation Post-Flight

Figure 9-2. Proprioceptive illusions experienced when pushing against wall (top) or floor (bottom).

rium have been among the most consistent findings related to the human response to space flight, and may provide a key to understanding how an individual adapts to the unique environment of microgravity.

Maintenance of posture requires the constant interaction of sensory input and motor output. Disturbance of either results in inappropriate postural responses. The sensory input required to maintain posture is the integrated response of visual, vestibular, somatosensory, and proprioceptive receptors. Microgravity results in new weighting, or reinterpretation, of sensory information from these receptors.

The effects of weightlessness on posture have been examined using three principal methods: crewmembers' reports of changes in sensations, performance on balance rails and moving platforms, and mea-

surement of muscle potentials from the major antigravity and weight-bearing muscles.

Crewmembers from Mercury through Shuttle flights have reported one or more of four basic unusual sensations during the first few hours after landing (Figure 9-3). These include the sensation of turning while attempting to walk a straight path. Overcompensating for this, many crewmembers actually walked in a curved path in the opposite direction. Second, some crewmembers have reported sudden loss of postural stability, much as though they had been pushed to one side by a "giant hand." Usually this was experienced while attempting to walk around a corner. Third, the pitching and rolling head motions that accompany normal walking were perceived as greatly exaggerated. Finally, in a visual environment that is not well structured, some crewmembers experienced a sudden loss of orientation and pitched forward, or began a tumbling movement before position awareness was regained.

Postural tests performed immediately postflight have enhanced understanding of inflight adaptation. The ability of astro-

nauts to stand on narrow rails was reduced after landing (Homick et al., 1977; Kenyon and Young, 1986). This decrement was more pronounced with the eyes closed, and greater after longer flights. Other postural performance tests have relied on platforms that move parallel to the Earth

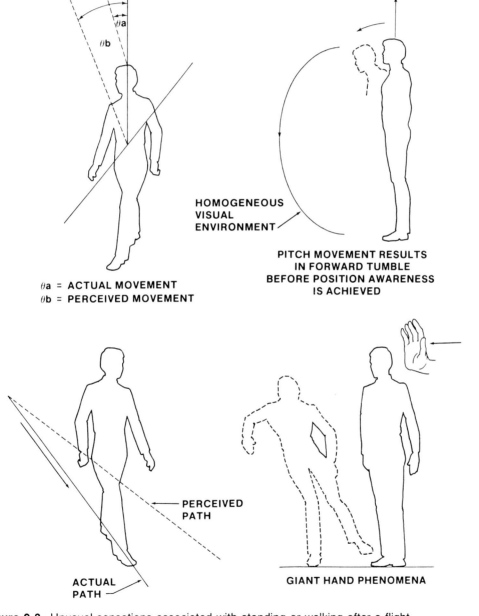

θa = ACTUAL MOVEMENT
θb = PERCEIVED MOVEMENT

HOMOGENEOUS
VISUAL
ENVIRONMENT

PITCH MOVEMENT RESULTS
IN FORWARD TUMBLE
BEFORE POSITION AWARENESS
IS ACHIEVED

PERCEIVED
PATH

ACTUAL
PATH

GIANT HAND PHENOMENA

Figure 9-3. Unusual sensations associated with standing or walking after a flight.

(Anderson et al., 1986) and tilting platforms (Kenyon and Young, 1986). Overall, results of postural performance tests suggest that astronauts adapt to weightlessness by increasing their reliance on vision.

Soviet investigators have also examined postural performance postflight. One test evaluated the ability of crewmembers to retain balance following a disturbance (in this case, a push against the chest). The results indicated that performance did not return to preflight levels for as long as 42 days after landing (Yegorov, 1979).

Postflight postural instability has been assessed quantitatively by recording body position and muscle potentials after disturbing crewmembers' postural equilibrium by exposing them to unexpected movements. Four such tests were part of the first Spacelab postflight biomedical test battery. Reschke and his colleagues (1986) examined the effects of weightlessness on a monosynaptic spinal reflex— the Hoffmann reflex (H reflex). This reflex can be modulated by a nerve pathway from the otolith receptors. Activity in this otolith pathway was elicited by exposing the subjects to unexpected drops (falls). Changes in the brain's interpretation of information from the otolith receptor was revealed by changes in the H reflex. During flight, the effect of otolith stimulation on the H reflex gradually declined. Return to preflight levels of response occurred gradually during the postflight test sessions. Otolith modulation of the H reflex is lost because this modulation has no adaptive value for the astronaut in weightlessness. Self-motion sensations were reported after the drops; early inflight drops were perceived in the same manner as preflight. Drops late in the flight were described as sudden, fast, hard, and translational in nature. Immediately postflight, the drops were perceived like those late in flight, and the astronauts stated that they did not feel as though they were falling, but rather that the floor was rising to meet them.

In a related Spacelab 1 experiment (Watt et al., 1985), otolith-spinal reflexes were elicited by sudden, unexpected Earth vertical falls (like the H reflex experiment, falls were executed in flight by pulling subjects to the deck of the Spacelab using elastic cords). EMG activity recorded early in flight from the gastrocnemius-soleus during the fall was lower than preflight and continued to decline as the flight progressed. Postflight, EMG amplitude had returned to normal prior to the first opportunity for measurement.

Following the first Spacelab flight, posture measurements were made using a dynamic platform which could be moved parallel to the floor in both predictable and unpredictable patterns. In this experiment (Anderson et al., 1986), EMG data were obtained from the soleus and anterior tibialis muscles, and hip and shoulder movements were recorded with digital line-scan cameras. When the eyes were open and the platform was moved with a backward step function, the subject's response as he attempted to maintain equilibrium showed an overshoot with the shoulders and an undershoot with the hips. Also, the time required to assume a new stable position was greater after flight than before. (Surprisingly, vision appeared to deter postural stability.) The EMG data indicated that soleus muscle latency was greater postflight.

In another posture platform test (Kenyon and Young, 1986), one Spacelab 1 crewmember's erect posture was tested by pitching the platform base unexpectedly about the ankle joint. EMG activity from the tibialis anterior and gastrocnemius muscles was measured with the eyes open and closed. Early EMG activity (first 500 ms) did not change in latency or amplitude when the platform was pitched. However, EMG activity which occurred later than 500 ms showed higher amplitudes than those obtained preflight.

In a joint French and Soviet experiment (Clement et al., 1984), adaptation of motor control to space flight was investigated. Control of upright posture was examined during voluntary upward movement of the arm and voluntary raising on tiptoe. Results showed that early inflight postural attitude was similar to that on Earth, but that as the flight progressed there was a forward inclination of the body which increased with vision stabilized. Muscle responses to sudden voluntary perturbations indicated a redistribution of tonic activity between extensor and flexor muscles of the ankle, and a general reduction of extensor tone.

In summary, posture experiments suggest that the sensory-motor programs which have evolved on Earth are not appropriate for orientation and locomotion in a microgravity environment. The new posture programs developed during space flight are equally inappropriate for locomotion upon return to Earth. Vision is an important factor in the adaptation process.

Currently, there is no single posture test or group of tests that explores all the changes that have been measured or experienced by astronauts. Most tests have concentrated on the effects of vision and otolith function. Because of the importance of posture for returning astronauts, it is necessary to develop tests that measure the full range of responses, including those currently expressed as sensations and feelings of instability.

MOTOR PERFORMANCE

The Skylab Program offered American scientists their first opportunity to study astronaut performance in detail during extended exposure to weightlessness. Kubis et al. (1977) photographed activities such as using the Lower Body Negative Pressure Device, exercising on the ergometer, assembling and using photometer and camera systems, maintaining hardware assemblies, donning and doffing an EVA space suit, and all activities involved in the preparation of food. These studies produced no evidence of performance deterioration that could be attributed to the effects of long-duration exposure to the space environment. The first inflight performance of a task generally took longer than the last preflight performance. This was probably due to several factors, including development of space motion sickness symptoms, which are exacerbated by head movements. However, recovery of skilled performance was quite rapid, and by the end of the second trial approximately half of all tasks were completed within the time recorded for the last preflight trial.

SLEEP

Although sleep is clearly possible in space, astronauts frequently report sleep disturbances. United States researchers first obtained objective measures of sleep during the Gemini 7 flight. This type of study was continued in the Skylab Program; measurements were made of the quality of astronauts' sleep (Frost et al., 1977), including electroencephalograms, electrooculograms, and head motions while sleeping.

The Skylab experiments did not show any major adverse changes in sleep as a result of prolonged space flight. Only during the 84-day flight did one subject experience any real difficulty sleeping. Even here, the problem diminished with time, although sleeping medication was required on occasion. The most significant changes occurred postflight, with alterations more of sleep quality than quantity. It appears that readaptation to one gravity is more disruptive to sleep than adaptation to microgravity.

Careful recordings of eye movements during sleep were obtained from one Spacelab 1 crewmember pre-, in-, and postflight (Quadens and Green, 1984). The results suggest that initial exposure to weightlessness is associated with an approximately fourfold increase in the number of eye movements, with rapid eye movements (REMs) predominating (Figure 9-4). Previous research indicates that REM may reflect learning and retention of new information. Quadens and Green suggested that the increased REM observed during the initial sleep period following launch reflected learning processes as the astronaut started adapting to the new environment.

Santy et al. (1987) reviewed sleep-related problems with 58 Shuttle crewmembers during postflight debriefings. Although none used medication on Earth, over 30 percent requested sleep medication while on orbit. Greatest disturbances were experienced during the first and last days of the mission. Among the factors reported to disturb sleep were space motion sickness, noise, and excitement. Sleep disturbance and the associated use of medication could have a detrimental impact on crew performance. Further study is needed to address this potential problem.

SUMMARY

Certain research suggests that performance might be degraded following prolonged exposure to microgravity. For example, data from four Shuttle astronauts showed changes in reaction times and time perception (Ratino et al., 1986). This, coupled with the potential sensory-motor changes discussed above and the gradual loss of muscle function, could limit the ability to perform certain manual tasks.

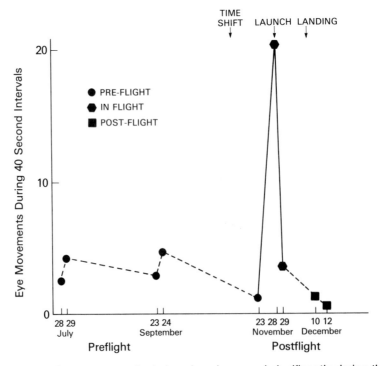

Figure 9-4. Number of eye movements during sleep increased significantly during the first night of sleep on orbit relative to pre- and postflight observations.

However, results of performance studies by American and Soviet investigators are usually interpreted as supporting the view that neither sensory-motor nor sleep disturbances are likely to compromise future advanced space operations. In addition, complex motor activities, such as operation of the remote manipulator arm of the Space Shuttle, can be performed with precision and efficiency.

REFERENCES

Anderson, D.J., Reschke, M.F., Homick, J.E., and Werness, S.A.S. Dynamic posture analysis of Spacelab crewmembers. Experimental Brain Research. 64:380–391, 1986.

Clement, G., Gurfinkel, V.S., Lestienne, F., Lipshits, M.I., and Popov, K.E. Adaptation of posture control to weightlessness. Experimental Brain Research. 57:61–72, 1984.

Draeger, J., Wirt, H., Schwartz, R., and Tomex, R. Messung Des Augeninnendrucks Unter MG-Bedingungen. Naturwissenschaften 73:450–452, 1986.

Duntley, S.Q., Austin, R.W., Taylor, J.H., and Harris, J.L. Experiment S-8/D-13, visual acuity and astronaut visibility. In: Gemini Midprogram Conference (NASA SP-121). U.S. Government Printing Office, Washington, D.C., 1966.

Frost, J.D., Jr., Shumate, W.H., Salamy, J.G., and Booher, C.R. Experiment M133. Sleep monitoring on Skylab. In: Biomedical Results from Skylab (NASA SP-377). Edited by R.S. Johnston and L.F. Dietlein. U.S. Government Printing Office, Washington, D.C., 1977.

Ginsburg, A.P., Vanderploeg, J. Vision in Space: Near vision acuity and contrast sensitivity. NASA Interim Report: Space Shuttle Medical DSOs, Johnson Space Center, Houston, TX, 1986.

Graybiel, A., Miller, E.F., and Homick, J.L. Experiment M131. Human vestibular function. In: Biomedical Results from Skylab (NASA SP-377). Edited by R.S. Johnston and L.F. Dietlein. U.S. Government Printing Office, Washington, D.C., 1977.

Grigoriev, R.A., Gazenko, O.G., Kozlovskaya, I.B., Barmin, V.A., and Kreidich, Y.V. Vestibulo-cerebellar regulation of oculomotor reactions in microgravity conditions. In: Adaptive Processes in Visual and Oculomotor Systems. Edited by E.L. Keller and D.S. Zee, New York, Pergamon Press, 1986.

Hawkins, W.R., and Zieglschmid, J.F. Clinical aspects of crew health. In: Biomedical Results of Apollo (NASA SP-369). Edited by R.S. Johnston, L.F. Dietlein, and C.A. Berry. U.S. Government Printing Office, Washington, D.C., 1975.

Hoffman, R.A., Pinsky, L.S., Osborne, W.Z., and Bailey, J.V. Visual light flash observations on Skylab 4. In: Biomedical Results from Skylab (NASA SP-377). Edited by R.S. Johnston and C.F. Dietlein. U.S. Government Printing Office, Washington, D.C., 1977.

Homick, J.F., Reschke, M.F., and Miller, E.F., II. Effects of prolonged exposure to weightlessness on postural equilibrium. In: Biomedical Results from Skylab (NASA SP-377). Edited by R.S. Johnston and L.F. Dietlein, U.S. Government Printing Office, Washington, D.C., 1977.

Kenyon, R.V., and Young, L.R. MIT/Canadian vestibular experiments on Spacelab 1: Postural responses following exposure to weightlessness. Experimental Brain Research. 64:1986.

Kirsch, K., Haenel, F., Rocker, L., and Wicke, H.J. Venous pressure in microgravity. Naturwissenschaften 73:447–449, 1986.

Kubis, J.F., McLaughlin, E.J., Jackson, J.M., Rusnak, R., McBride, G.H., and Saxon, S.V. Task and work performance on Skylab missions 2, 3, and 4. Time and motion study—experiment M151. In: Biomedical Results from Skylab (NASA SP-377). Edited by R.S. Johnston and L.F. Dietlein. U.S. Government Printing Office, Washington, D.C., 1977.

Lackner, J.R. and Graybiel, A. Variations in gravitoinertial force level affect the gain of the vestibulo-ocular reflex: implications for the etiology of space motion sickness. Aviation Space and Environmental Medicine, 52:154, 1981.

Lazarev, A.I., Kovalenok, V.V., Ivanchenkov, A.S. and Avakyan, S.V. Atmosphere of Earth from Salyut-6. Translation of Atmosfera Zemli s Salyuta-6. Leningrad, Gidrometeoizdat, 1981.

Linder, B.J., and Trick, G.L. Simulation of space flight with whole-body head-down tilt: Influence on intraocular pressure and retinocortical processing. NASA Interim Report: Space Shuttle Medical DSOs, Johnson Space Center, Houston, TX, 1986.

Mittelstaedt, H. In search of the causes of the "inversion illusions." Presented at the VII International Man in Space Symposium, Houston, TX, Feb. 10–13, 1986.

Parker, D.E., Reschke, M.F., Arrott, A.P., Homick, J.L., and Lichtenberg, B.K. Otolith tilt-translation reinterpretation following prolonged weightlessness: implications for preflight training. Aviation Space and Environmental Medicine, 56: 601–606, 1985.

Quadens, O., and Green, H. Eye movements during sleep in weightlessness. Science, 225:221, July 1984.

Ratino, D.A., Repperger, D., Goodyear, C. Test battery to measure decision time and time perception under space flight conditions. Abstract of poster presented at IAA Man in Space Symposium, Houston, TX, 1986.

Reschke, M.F., Anderson, D.J., and Homick, J.L. Vestibulo-spinal response modification as determined with the H reflex during the Spacelab 1 flight. Experimental Brain Research. 64:367–379, 1986.

Reschke, M.F., and Parker, D.E. Effects of prolonged weightlessness on self-motion perception and eye movements evoked by roll and pitch. Aviation Space and Environmental Medicine. 58:(9) Sect. 11, Sept., 1987.

Ross, H.E., Schwartz, E., and Emmerson, P. Mass discrimination in weightlessness improves with arm movements of higher acceleration. Naturwissenschaften 73:453–454, 1986.

Santy, P.A., Kapanka, H., Davis, J.R., Stewart, D.F. Analysis of sleep on Shuttle missions. Presentation at the 1987 Aerospace Medical Association meeting, Las Vegas, Nevada, May, 1987.

Schmitt, H.H., and Reid, D.J. Anecdotal Information on Space Adaptation Syndrome. Johnson Space Center, Houston, TX, 1985.

Task, H.L., and Genco, L.Y. Effects of short-term space flight on several visual functions. NASA Interim Report: Space shuttle Medical DSOs, Johnson Space Center, Houston, TX, 1986.

Vieville, T., Clement, G., Lestienne, F., and Berthoz, A. Adaptive modifications of the optokinetic and vestibulo-ocular reflexes in microgravity. In: Adaptive Processes in Visual and Oculomotor Systems. Edited by E.L. Keller and D.S. Zee, New York, Pergamon Press, 1986.

Watt, D.G.D., Money, K.E., Bondar, R.L., Thirsk, R.B., Garneau, M., and Scully-Power, P. Canadian medical experiments on Shuttle flight 41-G. Canadian Aeronautics and Space Journal. 31:215–226, 1985.

Yakovleva, I.Ya., Kornilova, L.N., Tarasov, I.K., and Alekseyev, V.N. Results of studies of cosmonauts' vestibular function and spatial perception. Space Biology and Aerospace Medicine, 16(1):26–33 (JPRS 80323), 1982.

Yegorov, A.D. Results of medical studies during long-term manned flights on the orbital Salyut-6 and Soyuz complex. USSR Academy of Sciences, NASA TN–76014, 1979.

Young, L.R., Oman, C.M., Watt, D.G.D., Money, K.E., and Lichtenberg, B.K. Spatial orientation in weightlessness and readaptation to Earth's gravity. Science, 225:206, 1984.

10 The Cardiopulmonary System

MICHAEL W. BUNGO

The human cardiopulmonary system has evolved an array of specific mechanisms to counter the continuous pull of gravity. The species spends approximately two-thirds of its existence in an upright posture, and it is this position that evolution has described as the norm. To accommodate the weightlessness of space flight, the cardiopulmonary system undergoes substantial change. Some of these changes, such as cephalad-central fluid shifts, are the direct result of microgravity; others are concomitant adjustments; and still others may result from the unusual circumstances unique to the space environment. There is a vast library of research describing both animal and human responses to ground-based simulations of space flight conditions (Blomqvist and Stone, 1983). For the purposes of creating a manageable information source, this chapter will only report actual space flight data collected from humans. As a result, this will probably raise more questions than it answers, but in that respect it will honestly reflect the infancy of our knowledge in this area.

FLUID SHIFTS

The most visibly obvious alteration that occurs in the cardiovascular system upon exposure to weightlessness is the cephalad shift of fluid, estimated at 1.5 to 2.0 liters from the lower extremities and an unclear amount from the pelvic region. Evidence for this shift comes from a number of observations.

PHOTOGRAPHIC EVIDENCE

Photographs taken of the Skylab crew in flight show signs of periorbital puffiness, facial edema, and thickening of the eyelids (Thornton, Hoffler, and Rummel, 1977). The jugular veins and the veins in the temple, scalp, and forehead appear full and distended. Figure 10-1 shows photographs of the Skylab 3 Commander (CDR) taken in flight (a), and postflight (b). Although the inflight uplifting in the facial tissue may have been partly due to the absence of gravity, fluid shifts probably played a

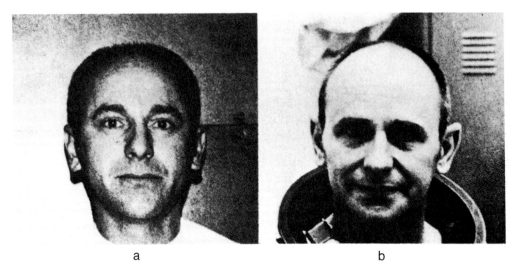

a   b

Figure 10-1. Skylab 3 Commander comparing the puffy face in flight (a) to the normal face preflight (b). (From Thornton, Hoffler, and Rummel, 1977).

significant role, particularly through venous engorgement. These photographs were taken near the end of the Skylab 3 mission (59 days), indicating that edema and venous engorgement do not subside even after some months in space. The crews' subjective observations of nasal stuffiness, head "fullness," and facial puffiness support the hypothesis of substantial fluid shifts.

CHANGES IN CALF GIRTH AND LEG VOLUME

Astronauts have typically shown inflight decrements in calf girth of up to 30 percent. For Skylab and Apollo-Soyuz, multiple circumferential measurements of the lower extremities were taken pre-, in-, and postflight to obtain volumetric estimates and ascertain the time course of fluid shifts. Figure 10-2 shows the measurement technique.

Figure 10-3 shows limb volume data for the Skylab 4 Commander, demonstrating that lower, but not upper, limb volumes decrease early in flight, and return rapidly

to preflight values upon return to Earth (Thornton, Hoffler, and Rummel, 1977). Figure 10-4 shows limb volume data from Apollo-Soyuz, in which it was possible to obtain measurements as early as 6 hours in flight from one crewmember. From these data, it appears that the major shift of fluids occurs rapidly upon insertion into orbit. The rate of this fluid shift appears to follow an exponential course, attaining a maximum within 24 hours and reaching a plateau or a new steady state within 3 to 5 days (Hoffler, Bergman, and Nicogossian, 1977). Calf volume measurements taken during long-term Soviet missions on board Salyut-6 showed a similar pattern of decrease, with values reaching a plateau on the 12th inflight day. Over 140-, 175-, and 185-day missions, fluctuations in leg volume followed a wavelike course of loss and recovery (Gazenko, Genin, and Yegorov, 1981a).

Changes in limb volume, particularly the rapid postflight recovery, combined with photographic evidence and crewmembers' subjective observations, indicate substantial cephalad fluid shifts in

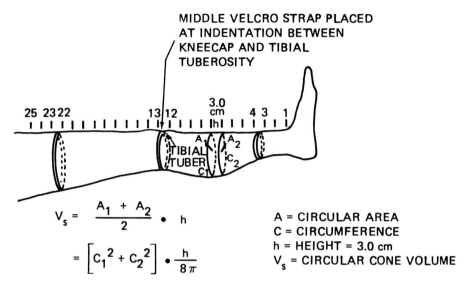

$$V_s = \frac{A_1 + A_2}{2} \cdot h$$

$$= \left[c_1{}^2 + c_2{}^2 \right] \cdot \frac{h}{8\pi}$$

A = CIRCULAR AREA
C = CIRCUMFERENCE
h = HEIGHT = 3.0 cm
V_s = CIRCULAR CONE VOLUME

Figure 10-2. Estimation of leg volume by measurement of multiple circumferences. Calculation is based on assumed circular geometry and summation of multiple, truncated, and conical volumes.

flight. On the basis of inferences drawn from the results of ground-based simulation studies (Burkovskaya et al., 1980; Katkov, Chestukhin et al., 1981; Nicogossian et al., 1979; Sandler, 1977) and inflight data (Gazenko, Genin and Yegorov, 1981b), it appears that these fluid shifts result in a number of physiological readjustments. One hypothesis is diagrammed in Figure 10-5; however, other theories support the role of an atrial natriuretic factor, and still other data fail to substantiate the expected diuresis. Serious questions have also been raised as to the validity of previous bed rest investigations in providing an adequate simulation of the microgravity condition. Granting the observation that similar alterations occur, is

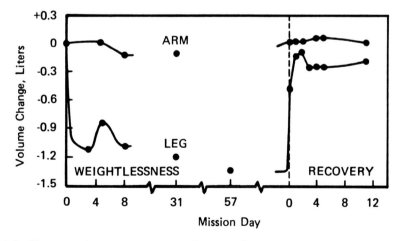

Figure 10-3. Change in left limb volumes of Skylab 4 Commander. (From Thornton, Hoffler, and Rummel, 1977).

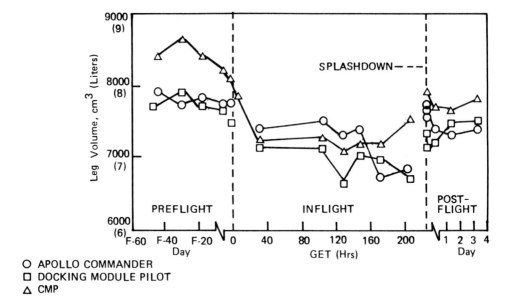

O APOLLO COMMANDER
□ DOCKING MODULE PILOT
△ CMP

Figure 10-4. Left leg volume measurements of U.S. crewmen in the Apollo-Soyuz Test Project. (From Hoffler, Bergman, and Nicogossian, 1977).

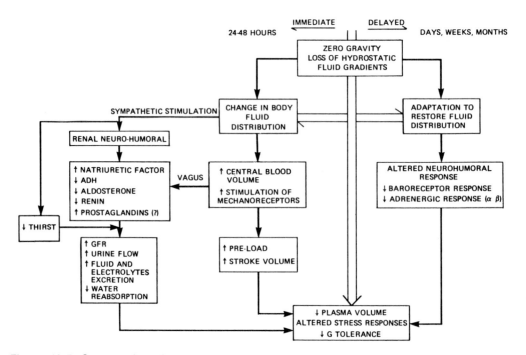

Figure 10-5. Suggested cardiovascular response to weightlessness.

the time course of these events similar and, therefore, are similar reflex mechanisms utilized? For example, Figure 10-6 demonstrates the inflight heart rate from a composite of both Soviet and U.S. space flights. Resting heart rate is nearly universally increased during exposure to weightlessness, regardless of mission duration. Figure 10-7 is the resting heart rate determined during a 6° head-down bed rest simulation of the U.S. Spacelab 1 mission, compared with heart rates measured on the French cosmonaut on board Salyut-6. The former is decreased below the norm and the latter is in line with the summary data presented in Figure 10-6.

DECREASED ORTHOSTATIC TOLERANCE

Decreased orthostatic tolerance has invariably been observed in both American and Soviet crewmembers postflight. Symptoms have ranged from increased heart rate and decreased pulse pressure to a tendency toward spontaneous syncope. The meth-

ods most widely used to quantify orthostatic tolerance include the tilt test, stand test, and lower body negative pressure (LBNP). Figure 10-8 shows the protocols for these tests, and the cardiovascular parameters measured.

PASSIVE TESTING

Gemini crewmen were tested for orthostatic tolerance utilizing a tilt table from a supine control position to a 70° head-up tilt. Figure 10-9 shows a typical response, which was aborted because of presyncopal symptoms. The stand test, in which the subject leans against a wall in a relaxed manner with his heels 15 cm from the wall, was used on some Apollo crewmen. Similar exaggerations in postflight cardiovascular responses are observed in this type of test (Hoffler and Johnson, 1975).

LOWER BODY NEGATIVE PRESSURE TEST

Lower body negative pressure (LBNP), shown in Figure 10-10, is a useful means

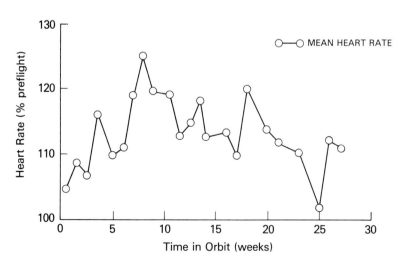

Figure 10-6. Weekly mean resting heart rate in orbit. (Composite data from Soviet and U.S. space flights).

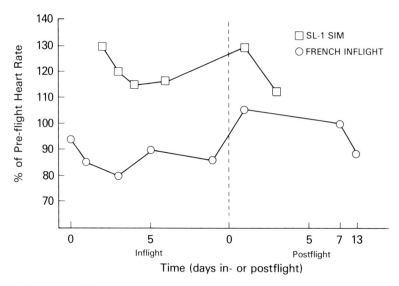

Figure 10-7. Response of heart rate to simulated and actual weightlessness. (U.S. Spacelab 1 mission simulation and Salyut 6 French cosmonaut data).

of assessing orthostatic tolerance because, unlike passive methods, it can be used in zero gravity. Different levels of negative pressure can be applied to the lower portion of the body, resulting in footward displacement of body fluids (Wolthius et al., 1974). An appropriate protocol can simulate the effects of erect posture on the cardiovascular system in one gravity. Figure 10-11 shows a comparison of the pre- and postflight responses of the Apollo 8 Commander to the LBNP protocol.

LBNP tests were performed in flight at regular intervals of 3 days during Skylab missions, affording an opportunity to observe the time course of changes in physiological responses to this kind of orthostatic stress. Figure 10-12 shows a comparison of the responses of the Skylab 4 Scientist Pilot (SPT) for tests conducted 21 days prior to flight and for the first inflight test (mission day 6) (Johnson et al., 1977). Figure 10-13 shows resting and orthostatically stressed heart rates for the Skylab 4 pilot (PLT). Elevations in both parameters were evident in the first test (4 to 6 days in flight), and cardiovascular responses to LBNP continued to show in-

stability, especially during the first 3 weeks.

These results, along with corresponding Soviet findings (Gazenko et al., 1981b), indicate that inflight LBNP presents greater stress to the cardiovascular system than the same levels of LBNP preflight, apparently due to alterations attending the large cephalad migration of body fluids in flight. Diminishing total blood volume probably plays a significant role, but the time course of fluid loss in flight is not clearly defined. Nevertheless, an inverse relationship exists between changes in orthostatically stressed heart rates pre- versus postflight, and corresponding changes in blood volume.

This relationship is shown in Figure 10-14 as percent change from preflight reference values. Recent findings that rigorous inflight exercise (which moderates fluid loss and other aspects of deconditioning) normalizes certain parameters of the inflight response LBNP appear to corroborate this relationship (Yegorov et al., 1981). These data indicate that depleted blood volume is at least associated with the exaggerated cardiovascular responses to LBNP observed postflight, and perhaps with those observed in flight as well (Hoffler, 1977).

ORTHOSTATIC INTOLERANCE DURING SHUTTLE FLIGHTS

Orthostatic intolerance became of even greater concern when the United States embarked upon the Space Shuttle Program of the early 1980s. For the first time in the history of manned exploration of space, the returning crew would be subject to the stress of gravity along the body's Z axis (head-to-toe) during the critical reentry period, and would be manually piloting and landing the spacecraft. The stand test described earlier in this chapter was adopted as the easiest, yet readily reproducible and valid, provocative test of orthostatic intolerance.

Based on previous bed rest studies (P.C. Johnson, 1979), fluid loading with a liter

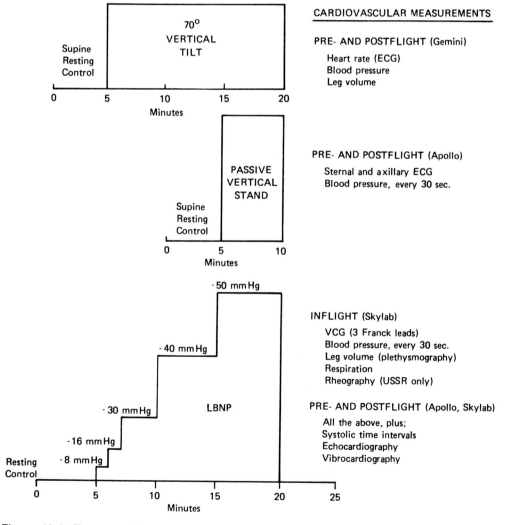

Figure 10-8. Tests used for assessing orthostatic tolerance.

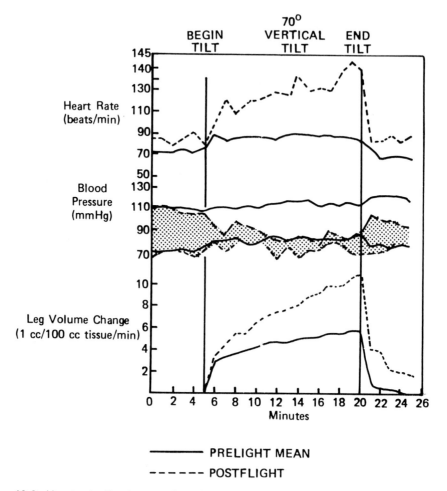

Figure 10-9. Heart rate (beats per minute), blood pressure (systolic and diastolic, in mmHg), and change in leg volume (in percentage) during a 25-minute, 70° tilt test protocol, the first and last 5 minutes being in the horizontal, supine position. Preflight mean curves are solid lines and the first postflight test values are dashed (or hatched). The crewman was the Command Pilot of the 14-day Gemini 7 flight. (After Berry and Catterson, 1967).

of normal saline prior to reexposure to gravitational stress would theoretically allow at least 40 percent of the loading volume to be maintained as increased plasma volume for at least 4 hours after oral ingestion of the solution. The results (Bungo et al., 1985) of this volume loading in Shuttle crewmembers are presented in Figures 10-15 and 10-16. Preflight supine resting heart rates of crewmembers utilizing the countermeasure were identical to those who did not. Postflight, however, it was clear (p < .005) that the countermeasure protected its user with a lower supine heart rate, lower standing heart rate, and the maintenance of mean blood pressure in comparison with a counterpart who used no countermeasure (heart rate and blood pressure being only one measure of orthostatic tolerance and orthostatic intol-

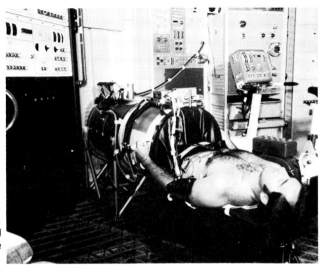

Figure 10-10. Subject undergoing test in lower body negative pressure device.

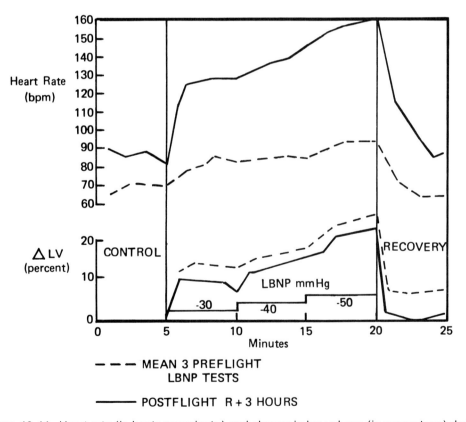

MEAN 3 PREFLIGHT
LBNP TESTS

POSTFLIGHT R + 3 HOURS

Figure 10-11. Heart rate (in beats per minute) and change in leg volume (in percentage) during a 25-minute LBNP test protocol. Preflight mean curves are dashed and the first postflight test data 3 hours after splashdown are solid lines. The crewman was Commander of the Apollo 8 flight.

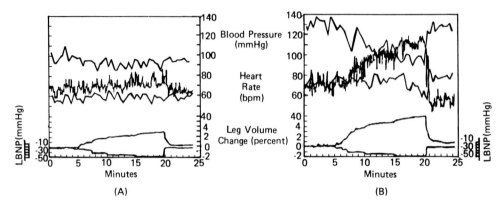

Figure 10-12. Cardiovascular responses of the Skylab 4 scientist pilot during the LBNP test 21 days prior to flight (A) and during the first inflight test on mission day 6 (B). (From Johnson et al., 1977).

erance being only one manifestation of cardiovascular deconditioning as it relates to space flight). Yet 33 percent of those Shuttle crewmembers not utilizing a cardiovascular countermeasure exhibited postflight syncope or presyncope during the stand test. Three percent (one individual) of those who used the fluid loading

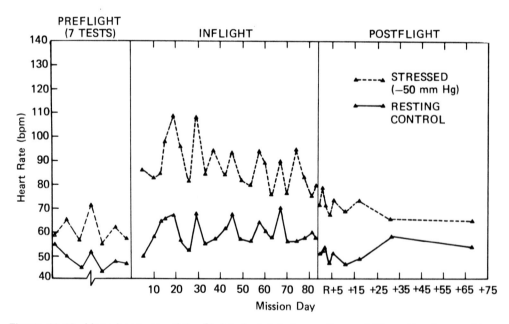

Figure 10-13. Mean heart rate of the Skylab 4 pilot during resting and 50 mmHg phases of lower body negative pressure. The high heart rates that appeared periodically declined in magnitude after the first month in flight. A slight downward trend in stressed heart rates was apparent during the latter period. A presyncopal episode on mission day 10 may have been associated with the lower mean stressed heart rate on that day. (From Johnson et al., 1977).

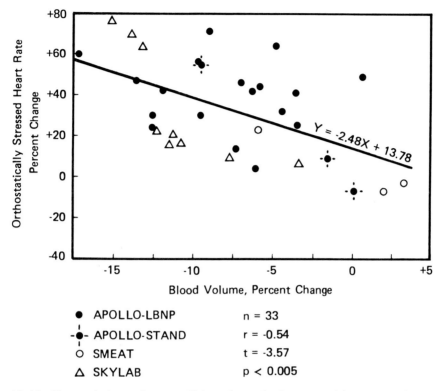

$$Y = -2.48X + 13.78$$

● APOLLO-LBNP	n = 33
-●- APOLLO-STAND	r = -0.54
○ SMEAT	t = -3.57
△ SKYLAB	p < 0.005

Figure 10-14. Change in immediate postflight orthostatically stressed heart rates from preflight mean reference values as a function of change in corresponding pre- and postflight total blood volumes (measured by radioisotope dilution methods). Both LBNP and passive 90° standing orthostatic stress techniques are included. The equation of the best-fit linear regression through all 33 data points is given, and the r value of −0.54 is statistically significant (p < 0.005).

countermeasure had a postflight syncopal episode not related to the stand test provocation.

BLOOD FLOW

Using an arm pressure cuff and a leg band plethysmograph, it was possible to obtain inflight measurements of calf blood flow on Skylab 4 (Thornton and Hoffler, 1977). Figure 10-17 shows measurements obtained from preflight, inflight, and postflight tests for each crewmember. Although there is great individual variability, it appears clear that leg blood flow significantly increased in flight. Measure-

ments rapidly reverted to preflight levels upon recovery. Transient increases in intrathoracic venous pressure, increased cardiac output, or reduced peripheral resistance may have accounted for the blood flow changes noted in flight.

VENOUS COMPLIANCE

Measures of venous compliance in the lower extremities were obtained in conjunction with measures of blood flow on Skylab 4. Figure 10-18 shows vascular compliance change (in volume percent) for tests conducted preflight, inflight, and postflight. Vascular compliance increased

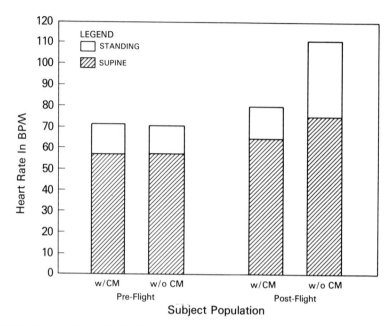

Figure 10-15. Pre- and post-flight heart rate in Shuttle crewmembers with and without saline loading countermeasures.

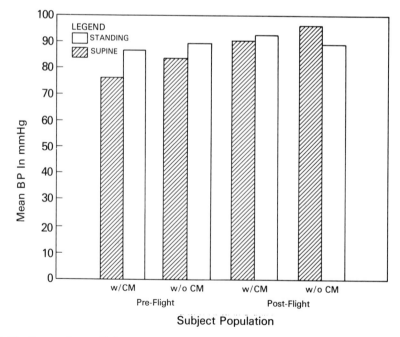

Figure 10-16. Pre- and post-flight mean blood pressure in Shuttle crewmembers with and without saline loading countermeasures.

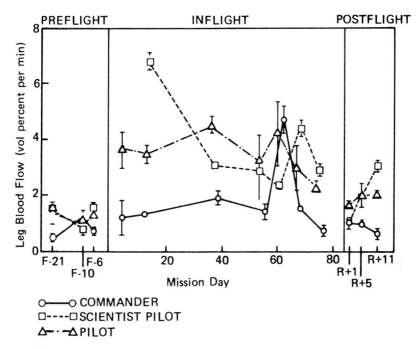

Figure 10-17. Skylab 4 crew leg blood flow measurements, −50 mmHg. (From Thornton and Hoffler, 1977).

in flight, and did not reach maximum values for at least 10 days. In the later weeks of the flight, compliance appeared to reverse this trend, and rapidly returned to preflight levels after recovery. Changes in venous compliance combined with cephalad fluid shifts and depleted blood volume appear to contribute to the stressful effects of inflight LBNP (Thornton and Hoffler, 1977).

CARDIAC DYNAMICS AND ELECTROMECHANICS

A variety of measures have been obtained to ascertain the effects of space flight on cardiac dynamics and electromechanics, including studies of cardiac size, systolic time intervals, echocardiography, rheography, and vectorcardiography.

CARDIAC SIZE

Standard posterior-anterior chest X-rays were taken before and after each U.S. space flight, and these films have provided a base for determining changes in cardiac silhouette size. Each of the nine Skylab crewmembers showed modest decreases in cardiothoracic (C/T) ratios (Nicogossian et al., 1976). Combining the data from 4 Mercury, 18 Gemini, 30 Apollo, and 9 Skylab crewmen, postflight decrements in C/T ratio averaged −.018.

SYSTOLIC TIME INTERVALS

To assess ventricular function pre- and postflight, systolic time intervals were obtained during rest and LBNP stress. Figure 10-19 shows the average ratios of pre-ejection period (PEP) over left ventricular

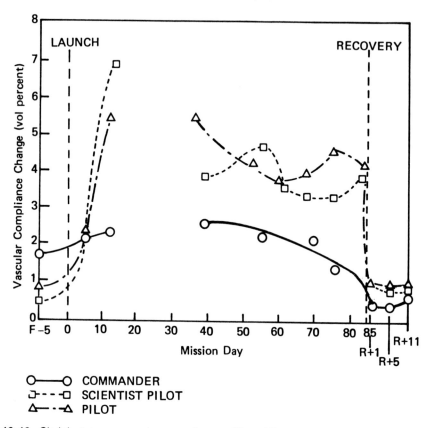

Figure 10-18. Skylab 4 crew vascular compliance. (From Thornton and Hoffler, 1977).

ejection time (ET) for the Skylab 4 crewmen. The postflight changes in PEP/ET ratio are probably due to markedly decreased ventricular filling and diminished total blood volume, although decreased contractility cannot be excluded (Bergman et al., 1977; Hoffler, 1977). Due to the multiplicity of explanations which can be invoked to interpret systolic time intervals, this technique has largely been discontinued.

ECHOCARDIOGRAPHY

Echocardiograms (ECGs) were obtained pre- and postflight for the Skylab 4 crewmen during rest and LBNP stress in order to further assess ventricular function.

These studies demonstrated postflight decreases in stroke volume, left ventricular end-diastolic volume, and estimated left ventricular mass. Ventricular function curves were constructed by plotting left ventricular end diastolic volume versus stroke volume. Pre- and postflight curves for the Commander are shown in Figure 10-20. Since the curves fall on a straight line, it appears that cardiac function and myocardial contractility did not deteriorate, despite decreases in cardiac size and stroke volume (Henry et al., 1977). Additional studies concluded in conjunction with the Salyut-6 missions tend to corroborate the above findings (Gazenko et al., 1981b). Pre- and postflight echocardiographic measurements were continued (Bungo et al., 1987) during U.S. Shuttle

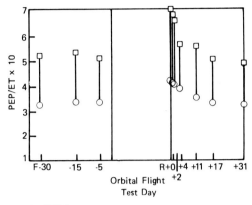

O REST

□ -50 mmHg
(LBNP)

Figure 10-19. Resting and LBNP-stressed, pre-ejection period / ejection time (PEP / ET): mean values for Skylab 4 crewmen. (From Bergman, Johnson, and Hoffler, 1977).

flights and obtained on one French cosmonaut during Salyut 6. Shuttle data presented in Figure 10-21 continue to show decreases of 16 percent in the left ventricular volume index immediately postflight, while systolic volume is changed little. The net result is a decrease in stroke volume, but when coupled with the increased heart rate, this results in no change in cardiac index (cardiac output normalized to body surface area).

Cardiac wall thickness is not changed and, as seen in Skylab, this implies an overall decrease of approximately 11 percent in left ventricular mass. The rapid recovery of this mass deficit (Figure 10-22) appears to lead to the hypothesis that it may be intracellular or interstitial myocardial hydration that is altered, yet the precise explanation is not known. Ground-based studies have shown changes in myocardial ultrastructure and biochemistry, but the applicability of this data to the clinical description in space medicine is not defined. This data was further enhanced by inflight echocardiographic data ob-

tained on four crewmembers during Shuttle flight 51-D. Measurements were made as early as 4 hours into the mission and compared with preflight values obtained in the resting supine left lateral decubitus position. Right ventricular dimension was decreased 30 percent throughout the duration of the 7-day mission and returned to preflight level immediately postflight (when an additional quart of saline was consumed as part of a countermeasure for orthostatic intolerance). Left ventricular diastolic volume index and stroke volume index were elevated on flight day 1 and then decreased to levels 15 percent below the preflight level. Heart rate (consistent with previous data) was elevated and mean blood pressure (both systolic and diastolic components) remained greater than preflight levels during the mission. Cardiac index was greatly accentuated during the first day of rapid fluid shifts and approached Earth level for the duration of the inflight study (Bungo et al., 1986). These data are graphically summarized in Figure 10-23. By a week postflight, nearly all Shuttle crewmembers showed return of preflight blood pressure values. However, as seen from both Fig-

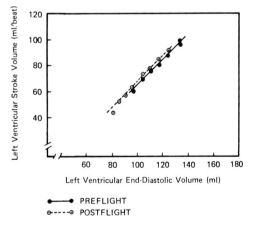

●——● PREFLIGHT
⊘----⊘ POSTFLIGHT

Figure 10-20. Ventricular function curve of Skylab 4 Commander. (From Henry et al., 1977).

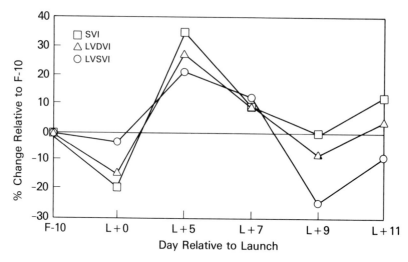

Figure 10-21. Preflight and postflight left ventricular volume indices in Space Shuttle crewmembers.

ures 10-21 and 10-22, most echocardiographically measured parameters went through a postflight oscillatory phase 5 days after return to Earth, before preflight values were once again recorded. This new description of postflight cardiovascular recovery does not immediately provoke a simple explanation. When these data were compared to inflight data obtained on Salyut 6 or on U.S. Shuttle mission 51-D, the postflight values are in excellent agreement. In contrast, values of left ventricular diastolic volume obtained during a bed rest simulation of Spacelab 1 (also Figure 10-24) show alterations "out-of-phase" with the flight data. Similar data were obtained

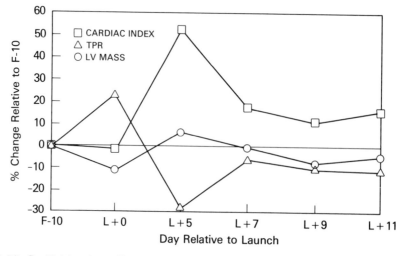

Figure 10-22. Preflight and postflight cardiac index, total peripheral resistance, and left ventricular mass in Space Shuttle crewmembers.

CARDIOVASCULAR EFFECTS OF SPACE FLIGHT

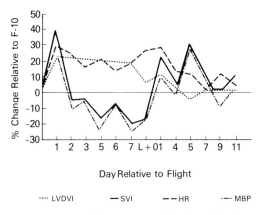

Figure 10-23. Time course of selected echocardiographic changes during and following (L+) space flight.

from the other echocardiographically measured volumes and calculated functional parameters.

RHEOGRAPHY

Soviet scientists use rheographic measurement of central and peripheral hemodynamic responses at rest to detail compensatory mechanisms in the adaptation to weightlessness. These data have consistently shown decreases in cardiac

stroke output, with a shorter isovolumetric contraction (Yegorov et al., 1981). In one study (Turchaninova and Domracheva, 1980), an initial increase in stroke volume was demonstrated, subsiding after the first week. Changes in all cardiovascular functions, as measured by this technique, are seen to vary phasically throughout a mission (Yegorov et al., 1981).

VECTORCARDIOGRAPHY

Table 10-1 presents a summary of the changes (as percent change from preflight resting values) in vectorcardiography determinations obtained from Skylab crewmen during rest and LBNP (Hoffler et al., 1977). One common observation was the increase in the QRS maximum vector in flight, a phenomenon that probably stems from the cephalad shift of fluid volume in weightlessness. The mechanism may be related to an augmented preload producing the Brody effect. Another observation was an inflight increase in the PR interval duration, a measure that provides an estimate of atrioventricular conduction time. This change may have been due to an increase in vagal tone (Hoffler et al., 1977; Smith et al., 1977).

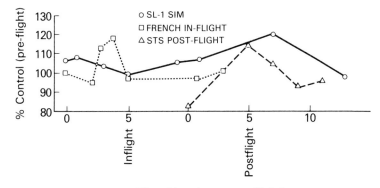

Time (days in- or post-flight)

Figure 10-24. Responses of left ventricular diastolic volume to simulated and actual weightlessness.

TABLE 10-1

PERCENT CHANGE AFTER DESIGNATED CONDITION FROM PREFLIGHT SUPINE RESTING REFERENCE VALUES

Vectorcardiogram Measurement	Condition = LBNP			Condition = Rest	
	Preflight	Inflight[a]	Postflight[a] R+O	Inflight	Postflight R+O
Heart rate (bpm)	+20[b]	+54	+57	+9	+2
PR interval (ms)	−11	−6	−5	+3[b]	+2
QRS duration (ms)	−6[b]	−6	−4	−3	+2
QT interval (ms)	−6[b]	−13	−14	−2	−1
QT_0 interval (ms)	+2[b]	+7	+7	+2[b]	+0
$P_{max}MAG$ (mV)	+27[b]	+78	+75	+24[b]	+16
$QRS_{max}MAG$ (mV)	−6[b]	+13	+12	+12[b]	+18[b]
PRS-E circ (mV)	+3	+24	+32	+19[b]	+21[b]
$ST_{max}MAG$ (mV)	−15[b]	−32	−37	−10	−6
J vector (mV)	+28[b]	+13	+26	+6	+18[b]
ST slope (mV/s)	−1	−21	−18	+5	−7
QRS-T angle (deg)	+61[b]	+13	+105	−17	+12

[a]Statistical tests were not performed.
[b]Statistically significant change from preflight reference values.
Adapted from Hoffler et al., 1977.

PULMONARY FUNCTION AND EXERCISE CAPACITY

Postflight pulmonary function tests have generally revealed no abnormalities. However, inflight decreases in vital capacity approaching 10 percent were observed in the Skylab 3 pilot and the entire Skylab 4 crew. Figure 10-25 shows the results of vital capacity tests for the three Skylab 4 crewmen. These inflight decreases may have been due to a combination of factors such as redistribution of body fluids into the thoracic cavity, cephalad shift of the diaphragm, or decrease in cabin ambient pressure to $\frac{1}{3}$ of sea-level pressure (Sawin et al., 1976).

Measures of postflight cardiopulmonary responses to exercise have consistently revealed decreases in exercise capacity. For example, measurements were obtained pre- and postflight on Apollo 7 through 11 (Rummel et al., 1973). These studies demonstrated significant decreases im-

mediately postflight in workload, oxygen consumption, systolic blood pressure, and diastolic blood pressure, at a heart rate of 160 beats/minute. Mechanical efficiency (oxygen required to perform a given amount of work) showed no gross changes postflight. Studies of Skylab crewmen revealed similar postflight decrements in exercise capacity, evidenced by decreases in oxygen uptake, pulse, cardiac output, and stroke volume (Michel et al., 1977). Most cardiovascular responses returned to normal within 3 weeks. Similar results were reported by Soviet investigators (Gazenko et al., 1981b; Gazenko, Kakurin, and Kuznetsov, 1976).

Studies on board both Skylab and Salyut-6, however, demonstrated that exercise capacity is not adversely affected in flight (Gazenko, Genin, and Yegorov, 1981a, 1981b; Michel et al., 1977). For example, Figure 10-26 shows Skylab preflight, inflight, and postflight heart rates during 75 percent maximum exercise. Most Skylab crewmen exhibited increased heart rates postflight relative to preflight baselines, but little changes in inflight heart rate during exercise. Similarly, Salyut cosmonauts have shown no change in inflight performance under physical load, as reflected in measures of oxygen efficacy. Crewmembers on the longer missions in both programs did not require more time for readaptation postflight. In Soviet missions lasting 96, 140, 175, and 185 days, readaptation time has not varied substantially. All cardiovascular parameters returned to normal in 18 to 21 days for the Skylab 2 crew (28-day mission), 5 days for the Skylab 3 crew (59-day mission), and 4 days for the Skylab 4 crew (84-day mission). Since the crew of Skylab 4 performed the most exercise in flight and the crew of Skylab 2 the least, it appears that the amount of exercise performed in flight is inversely related to the amount of time required for the cardiovascular system to readapt to the one-gravity environment. Of course, factors other than the amount of inflight exercise may have contributed to this apparent paradox concerning mission length and postflight recovery time. For example, high initial levels of conditioning may be a factor, especially if the vigorous inflight exercise required to maintain this level of conditioning is not performed. Loss of muscle mass might also contribute to this phenomenon, since significant losses and decreased strength will result in early fatigue and inability to complete the stress test protocols.

DYSRHYTHMIAS

Various levels of cardiac dysrhythmias have been seen throughout the U.S. space

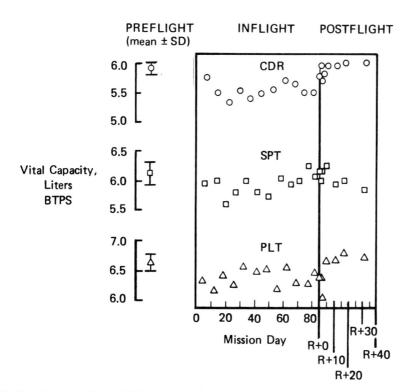

Figure 10-25. Vital capacities of Skylab 4 crewmen. (From Sawin et al., 1976).

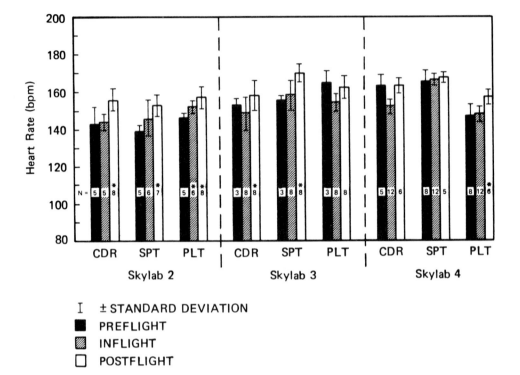

Figure 10-26. Heart rates pre-, in-, and postflight at 75 percent maximum exercise. (From Michel et al., 1977).

flight experience. During the Gemini and Apollo era, occasional premature ventricular contractions were seen and at least one episode of nonsustained atrial bigeminy was noted. At the time, these were attributed to possible hypokalemia, or considered to be within an acceptable "normal" range. During the Skylab series all crewmembers exhibited some form of rhythm disturbance. For the majority, these were rare PVCs; however, one crewmember exhibited a five-beat run of ventricular tachycardia during a lower body negative pressure testing protocol. A second crewmember had periods of wandering supraventricular pacemaker during rest and following exercise periods. Although attaching quantitative statistical significance to these findings becomes difficult,

it is clear that these levels of dysrhythmia were greater than any shown by these crewmen during their preflight ground testing over extended periods of time, and that they were also higher than would be expected in a "healthy" population studied at random in Air Force studies.

In the first Shuttle flights, the continued prevalence of dysrhythmias was again noted. During reentry, a Shuttle crewmember exhibited up to 16 PVCs per minute (Bungo et al., 1983), a tenfold increase over any previous data on this same individual. A subsequent crewmember also exhibited frequent PVCs during the reentry phase. Sustained ventricular bigeminy was noted on an additional crewmember in the course of extravehicular activity (EVA). During prior ground-based treadmill testing this individual exhibited frequent PVCs during the recovery phase of his exercise protocol. Another crewmember who showed no prior evidence of any dysrhythmias demonstrated sustained atrial quadrageminy during EVA.

The degree to which space flight and its many variables can be considered arrhythmogenic is not clear. Certainly it appears that more than casual attention should be given to this area, since many conditions such as gravitational stress, thermal load, electrolyte changes, and catecholamine alterations have been shown to play important roles in the Earth environment.

SUMMARY

In spite of over 25 years experience in manned space flight, our knowledge of physiologic alterations in microgravity is far from complete. To a great extent, this is due to the limited opportunities for medical experimentation on actual missions. Instead, data has been inferred from ground-based analogs such as bed rest and animal experiments. There is now some serious question as to the validity of these inferences.

From knowledge gained thus far, it can be stated that the cardiovascular system undergoes an acclimation to the microgravity environment, consisting of a fairly rapid redistribution of fluids followed by a "resetting" of several controlling mechanisms. The significance and time course of these alterations have been appreciated in the postflight period, where crewmembers required several weeks before cardiovascular performance indices returned to preflight levels. Since the cardiovascular system is more easily probed for "numerical" data than some of the other body systems, the first attempts to develop a countermeasure to cardiovascular deconditioning have also been tested.

With the Space Shuttle and the planned Space Station Freedom, humans will spend increasingly longer times in space. Answers to these pressing physiological clinical questions will evolve in accordance with opportunities to conduct meaningful, controlled studies in space and enhance the development of effective countermeasures.

REFERENCES

Bergman, S.A., Johnson, R.L., and Hoffler, G.W. Evaluation of the electromechanical properties of the cardiovascular system after prolonged weightlessness. In: Biomedical results from Skylab (NASA SP-377). Edited by R.S. Johnston and L.F. Dietlein. U.S. Government Printing Office, Washington, D.C., 1977.

Berry, C.A., and Catterson, A.D. Pre-Gemini medical predictions vs. Gemini flight results. In Gemini Summary Conference, February 1 and 2, 1967, Manned Spacecraft Center, Houston, Texas (NASA SP-138). Washington, D.C.: U.S. Government Printing Office, Washington, D.C. 1967.

Blomqvist, C.G., Stone, H.L. Cardiovascular Adjustments to Gravitational Stress. In: Handbook of Physiology; section 2 (the Cardiovascular System), Vol. III. Edited by J.T. Shepard and F.M. Abboud, Bethesda, Maryland, American Physiological Society, pp. 1025–1063, 1983.

Bungo, M.W., Johnson, P.C., Jr. Cardiovascular Examinations and Observations of Deconditioning During the Space Shuttle Orbital Flight Test Program. Aviation, Space, and Environmental Medicine. 54 (11):1001–1004, 1983.

Bungo, M.W., Charles, J.B., and Johnson, P.C., Jr. Cardiovascular deconditioning during space flight and the use of saline as a countermeasure to orthostatic intolerance. Aviation, Space, and Environmental Medicine. 56:985–990, 1985.

Bungo, M.W., Goldwater, D.J., Popp, R.L., Sandler, H. Echocardiographic evaluation of Space Shuttle crewmembers. J. Applied Physiol., 62:278–283, 1987.

Bungo, M.W., Charles, J.B., Riddle, J., Roesch, J., Wolf, D.A., Seddon, M.R. Echocardiographic investigation of the hemodynamics of weightlessness. Journal of the American College of Cardiology, Vol. 7, #2 192A:February 1986.

Burkovskaya, T.Ye., Ilyukhin, A.V., Lobachik, V.I., and Zhidkov, V.V. Erythrocyte balance during 182-day hypokinesia. From JPRS, U.S.S.R. Report: Space Biology and Aerospace Medicine, 14(5):75–80, 30 October 1980.

Gazenko, O.G., Kakurin, L.I., and Kuznetsov, A.G. (Eds.). Space flights onboard the spacecraft Soyuz. Moscow, Nauka, 1976.

Gazenko, O.G., Genin, A.M., and Yegorov, A.D. Major medical results of the Salyut-6/Soyuz 185-day space flight. NASA NDB 2747. Proceedings of the XXXII Congress of the International Astronautical Federation, Rome, Italy, 6–12 September, 1981a.

Gazenko, O.G., Genin, A.M., and Yegorov, A.D. Summary of medical investigations in the U.S.S.R. manned space missions. Acta Astronautica, 8(9–10):907–917, 1981b.

Golubchikova, Z.A., Yegorov, A.D., and Kalinichenko, V.V. Results of vectorcardiographic examinations during and after long-term space flights aboard the Salyut-6/Soyuz orbital complex. Space Biology and Aerospace Medicine, 15(1):31–35, 5 March 1981.

Henry, W.L., Epstein, S.E., Griffith, J.M., Goldstein, R.E., and Redwood, D.R. Effect of prolonged space flight on cardiac function and dimensions. In: Biomedical results from Skylab (NASA SP-377). Edited by R.S. Johnston and L.F. Dietlein, U.S. Government Printing Office, Washington, D.C., 1977.

Hoffler, G.W. Cardiovascular studies of U.S. space crews: An overview and perspective. In: Cardiovascular flow dynamics and measurements. Edited by N.H.C. Hwang and N.A. Normann, Baltimore, MD, University Park Press, 1977.

Hoffler, G.W., Bergman, S.A., and Nicogossian, A.E. Inflight lower limb volume measurement. In: The Apollo-Soyuz Test Project medical report (NASA SP-411). Edited by A.E. Nicogossian, U.S. Government Printing Office, Washington, D.C., 1977.

Hoffler, G.W., and Johnson, R.L. Apollo flight crew cardiovascular evaluations. In: Biomedical results of Apollo (NASA SP-368). Edited by R.S. Johnston, L.F. Dietlein, and C.A. Berry, U.S. Government Printing Office, Washington, D.C., 1975.

Hoffler, G.W., Johnson, R.L., Nicogossian, A.E., Bergman, S.A., and Jackson, M.M. Vectorcardiographic results from Skylab medical experiment M092: Lower body negative pressure. In: Biomedical results from Skylab (NASA SP-377). Edited by R.S. Johnston and L.F. Dietlein, U.S. Government Printing Office, Washington, D.C., 1977.

Johnson, P.C., Jr. Fluid Volume Changes Induced by Space Flight. Acta Astronautica, 6:1335–1341, 1979.

Johnson, R.L., Hoffler, G.W., Nicogossian, A.E., Bergman, S.A., and Jackson, M.M. Lower body negative pressure: Third manned Skylab mission. In: Biomedical results from Skylab (NASA SP-377). Edited by R.S. Johnston and L.F. Dietlein, U.S. Government Printing Office, Washington, D.C., 1977.

Katkov, V.Ye., Chestukhin, V.V., Rumyantsev, V.V., Troshin, A.Z., and Zybin, O.Kh. Jugular, right atrial pressure and cerebral hemodynamics of healthy man submitted to postural tests. Space Biology and Aerospace Medicine, 15(5):68–73, 1981.

Michel, E.L., Rummel, J.A., Sawin, C.F., Buderer, M.C., and Lem, J.D. Results of Skylab medical experiment M171—metabolic activity. In: Biomedical results from Skylab (NASA SP-377). Edited by R.S. Johnston and L.F. Dietlein, U.S. Government Printing Office, Washington, D.C., 1977.

Nicogossian, A., Hoffler, G.W., Johnson, R.L., and Gowen, R.J. Determination of cardiac size following space missions of different durations: The second manned Skylab mission. Aviation, Space, and Environmental Medicine, 47(4):362–365, 1976.

Nicogossian, A.E., Whyte, A.A., Sandler, H., Leach, C.S., and Rambaut, P.C. (Eds.). Chronological summaries of United States, European, and Soviet bed rest studies. NASA, Washington, D.C., 1979.

Rummel, J.A., Michel, E.L., and Berry, C.A. Physiological responses to exercise after space flight—Apollo 7 to Apollo 11. Aerospace Medicine, 44:235–238, 1973.

Sandler, H. Cardiovascular effects of weightlessness. In: Progress in cardiology, Volume 6. Edited by P.M. Yu and J.F. Goodwin, Philadelphia, Lea and Febiger, 1977.

Sawin, C.F., Nicogossian, A.E., Rummel, J.A., and Michel, E.L. Pulmonary function evaluation during the Skylab and Apollo-Soyuz missions. Aviation, Space, and Environmental Medicine, 47(2):168–172, 1976.

Smith, R.F., Stanton, K., Stoop, D., Brown, D., Janusz, W., and King, P. Vectorcardiographic changes during extended space flight (M093): Observations at rest and during exercise. In: Biomedical results from Skylab (NASA SP-377). Edited by R.S. Johnston and L.F. Dietlein, U.S. Government Printing Office, Washington, D.C., 1977.

Thornton, W.E., and Hoffler, G.W. Hemodynamic studies of the legs under weightlessness. In: Biomedical results from Skylab (NASA SP-377). Edited by R.S. Johnston and L.F. Dietlein, U.S. Government Printing Office, Washington, D.C., 1977.

Thornton, W.E., Hoffler, G.W., and Rummel, J.A. Anthropometric changes and fluid shifts. In: Biomedical results from Skylab (NASA SP-377). Edited by R.S. Johnston and L.F. Dietlein, U.S. Government Printing Office, Washington, D.C., 1977.

Turchaninova, V.F., and Domracheva, M.V. Results of studies of pulsed blood flow and regional vas-cular tonus during flight in the first and second expeditions aboard the Salyut-6/Soyuz orbital complex. Space Biology and Aerospace Medicine, 14(3):11–14, 1980.

Wolthius, R.A., Bergman, S.A., and Nicogossian, A.E. Physiological effects of locally applied reduced pressure in man. Physiological Reviews, 54(3):566–595, 1974.

Yegorov, A.D., Itsekhovskiy, O.G., Kas'yan, I.I., Alferova, I.V., Polyakova, A.P., Turchaninova, V.F., Bernadskiy, V.I., Dororshev, V.G., and Kobzev, Ye.A. Study of hemodynamics and phase structure of cardiac cycle in second crew of the Salyut-6 orbital station at rest. Space Biology and Aerospace Medicine, 14(6):11–15, 1981.

11 Nutrition

PAUL C. RAMBAUT
PHILIP C. JOHNSON

In the last quarter century, man has extended his stay-time in space from a brief suborbital flight of 15 minutes to an orbital residence of almost 8 months. Complex spacecraft now routinely transport humans into an environment more forbidding than any previously encountered. These spacecraft must, to the greatest extent possible, simulate many essential characteristics of the home planet. Temperatures must be maintained, radiation shielded, wastes removed, and, especially important, water and food provided. This chapter briefly reviews the development of space food systems, and the nutritional and metabolic knowledge derived from experience using these systems.

SPACECRAFT FOOD SYSTEMS

From the beginning, the objective of a spacecraft food-supply system has been to provide nutritious food products in a form that allows easy manipulation in weightlessness and requires minimum time and effort for preparation and clean up. The shelf life of a space food must be considerably longer than the maximum flight length. Space foods must be processed well in advance of a mission in order to allow time for testing and packaging before shipment to the launch site, where they are usually stowed on board the spacecraft for an extended period.

MERCURY

Early researchers were concerned about the astronaut's ability to swallow in microgravity. Accordingly, foods for Mercury flights were formulated so that they would be easy to swallow and digest. Delivered via tubes inserted through the faceplate of the helmet, such foods included pureed meats, vegetables, and fruit packages in collapsible containers. There were also bite-sized, 1.9-centimeter cubes coated with an edible fat and, in the 34-hour Mercury 9 mission, freeze-dehydrated foods (Huber et al., 1972). The purpose of coating the cubes was to reduce crumbs and greasiness. Since these coatings were designed to be stable for 3 hours at 43°C, the cubes were unpalatable and poorly digested. When this temperature limitation was later lowered to 27°C the food tended to melt.

Mercury astronaut John Glenn was the first American to dine in orbit. He consumed 80 kcal of applesauce, 130 kcal of beef and gravy, and 60 kcal of beef and vegetables.

GEMINI

The volume and weight of the food used on Gemini were 2130 cubic centimeters and 726 grams per person per day, respectively. Approximately 2800 kcal was provided, consisting of 16 percent protein, 31 percent fat, and 53 percent carbohydrate. Three types of foods were used: bite-sized cubes of meat, fruit, dessert, and bread with a uniform caloric density of 5 kcal per gram; intermediate moisture foods; and rehydratable fruits, salads, meats, soups, desserts, and beverages. Dehydrated foods were used primarily for reducing weight and extending shelf life. The slow process of rehydration of foods on Gemini detracted from their acceptability.

On the 4-day Gemini 4 mission, crewmembers were furnished 2500 kcal in four meals. The crew consumed all the food available. On Gemini 5 (8 days), the crew was furnished three meals per day and 2750 kcal. Average daily intake varied around 1000 kcal. About 2450 kcal per day were furnished for the 14-day mission and the crew consumed about 2200 kcal per day (Huber et al., 1972).

APOLLO

Initially, the Apollo food system was comprised primarily of the same types of food used on Gemini (Huber et al., 1972): bite-sized cubes and rehydratables. As in Gem-

ini, crewmembers ate with their fingers or through a tube built into the package. Nonflammable, fluorohydrocarbon overwraps were provided to reduce the flammability hazard inside the spacecraft. Greater variety was available and hot water at 65°C was provided in the Command Module, but not in the Lunar Module.

On later Apollo flights, thermostabilized foods in flexible foil-laminated pouches were introduced. Thermostabilized foods contained a normal amount of moisture and thus did not have to be rehydrated. In general, crews preferred these foods to dehydrated or rehydratable.

Irradiation, as a method of food preservation, was used for the first time on Apollo. Bread made from irradiated flour had a minimum shelf life of 4 weeks and was used to make sandwiches throughout the multi-day missions.

Astronauts working in space suits on the lunar surface were supplied with a fruit bar, as well as water and fruit-flavored beverages.

SKYLAB

As a result of metabolic balance studies, nutrient composition of food consumed by Skylab crews was closely regulated (Huber et al., 1972). As in previous missions dehydrated, thermostabilized, and irradiated foods were included in the Skylab food system: 49 percent were rehydratable, 24 percent thermostabilized, 15 percent natural-form or ready-to-eat, 11 percent frozen, and 1 percent irradiated. In addition, some foods were precooked and frozen. Items were packed individually in aluminum cans. A plastic membrane under the lid served to keep most thermostabilized and frozen foods in the can when the lid was opened in the weightless environment. Rehydratable foods were packaged in a flexible container enclosed within an aluminum can. Beverages were packaged in a bellows-like polyethylene container with a nylon valve at the neck of the bellows.

Individual food cans were sealed in aluminum canisters at an internal pressure of 5 psi. These overcans protected individual food items during launch. Facilities were provided to rehydrate food and heat certain items. Complaints of blandness spurred the provision of extra condiments for the last two missions.

Skylab astronauts were subjected to strict dietary controls beginning 21 days preflight and continuing for 18 days after landing. Intakes of sodium, potassium, phosphorus, calcium, nitrogen, and magnesium were controlled to within 2 percent. The daily nutrient content was 90–125 g protein, 750–850 mg calcium, 1500–1700 mg phosphorus, 36 g sodium, 300–400 mg magnesium, and 3945 mg potassium. Crewmembers were able to gain additional calories through snacks which were low in the prescribed nutrients.

The crew reported any food not eaten. Ground personnel calculated the amount of the controlled nutrients that were not consumed, and mineral supplements were prescribed to make up for any deficits. Water intake was also recorded to an accuracy of 1 percent. A vitamin pill was also taken daily during each of the three Skylab missions.

SPACE SHUTTLE

Foods used on the Space Shuttle include thermostabilized, rehydratable, irradiated, natural-form, and intermediate moisture. From a weight standpoint, it continues to be advantageous to store foods in dry form at launch and utilize the water produced in flight by the fuel cells for rehydration. A completely hydrated 3000 kcal food system weighs almost 6.5 lbs. before pack-

aging; dehydrated it weighs less than 3 lbs. (Stadler et al., 1982)

On some missions a galley is installed in the middeck of the Shuttle. This galley features dispensers for hot and cold water, serving trays, personal hygiene facilities, storage compartments, and a forced-air convection oven for warming food.

During Shuttle flights, preassembled standard menus provide three meals and 3000 kcal/person/day. Nutritional requirements for Shuttle crewmembers are essentially those designated in the Recommended Dietary Allowances published by the Food and Nutrition Board of the National Academy of Sciences. No allowances are made for any special influences of weightlessness.

Unlike those used in previous programs, foods on the Shuttle consist mainly of commercially available food, packaged in metal cans which have been flushed with nitrogen. The package used for rehydratable foods with beverages consists of a molded, high-density polyethylene base covered with a thermoformed laminated film lid which has been heat-sealed to the base. The package has a needle septum for adding water. Other packages include flexible aluminum pouches, cans for thermostabilized foods, and plastic pouches for such natural-form foods as nuts and cookies.

No direct measurements or estimates of an individual's consumption of food and water are available, since these quantities are not recorded, and any crewmember can eat any food item desired.

U.S.S.R. SPACECRAFT

On the first manned orbital flight, which lasted only 108 minutes, cosmonaut Yuri Gagarin became the first person to eat and drink in weightlessness.

Diets on the first two Soviet space flights consisted of pureed and liquid foods. From the third flight on, semi-solid and perishable foods were added to the menu. A diet of 2500 kcal was used on the Voskhod flights, with over 150 g of protein and over 400 g of carbohydrate, and a total caloric value of 3600 kcal. Weight loss was a universal finding and was believed to be a result of dehydration, since water loading experiments conducted postflight showed temporal delays in excretion of ingested water.

Soyuz missions featured a diet of 2800 kcal, with about 140 g of protein and 345 g of carbohydrates. A four-meal-per-day schedule was used. Salyut 6 space station crews remained on orbit for up to 185 days, and crewmembers generally consumed about 3000 kcal per day of the 3150 offered. When visiting crews were on board, food intake tended to increase. The 185-day crew requested and were given fresh apples, cucumbers, tomatoes, lemons, onions, and garlic, delivered by the Progress supply ships and the Soyuz spacecraft carrying the visiting crews. Since water was regenerated, dehydrated foods were particularly advantageous.

U.S. SPACE STATION

The next 10 years of the U.S. space program are expected to include the development and launch of a Space Station that will operate permanently in low Earth orbit. The Space Station will undoubtedly employ life-support systems that minimize usage of consumables. The first step in this direction will be the development of relatively simple physicochemical approaches to onboard water purification and air regeneration. However, cost factors and the prospect of permanent station operations will provide incentives to investigate and adopt increasingly sophisticated life support approaches.

PHYSIOLOGICAL CONSIDERATIONS

SWALLOWING AND DIGESTION

Initially, there was concern for the mechanics of eating and eliminating in weightless flight. The space flight experiences of American and Soviet pilots in the early 1960s largely dispelled these fears. Observations on these early missions validated previous findings on aircraft flying parabolic maneuvers that the physiological mechanisms of food ingestion were not sensitive to gravity. Although the absence of gravity restricted food selection and constrained package design, once food was in the mouth the subsequent steps of swallowing, digestion, and elimination appeared to proceed normally (Nanz et al., 1977; Rambaut et al., 1977).

TASTE AND AROMA

Anecdotal reports of changes in the response to taste or aroma during weightless flight have been provided by both American and Soviet crews. Indeed, diminished sensitivity to odors might be expected to result from the passive nasal congestion which has been frequently reported. Another possible factor which might be hypothesized to cause taste shifts in weightlessness is reduced stimulation of taste buds as a result of changes in convective activity in zero gravity.

REQUIREMENT FOR ENERGY

Determination of human energy requirements in zero gravity is crucial to the design of life-support systems and the overall assessment of a person's ability to live and work productively in weightlessness. The need for relatively nonspecific sources of energy determines the weight and volume of the food supply and sets the requirement for oxygen.

It might seem logical to assume that activity in a weightless environment would require less energy than in one gravity, since work associated with counteracting the force of gravity is eliminated. However, while locomotion in reduced gravity demands less energy than in one gravity, those tasks which ordinarily depend on friction for the reactive force require muscular work to supply that force. In addition, it can be argued that very little of man's basal energy expenditure is attributable to direct gravity effects.

Prior to Skylab, several investigators observed that the energetic cost of life in space is much higher than indicated by the actual total energy content of the food consumed (Johnson et al., 1973; Vanderveen and Allen, 1972). Data acquired during the Skylab missions revealed that the overall energy consumption in flight was not statistically different from that observed on the ground. However, as might be expected, the secondary effects of weightlessness grew progressively more pronounced as time in flight increased (Rambaut et al., 1977). Such secondary effects may include reduction in body mass, muscle atrophy from disuse, changes in tissue hydration, and altered endocrinological status.

All crewmembers lost weight during the first month of the Skylab mission. During the second month and continuing into the third, this trend slowed and then reversed. Protein was lost continuously in the first month only. Fat, equivalent to the difference between total body mass and mass of protein and water, was lost during each month. A similar trend was noted for body water, which was estimated by balance procedures and isotopic dilution.

Average daily net energy input for each period was computed by dividing daily net energy input for each crewmember by estimated quantity of potassium his body contained on the last day of each period. This type of analysis revealed that the mean value during the first inflight period was significantly lower than the mean value obtained preflight, whereas during the second period the mean value was significantly higher. This trend appeared to continue into the third inflight period as well.

The energy utilization rate of Skylab crewmembers at the beginning of their 3-month flight was 43.7 kcal/kg per day. This increased approximately 1.6 percent per month. The average increase in "normalized" rate was about 3.7 percent per month.

The gradual elevation in energy input in flight is presumptive evidence of either increasing energy output or decreasing metabolic efficiency. Quantitative measurements of energy output were not made on a continuous basis during Skylab. However, while performing a standardized level of work on a bicycle ergometer, the ratio of carbon dioxide produced to oxygen consumed did increase by an average of about 3 percent in flight (Michel et al., 1974). This finding is probably attributable to an increase in carbohydrate intake of about 14 percent and an inflight decrease in fat intake of about 21 percent compared to preflight. The apparent increases in thyroxine following recovery from Apollo and Skylab missions lend some support to the concept that metabolic efficiency may have diminished in flight (Sheinfeld et al., 1974). This is perhaps attributable to the proportionately greater work demanded of a diminishing muscle mass. Supporting evidence for decreasing metabolic activity was also obtained on some of the Soviet Cosmos Biosatellite flights, where it was found that the rate at which young rats gained weight in flight was less per gram of food intake than for control rats on the ground.

In the case of the Skylab astronauts, it was apparent that much of the additional energy used in flight was derived from catabolism of the body's endogenous fat. Although this estimate of the change in body fat was obtained indirectly, supporting evidence was provided through various indirect, though nonquantitative, estimates of body fat. Density, for instance, generally increased during the course of the flight, indicating a loss of adipose tissue. Analysis of various cross sections of the body, measured by stereophotogrammetry, showed marked losses in the volume of the abdomen, buttocks, and calves. In the 84-day flight, the thickness of folds of skin at six points on the body surface was measured by the same observer. The crew, as a whole, lost about 10 percent of the skin-fold thickness over the triceps (Whittle et al., 1974).

REQUIREMENT FOR FAT

In conventional diets, calories are derived from a mixture of protein, fat, and carbohydrate. As long as conventional foods are carried into space, it is unlikely that one or another of these energy sources will be excluded. If, on the other hand, food is one day regenerated wholly or in part, the regenerable products could result in extreme departures from the normal mixture. In the future there will be some concern for minimum and maximum limits for fat. The minimum need can probably be met by a diet in which 1 percent of total calories is provided by linoleic acid. As for the maximum limit, people often complain when fat intake exceeds about 150 g per day, although tolerance varies widely and those who are able to tolerate the initial discomfort often adjust to the diet.

REQUIREMENT FOR CARBOHYDRATE

The maximum tolerance for carbohydrate is unknown, but varies both for individuals and specific carbohydrates. Blood levels of lipids become undesirably high only when carbohydrate exceeds 85–90 percent of total calories. Dietary carbohydrates of differing chemical structure are known to differentially influence work output in human subjects and to affect the central nervous system. It would be advantageous to utilize the most appropriate types of carbohydrates in the design of space food systems.

REQUIREMENT FOR PROTEIN

During the Gemini and Apollo Programs, diets were formulated to provide 16–17 percent of total calories from protein. Because food diaries were kept throughout the Apollo missions, it is possible to estimate the protein intake of the crews even though the amount of food consumed was left to the discretion of the individual crewmember. During Apollo, daily intake of protein varied from 52 g/day to 126 g/day. The mean daily intake was 76 g. More precise records were kept for experimental purposes on Skylab, and protein intake was maintained between 90 and 125 g/day.

In Space Shuttle missions, crews are provided at least the recommended dietary allowance of high quality protein. Protein intake during the first few Shuttle missions was estimated at between 66 and 107 g/day. The higher values resulted from substitutions by crewmembers in their individual menus.

It is debatable whether additional protein would be beneficial. Such an increase would not likely offset protein loss due to muscle atrophy, and would result in additional water loss and reduced organic products in the urine. Unless new information is forthcoming, the dietary protein offered Space Station crews will be very similar to that used on the Shuttle.

A metabolic balance study undertaken in conjunction with the 14-day flight of Gemini 7 showed decreased nitrogen retention (Lutwak et al., 1969). During the flight of Apollo 16, urine nitrogen was observed to be elevated (Johnson et al., 1974), and similar elevations were noted during the balance study conducted on Apollo 17 (Rambaut et al., 1975). Carefully planned and implemented inflight dietary controls and metabolic collections during the 28-, 59-, and 84-day Skylab flights confirmed and extended these findings. Increased excretion of nitrogen and phosphorus in flight indicated appreciable loss of muscle tissue in all three crewmembers. It is likely that the losses in nitrogen and phosphorus primarily reflect muscle atrophy in weightlessness rather than loss of bone. Calcium loss was closely correlated with flight duration, while losses of nitrogen and phosphorus are closely correlated with each other.

In contrast to the continuous inflight loss of calcium, nitrogen appeared to reach a plateau. Sustained increases in plasma cortisol and the rate of excretion of hydroxyproline and hydroxylysine were also observed.

Loss of muscle mass was evidenced by changes in limb girth and muscle strength, although these changes tended to abate with progressively longer missions. The latter tendency and the nitrogen balance data are consistent with the progressive increase in level of exercise over the 28-, 59-, and 84-day flights.

Following flight of any duration, crewmembers tend to be unable to perform programmed postflight exercise with the same physiological effectiveness as they did before and during flight. The most significant changes are elevated heart rates and elevated oxygen consumption. These effects become reversible in 24 to 36 hours.

REQUIREMENT FOR MACROMINERALS

The metabolic balance study undertaken in conjunction with the 14-day flight of Gemini 7 showed decreased retention of calcium and phosphorus, in addition to an absolute loss in bone mass measured by X-ray densitometry (Lutwak et al., 1969). During the balance study conducted on Apollo 17, the disproportionate increase in fecal calcium indicated the possibility of calcium malabsorption developing in flight (Rambaut et al., 1975).

Whedon et al. reported a gradual increase in urinary calcium during the 28-day Skylab 2 flight (Whedon et al., 1975). Urinary calcium excretion in the latter part of the flight was double preflight levels. Fecal calcium excretion did not change significantly, but calcium balance, owing to the urinary calcium rise, became either negative or less positive than in preflight measurements.

In the 59-day Skylab flight, urinary calcium rose significantly in flight with considerable variations among individuals (Whedon et al., 1976). Urinary calcium increased by about 50 percent in two crewmembers, more than doubled in the third, and remained elevated for all three crewmembers throughout flight. It did not decline until the recovery phase began.

Examination of the data obtained from all nine Skylab crewmembers revealed that calcium was lost exponentially as a function of time in flight: an average of 50 mg per day was lost on the 10th day, while an average of 300 mg was lost on the 84th day. The cumulative loss reveals that an average of 25 g of calcium was lost from the body during the 84-day flight. Assuming a total body calcium content of about 1 kg, it is evident that the pool was diminished by approximately 2.5 percent.

When fecal and urinary losses of calcium are plotted independently (see Chapter 12, Figure 12-2), two kinetically different trends are discernible. Urinary calcium rises rapidly following launch and within 30 days reaches a level approximately 100 percent above baseline, which is maintained for the remainder of the flight. Fecal calcium, on the other hand, does not begin to rise for 2 to 3 weeks following launch, at which time it rises at a constant rate for the remainder of the flight.

Apparently, two processes are occurring simultaneously. Calcium is mobilized from the bones, effecting a sustained rise in the serum calcium concentration. This is accompanied at first by slight elevations and thereafter by sustained depressions in serum parathyroid hormone and calcitonin (Grigoriev et al., 1985). At approximately the same time that bone mineral is mobilizing, increasingly less calcium is being absorbed from the gastrointestinal tract. Although normally sufficient quantities of vitamin D_2 are ingested, it is likely that a deficiency is developed in the conversion of vitamin D_2 to the 1,2, dihydroxycholecalciferol required to effect the absorption of the approximately 800 mg of dietary calcium present in the daily ration (Rambaut et al., 1977).

During the postflight portion of the Skylab flights, fecal calcium tended to decrease. The change was moderate, but fecal calcium remained elevated throughout the postflight periods. Serum and urine calcium fell rapidly during this period, and calcaneus mineral increased.

Skylab observations support the contention that long-term bed rest and space flight have similar consequences for the musculoskeletal system. For periods up to 9 months, bed-rested subjects have demonstrated unrelenting losses in calcium and nitrogen. Several ways of ameliorating the losses have been investigated in bed rest studies. Protocols involving exercise, compression suits, lower body negative pressure, and thyrocalcitonin administration have had little effect in moderating the losses.

Changes in dietary intake, particularly reductions in protein and elevated intakes of disphosphonates, calcium, and phosphorus have had slight remedial efficacy and point the way to the manipulation of nutritional intake as an important therapeutic tool in counteracting adverse effects of prolonged weightlessness (Rambaut et al., 1977).

The increased excretion of calcium derived from bone probably cannot be ameliorated by simply administering vitamin D. However, adequate amounts of this vitamin must be present to maintain inflow of calcium through the gastrointestinal tract. It is of interest to note that the current Soviet space station, Mir, is equipped with portholes transparent to ultraviolet light. When ultraviolet rays strike the skin's surface, they transform provitamin D, secreted by the skin, into vitamin D, which is then absorbed into the body.

It is clear that anyone exposed to microgravity for a period of time will lose mineral salt from bones involved in posture and locomotion. This salt is excreted in the urine, increasing the risk for renal stone formation. Pain attendant on the passage of a renal stone is of great clinical concern. No U.S. crewmember has developed symptoms of renal stone formation while in space. This is probably attributable both to the rather stringent medical selection criteria and the relative brevity of missions to date. Consequently, hypercalciuria has not yet peaked, and with the decreased dietary intake that results from space adaptation syndrome, there is a below-normal gastrointestinal calcium load.

Selection procedures eliminate candidates who have ever had a renal stone or are suspected of having a genetic abnormality or tendency to form stones. Thus, cystine-containing stones would not be expected, although uric acid-containing stones might occur as a result of muscle atrophy and red blood cell loss. Urate excretion was not statistically decreased in the Skylab studies. There are no available data on urine pH, although increased aldosterone excretion would be associated with systemic alkalosis. Urinary osmolality increased, suggesting a more concentrated urine. Increases in urine sodium and chloride partially explain the increase in osmolality.

REQUIREMENT FOR ELECTROLYTES

In the day following recovery from the 84-day Skylab flight, crewmembers showed a deficit of nearly 1 liter of body fluid in the lower limbs, which decreased to about 600 ml the following day, and further diminished to about 300 ml 3 days later. Both calf and thigh volume had returned to preflight values when measurements were made 30 days following recovery. It is clear from this that fluid loss represents at least part of the deficient volume. Some fluid volume is replaced after a day or two of recovery, but the remainder probably reflects atrophic changes.

Very low urine sodium and potassium concentrations have been observed consistently after space missions, signifying probable depletion of these electrolytes inflight. Blood potassium is slightly decreased postflight and, following the Skylab missions, decreases in total body potassium were observed, measured by changes in the abundance of potassium-40 or in the dilutional concentration of potassium-42.

Two crewmembers exhibited signs of cardiac arrhythmia during the Apollo 15 mission, and deteriorations in exercise and cardiovascular performance postflight. Added to these observations, a marginal dietary intake of potassium raised the possibility that significant quantities of potassium had been lost from the body.

In the final two Apollo flights, the diet was supplemented with potassium to a level of at least 100 mEq per day, and measures were adopted to ensure adequate intake of this electrolyte. Nevertheless, losses in total body potassium continued, although other signs attributable to potassium deficiency did not recur. The etiology of the difficulties experienced in Apollo 15 remains obscure, although it is speculated that severe fatigue following rigorous lunar surface activities was involved.

Skylab potassium balances became slightly less positive in flight, in line with other measurements suggesting potassium loss from the body. There was also a significant retention of the element in the recovery phase. Plasma potassium tended to increase in flight and remain high in the sample obtained immediately after recovery. A net loss in potassium was evidenced by a decrease in total body exchangeable potassium of about 6.3 percent for all crewmembers. There was also a modest negative shift for sodium during flight. Sharp sodium retention occurred in all crewmembers during the first few days following recovery on each flight (Leach and Rambaut, 1974).

As noted earlier, moderate dehydration was noted in all Apollo missions following recovery. In Skylab, water loss was evidenced by rapid weight loss in the first few days of flight and a reciprocal gain following recovery. Dehydration was of particular concern in Apollo because of food deprivation. Unlike Apollo, dehydration in Skylab was probably not due to decreased nutrient intake, but to changes in water balance presumed to accompany shifts in body fluid toward the thorax, thereby triggering the Gauer-Henry reflex. Actual water balance measurements substantiated the water loss in the early days of each Skylab mission, but revealed that it was the immediate consequence of decreased water intake rather than increased excretion.

GENERAL NUTRITIONAL CONSIDERATIONS

Although the diets used in space have always been nutritionally adequate by conventional criteria, marginal deficiency must still be suspected as a result either of inadequate intake or the extra demands exerted by space flight conditions for certain nutrients. As previously indicated, reduced appetites among crewmembers may have resulted in less than adequate consumption of a number of nutrients. One possible result of such a marginal deficiency (namely in the cases of Gemini 7, Apollo 16 and 17, and the three Skylab missions) is that no effort has been made to quantitate food consumption or acquire precise analytical information on the foods employed. Therefore, it is not possible to accurately estimate nutrient consumption for most flights.

On Skylab, each of the 70 or so individual foods employed was analyzed for all known nutrients, including individual amino and fatty acids. In addition, through a system of positive reporting and daily encouragement, food allotments for most days were consumed completely. Daily intake was held nearly constant for calcium, phosphorus, magnesium, sodium, and potassium. This was achieved through careful menu formation and the use of mineral supplements. Protein intakes were generally identical preflight, in flight, and postflight for any particular individual. They ranged from about 80 g in one individual to 160 g in another. The protein employed was of high quality, judged not only on the basis of the ingredients used but also on the basis of actual amino acid analysis.

Despite careful control of dietary intake, some differences between inflight and ground-based intakes were unavoidable. Carbohydrate consumption was generally higher in flight than on the ground, with averages of 400 g/day and 350 g/day respectively. Fat intake was lower on an isocaloric basis. Crude fiber intakes were about 5–10 g/day in flight and on the ground.

Vitamin A intakes exceeded the Recommended Dietary Allowances (RDA) by a wide margin, with greater values generally occurring in flight. Although vitamin D_2 was low or absent in Skylab foods, it was provided in the two longer flights by a multivitamin supplement containing 100 percent of the RDA.

In light of Soviet reports of increased losses of vitamins B and C from cosmonauts' blood under low-frequency vibration conditions, it is interesting to note that both vitamins were present at almost 10 times the RDA, even though there is little evidence to infer that space flight alters requirements for either vitamin.

Intake of folic acid is of some concern in view of the decreases in red cell mass of about 10 percent observed in any space mission, regardless of duration. The provision of about 200 percent of the RDA of folic acid in the two longer Skylab flights and the adequate intake of copper, zinc, and iron render a nutritional deficit an improbable causative factor for red blood cell loss.

SUMMARY

It is likely that low caloric intakes contributed partially to the biochemical and physiological changes observed in many early flights. It is also probable that certain deteriorative or adaptive processes accompanying space flight can affect nutritional requirements in such a way that intakes that are appropriate under ground-based conditions are suboptimal in flight.

It now seems clear that, despite the intake of adequate energy, man does not reach equilibrium with the weightless environment at least within a period of 84 days. Body mass continues to decline and the elemental constituents of bone and muscle continue to be lost. The relatively crude observations made thus far reveal these processes, but certainly do not preclude the existence of many other non-equilibrium states which are either too slow to detect or involve elements that have not yet been measured.

Nutritional research in the future must provide specifications for the design of space food systems. It is a fundamental requirement of all such systems that they be nutritionally and psychologically adequate at minimum mass. As with other life support expendables, the mass of the food system increases linearly with mission length and crew size. To minimize this mass, nutrient material must be provided to each crewmember in precise accordance with its expenditure. Ultimately, however, in addition to systems that recycle water and oxygen, a system that recycles some nutrient material must be developed. Such synthetic systems must tailor foods to unique nutritional specifications based on firm knowledge of the specific metabolic requirements generated by exposure to weightlessness.

The prevailing assumption that humans require a diet of great variety must be reexamined in terms of the Space Station and future missions. In many areas of the world people live on diets consisting of only a few types of food with no apparent ill effects, provided basic nutritional requirements are satisfied. Experimental evidence from many sources shows that individuals can be kept on a simple nutrient source for many years without suffering ill effects. There is also a strong possibility that a formula diet of greater acceptability than those used today will be developed.

Products of these various systems could be given a more appetizing taste and odor by special additives or processing. Powdered substances can be converted into gelatins, which are more convenient to eat, with the use of synthetic polymer compounds. We must be aware, however, that sensory properties of food are not the sole determinants of acceptability. Acceptability is an evasive concept largely determined by conditioning and internal chemistry.

All potential onboard food production systems must meet the nutritional needs of humans living and working in space for extended periods. These nutritional needs are, in fact, the gross chemical specifications of any diet, whether developed from stored or recycled materials, or a combination of both.

The ideal space food probably lies somewhere between a simple formula diet, closely controlled, and a diet of great variety. In any event, technologically expedient solutions should be considered with caution. Much effort has been devoted in the U.S. and Soviet space programs to determine the optimum diet for space missions. Research will undoubtedly continue through the years to design a space food system that is simple, controlled, and offers great variety while meeting the nutritional and energy requirements of space crews.

REFERENCES

Grigoriev, A.I. et al. Kosmicheskaya Biologii i Avia-kosmicheskaya Meditsina 3:21–27, 1985.

Huber, C.S., Heidelbaugh, N.D., Smith, M.C., and Klicka, M. Space Foods. In: Health and Foods. Edited by Birch, G.G., Green, L.F., and Plaskett, L.G. John Wiley and Sons, pp. 130–150, 1972.

Johnson, P.C., Leach, C.S., Rambaut, P.C. Apollo 16 bioenergetic considerations. Nutr. Metabol. 16:529–534, 1974.

Leach, C.S., and Rambaut, P.C. In: Proceedings of the Skylab Life Sciences Symposium (NASA TM X-58154). Edited by Johnston, R.S., and Dietlein, L.F., p. 427, Houston, TX, 1974.

Lutwak, L., Whedon, G.D., LaChance, P.A., Reid, J.M., and Lipscomb, H.J. Mineral, electrolyte and nitrogen balance studies of the Gemini VII 14-day orbital space flight. J. Clin. Endocrinol. and Metab. 29: 1140–1156, 1969.

Michel, E.L., Rummel, J.A., Sawin, C.F., Buderer, M.C., and Lem, J.D. In: Proceedings of the Skylab Life Sciences Symposium (NASA TM X-58154). Edited by Johnston, R.S., and Dietlein, L.F., p. 723, Houston, TX, 1974.

Nanz, R.A., Michel, E.L., and LaChance, P.A. Evolution of space feeding concepts. Food Technology, 21:1596–1601, 1977.

Rambaut, P.C., Leach, C.S., and Johnson, P.C. Calcium and phosphorus changes of the Apollo 17 crewmembers. Nutr. Metabol. 18:62–69. 1975.

Rambaut, P.C., Smith, M.C., Leach, C.S., Whedon, G.D., and Reid, J. Nutrition and responses to zero gravity. Federation Proceedings 36:1678–1682, 1977.

Rambaut, P.C., Leach, C.S., and Leonard, J.I. Observations in energy balance in man during space flight. Am. J. Physiol. 233:R208–R212, 1977.

Sheinfeld, M., Leach, C.S., and Johnson, P.C. Plasma thyroxine changes of the Apollo crewmen. Aviat. Space Environ. Med. 46:47–49, 1975.

Stadler, C.R., Bourland, C.T., Rapp, R.M., and Sauer, R.L. Food system for Space Shuttle Columbia. J. Am. Diet. Assoc., 30:108–114, 1982.

Thornton, W.E., and Rummel, J.A. Muscular deconditioning and its prevention in space flight. In: Biomedical results from Skylab (NASA SP-377). Edited by Johnston, R.S., and Dietlein, L.F. U.S. Government Printing Office, Washington, D.C., pp. 191–197, 1977.

Vanderveen, J.E., and Allen, T.H. In: Life Sciences and Space Research. Berlin, Akademie-Verlag, p. 105, 1972.

Whedon, G.D., Lutwak, L., Reid, J., Rambaut, P.C., Whittle, M., Smith, M., and Leach, C.S. Mineral and nitrogen balance study—results of metabolic observations on Skylab II 28-day orbital mission. Acta Astronautica 2, 297–309, 1975.

Whedon, G.D., Lutwak, L., Rambaut, P.C., Whittle, M.W., Reid, J., Smith, M.C., Leach, C.S., Stadler, C.R., and Sanford, D.D. Mineral and nitrogen balance study observations: the second manned Skylab mission. Aviat. Space Environ. Med. 47:391–396, 1976.

Whittle, M., Herron, R., and Cuzzi, J. In: Proceedings of the Skylab Life Sciences Symposium (NASA TM X-58154). Edited by Johnston, R.S., and Dietlein, L.F. Houston, TX, 1974.

12 Bone and Mineral Metabolism

VICTOR S. SCHNEIDER
ADRIAN LEBLANC
PAUL C. RAMBAUT

Biomedical data from multiple U.S. and Soviet space missions have made it clear that the weightlessness of space flight induces continuous and possibly progressive changes in the musculoskeletal system. These changes are manifested in the way the body conserves calcium and other minerals which are normally stored in the skeleton. Skeletal changes and loss of total body calcium have been observed in both humans and animals who have flown from 1 week to more than 237 days in space. These alterations in bone and mineral metabolism may be among the most profound biomedical changes associated with space flight.

BONE DENSITY STUDIES

During the Apollo and Skylab Programs, a precise method of photon absorptiometry was used to assess pre- and postflight bone mineral mass. Figure 12-1 shows the results of measurements of the central os calcis, which is almost wholly composed of trabecular bone, taken during the Skylab Program (Rambaut and Johnston, 1979). Greatest losses were observed in the Skylab 4 crew after 84 days of weightlessness. Bone mineral losses were not observed from the distal compact radius, however. Although these measurements were taken from different types of bone (compact and trabecular) they do not reveal whether mineral loss during space flight occurs solely in weight-bearing bones. Some suggestions may be found in Soviet space flight measurements in which mineral loss was determined from the tubercle and planter areas of the os calcis, predominately compact bone. Bone loss seemed to increase in rough proportion to mission length, and ranged from −0.9 percent to −19.8 percent over periods from 75 to 184 days (Stupakov et al., 1984). Thus, both compact and trabecular bone is lost from the heel (os calcis). Calcaneal

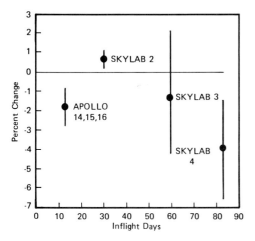

Figure 12-1. Postflight bone mineral changes in space flight crew (mean ± SE). (From Rambaut and Johnston, 1979).

mineral recovery is gradual and appears to take about the same length of time as loss (Vogel and Whittle, 1976). This measured recovery was incomplete in at least one Skylab 4 astronaut; only half his loss was replaced after 90 days postflight. Although the Soviets suggest that calcaneal recovery is complete, spine mineral loss was observed in cosmonauts (using an X-ray computerized tomography technique) during 6 months following flight (Cann, 1981).

CALCIUM BALANCE STUDIES

Studies of metabolic balance were conducted on Skylab missions where dietary intake and urinary and fecal excretion were monitored. Daily reports of food consumed by individual crewmembers were communicated to dietary personnel, who calculated daily intake of calories, minerals, and other nutrients. Urine was collected on a 24-hour basis; urine samples were mixed with a known quantity of a marker, and an aliquot was obtained for

analysis on Earth. Stools were collected and returned for analysis (however, enemas were used just prior to launch and the excreta discarded). Minerals in perspiration were not measured, nor were corrections made for perspiration losses. In spite of the problems in balance technique, Skylab balance studies were more accurate than the studies conducted with crewmembers on the Gemini and Apollo missions. Skylab studies positively demonstrated that space flight is accompanied by increased excretion of calcium and phosphorus.

Figure 12-2 shows the changes in urine and fecal calcium content in flight during Skylab IV (Rambaut and Johnston, 1979). Urine calcium content increased rapidly, but reached a plateau after 30 days in flight. A small fecal calcium increase was noted over the duration of the flight. Within 10 days in flight, preflight positive calcium balances became less positive until the body as a whole began to lose calcium. Rate of loss was slow at first, but increased to almost 300 mg per day by the 84th day of flight. For the three Skylab 4 crewmen, the average loss was 25 g of calcium from the overall body pool (about 1,250 g). Based on the trends in calcium loss during the first 30 days in flight, Rambaut and Johnston (1979) calculated that 1 year in flight might result in the loss of sufficient mineral to undermine bone strength. Similar conclusions can be drawn from Soviet research (Gazenko, Grigor'yev et al., 1980), in which increased calcium excretion is attributed to weightlessness.

Skylab calcium balance studies suggest that losses in bone mineral from the os calcis contribute relatively little to the overall calcium loss. The 4 percent loss observed in the os calcis after the 84-day mission represents a loss of only about 100 mg of calcium, while overall calcium losses for this mission were 250 times greater. Significant loss of os calcis mass was also seen in one Soviet mission which involved

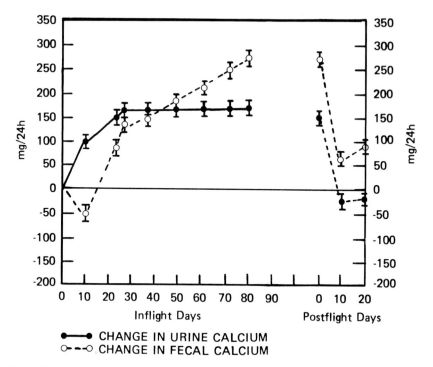

Figure 12-2. Changes in urine and fecal calcium as a function of Skylab flight duration (mean ± SE). (From Rambaut and Johnston, 1979).

substantial exercise by the cosmonauts, although the Soviets have indicated that extensive exercise programs in later missions decreased skeletal loss (Gazenko, Genin, and Yegorov, 1981). Thus, it is clear that other weight-bearing skeletal sites account for the major portion of the depleted mineral. Bone loss from other skeletal sites has not been reported.

Recovery of the lost calcium begins soon after return to one gravity. Urine calcium content dropped below preflight baseline by day 10 postflight, but fecal calcium content had not dropped to preflight levels by 20 days postflight. The markedly negative calcium balance also had not returned to zero by day 20. Evidence from studies on recovery of os calcis mineral content after space flight, and evidence from bed rest studies, suggests that after a period of weeks or months astronauts' os calcis bone

mineral content would return to normal. Nevertheless, it is possible that calcium balance could return to zero long before losses from space flight could be replaced resulting in irreversible damage to the skeleton.

BIOCHEMICAL ANALYSES

Analyses of inflight urine, fecal, and plasma samples from Skylab missions revealed changes in a number of biochemical parameters. Urinary output of hydroxyproline gradually increased, indicating deterioration of the collagenous matrix substance of weight-bearing bones. Output of nitrogen, reflecting muscle atrophy, also increased. The proportion of stearic acid in the total fecal fat increased throughout the flight as more and more calcium became available to form nonabsorbable salts. Urinary levels of catecholamines decreased, but urinary cortisol increased during space flight. Analyses of plasma revealed inflight increases in calcium and phosphate; inflight PTH levels never increased, but decreased from preflight or early flight levels (Whedon et al., 1977; Rambaut and Johnston, 1979; Leach, 1981).

GROUND-BASED SIMULATION MODELS

Bed rest provides a useful model for the effects of weightlessness on bone and mineral, since the force of gravity on the longitudinal skeleton is reduced from one to one-sixth gravity. Although results from space flight balance studies are not completely identical to the bed rest model, a number of factors must be considered. These include the ability to perform a greater number of studies on Earth, thereby minimizing individual variations; more critical monitoring of subjects; minimization of mineral losses from perspiration and vomitus during ambulatory control, bed rest, and recovery (compared to the lack of these controls in the astronauts preflight, and inflight with early space motion discomfort or later exercise periods, and postflight during physiologic recovery). Lack of measurement of these mineral losses could become a standard error of balance studies during space flight. Balances would initially appear positive and remain positive during space flight, although less so. If mineral losses from perspiration and vomitus were not measured throughout the entire flight to account for variations in cabin temperature, space motion discomfort or exercise effort,

mineral balance would appear to be inconsistent. Thus, inflight balance studies offer preliminary indications, but must be interpreted with caution. Bed rest studies offer reliable and reproducible results which have allowed the determination that bone loss continues unabated for at least 36 weeks, with no evidence that the expected new steady state is produced. Total body calcium stores decrease by 6 grams per month after the first month of bed rest, and by the end of 9 months at least 50 grams of calcium have been lost. Additionally, results of bed rest studies provide information on mechanisms underlying bone loss during hypokinesic states.

Bed rest studies have suggested a means to predict the amount of mineral that will be lost from the os calcis during bed rest or in space (Donaldson et al., 1970; Lockwood et al., 1973; Smith et al., 1977; Volozhin et al., 1981; Schneider and McDonald, 1984). The wide variability in the amount of lost mineral in bed-rested subjects can be partially explained by two other variables: (1) initial os calcis mineral content and (2) urinary hydroxyproline excretion rate (corrected for creatinine excretion). Figure 12-3 shows the regression of the prediction term (initial mineral divided by urinary hydroxyproline excretion rate) on the amount of mineral loss in subjects bed rested for 59 days (Vogel and Whittle, 1976). Data from two of the Skylab 3 astronauts are consistent (open circles), suggesting that these variables also can be used to predict the effects of space flight on os calcis mineral content.

Studies of animals with immobilized limbs have suggested that disuse produces changes in both bone formation and resorption, depending upon the duration of immobilization. For example, Landry and Fleisch (1964) used osseous tetracycline incorporation corrected by changes in bone weight as a direct index of bone formation and as an indirect index of bone resorption.

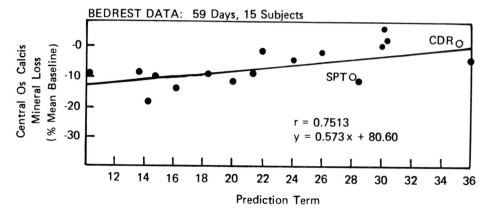

Figure 12-3. Os calcis mineral loss for varying prediction terms during 59 days of bed rest (solid circles) or space flight (open circles). (From Vogel and Whittle, 1976).

They found a short initial phase during which formation decreased, and a second phase in which formation increased while bone weight decreased, indicating an even greater increase in resorption. After 49 days of immobilization, formation again decreased below normal levels.

Young et al. (1986) couched monkeys (Macaca nemestrina) long term and demonstrated loss of trabecular and cortical bone in the weight-bearing areas. Moreover, recovery of the cortical bone deficiencies may not have been complete even after 40 months of ad libitum activity following restraint.

Didenko and Volozhin (1981) exposed rabbits to 30 days of confinement in order to study changes in bone mineral composition. Levels of calcium in bone did not change, although calcium excretion increased. This was attributed to an inhibition of bone reorganization in which bone mass was reduced without a corresponding alteration of crystalline structure.

The most pronounced changes are seen in weight-bearing bones. Mechanical stimulation apparently has a critical effect on bone structure and metabolism, as numerous studies involving bone strain measurement have shown (Hinsenkamp et al., 1981). There also appears to be an age-dependent variation in the relative rates of bone formation and resorption (Novikov and Il'yin, 1981), with older animals showing the highest net rate of bone loss during immobilization.

These and other results indicate that immobilization produces a number of time-dependent changes in bone accretion and resorption, and suggest proportionately larger increases in resorption as a key factor in loss of bone mineral mass. Skeletal losses in space are likely due to relatively larger increases in bone resorption compared to bone formation (except in immature growing animals). Autopsies of the three Soviet cosmonauts who died after a 3-week flight revealed "a good number of unusually wide osteocytic lacunae," which may have been due to increased bone resorption.

INFLIGHT ANIMAL EXPERIMENTS

Studies of animals flown on board the Cosmos biosatellites and Spacelab have also revealed changes in bone mineral content. Monkeys experiencing 8.8 days of weightlessness showed larger losses in bone mineral than ground controls (Mack, 1971). Spacelab 3 rat studies, as well as previous studies flown on the Cosmos biosatellites, revealed marked skeletal changes. Skeletal changes in rats exposed to as little as 7 days of space flight on Spacelab 3 included decreased bone growth, decreased mineralization, decreased bending strength, and decreased weight of the lumbar spines (L3) (Wronski et al., 1985; Duke et al., 1985). Flight rats after 18.5 days in the Cosmos experiment showed a 30 percent decrease in mechanical bending strength (Gazenko, Il'in, et al., 1980) compared to a 28 percent reduction after just 7 days on board Spacelab 3 (Buckendahl et al., 1985). In addition to these changes, other functional rearrangements have been documented, such as depression in bone cell size and number at the bone surface (Doty, 1985). However, no changes were seen in either qualitative or quantitative function of rat kidney calcitriol receptors, suggesting an absence of causal or effectual roles of this system in regulating renal calcium loss (Mangelsdorf et al., 1985). These and other studies suggest that the loss of bone mineral in growing rats might be due primarily to inhibited bone formation, rather than increased bone resorption (Morey and Baylink, 1978; Yagodovsky et al., 1976). Rats on the 22-day Cosmos 605 flight showed decreased metaphyseal bone in the vicinity of the epiphyseal cartilaginous plate, suggesting an inhibition of bone growth during flight. It is not yet possible to integrate these findings with those from hypokinesia studies on humans and animals in one gravity, because of such complicating factors as time-dependent changes, species differences, and potential differences in the mechanisms by which bone is lost in space and during bed rest or immobilization.

COUNTERMEASURES

The major countermeasures being explored to reduce the skeletal effects of space flight include various weight-loading, exercise, or artificial gravity regimens that counteract the loss of gravitational loading and muscular stress, and nutritional and pharmacological manipulations. The crews of Skylab 3 and 4 exercised heavily in flight. Three of these six crewmembers showed substantial mineral losses, which casts doubt on the effectiveness of the particular exercises used as a countermeasure. Soviet findings on the effect of inflight exercise during long-duration space flights have been inconsistent (Gazenko, Genin, and Yegorov, 1981). Nutritional supplements of calcium and phosphorus for brief periods of time, and drugs such as fluoride or clodronate (a diphosphonate) have shown promise in bed rest studies, and may prove effective as countermeasures for skeletal effects of space flight. Due to technical and hardware constraints, artificial gravity has so far been employed only in animal studies, but results have been encouraging. Centrifugation has been shown to prevent changes in calcium and phosphorus content of rat long bones (Gazenko, Il'in, et al., 1980), and to prevent osteoporosis (Stupakov, 1981).

SUMMARY

Based on the information obtained from space missions, particularly Skylab and the longer Salyut missions, it is clear that bone and mineral metabolism is substantially altered during space flight. Calcium balance becomes increasingly negative throughout flight, and bone mineral content of the os calcis declines. The major health hazards associated with skeletal changes include signs and symptoms of hypercalcemia with rapid bone turnover, risk of kidney stones due to hypercalciuria, lengthy recovery of lost bone mass postflight, possibility of irreversible bone loss (particularly the trabecular bone), possible effects of calcification in the soft tissues, and possible increase in fracture potential.

For these reasons, major research efforts are currently being directed toward elucidating the fundamental mechanisms by which bone is lost in space and developing more effective countermeasures to prevent both short-term and long-term complications.

REFERENCES

Buckendahl, P.E., Cann, C.E., Grindeland, R.E., Martin, R.B., Mechanic, G., and Arnaud, S.B. Osteocalcin as an indicator of bone metabolism during space flight. The Physiologist, 28(4):379, 1985.

Cann, C. Determination of spine mineral density using computerized tomography: a report. XII US/ USSR Joint Working Group Meeting on Space Biology and Medicine, Washington, D.C. November 9–22, 1981.

Didenko, I.Ye., and Volozhin, A.I. Chemical composition of mineral component of rabbit bones as related to 30-day hypokinesia. Space Biology and Aerospace Medicine, 15(1):123–127, 1981.

Donaldson, C.L., Hulley, S.B., Vogel, J.M., Hatner, R.S., Bayers, J.H., and McMillian, D.E. Effect of prolonged bed rest on bone mineral. Metabolism, 19:1071–1084, 1970.

Doty, S.B. Morphologic and histochemical studies of bone cells from SL-3 rats. The Physiologist, 28(4):379, 1985.

Duke, J., Janer, L., and Campbell, M. Microprobe analyses of epiphyseal plates from Spacelab 3 rats. The Physiologist, 28(4):378, 1985.

Gazenko, O.G., Genin, A.M., and Yegorov, A.D. Major medical results of the Salyut-6/Soyuz 185-day space flight. NASA NDB 2747. Proceedings of the XXXII Congress of the International Astronautical Federation. Rome, Italy, 6–12, 1981.

Gazenko, O.G., Grigor'yev, A.I., and Natochin, Yu.V. Fluid-electrolyte homeostasis and weightlessness. Space Biology and Aerospace Medicine, 14(5):1–11, 1980.

Gazenko, O.G., Il'in, Ye.A., Genin, A.M., Kotovskaya, A.R., Korol'kov, V.I., Tigranyan, R.A., and Portugalov, V.V. Principal results of physiological experiments with mammals aboard the Cosmos-936 biosatellite. Space Biology and Aerospace Medicine, 14(2):33–37, 1980.

Hinsenkamp, M., Burny, F., Bourgois, R., and Donkerwolcke, M. In vivo bone strain measurements: Clinical results, animal experiments, and a proposal for a study of bone demineralization in weightlessness. Aviation, Space, and Environmental Medicine, 52(2):95–103, 1981.

Kaplanskiy, A.S., Savina, Ye.A., Portugalov, V.V., Il'ina- Kakuyeva, Ye.I., Alexeyev, Ye.I., Durnova, G.N., Pankova, A.S., Plakhuta-Plakutina, G.I., Shvets, V.N., and Yakovleva, V.I. Results of morphological investigations aboard Cosmos biosatellites. The Physiologist (Supplement), 23(6):S51–S54, 1980.

Landry, M., and Fleisch, H. The influence of immobilization on bone formation as evaluated by osseous incorporation of tetracycline. Journal of Bone and Joint Surgery (British), 46B(4):764–771, 1964.

Leach, C.S. An overview of the endocrine and metabolic changes in manned space flight. Acta Astronautica, 8(9–10):977–986, 1981.

Leach, C.S., and Rambaut, P.C. Biochemical responses of the Skylab crewmen: An overview. In: Biomedical results from Skylab (NASA SP-377). Edited by R.S. Johnston and L.F. Dietlein. U.S. Government Printing Office, Washington, D.C., 1977.

Lockwood, D.R., Lammert, J.E., Vogel, J.M., and Hulley, S.B. Bone mineral loss during bed rest. In Clinical Aspects of Metabolic Bone Disease. Excerpta Medica, 261–265, 1973.

Mack, P.B., and Vogt, F.B. Roentgenographic bone density changes during representative Apollo space flight. American Journal of Roentgenology, 113:621–623, 1971.

Mangelsdorf, D.J., Marion, S.L., Pike, J.W., and Haussler, M.R. 1,25-Dihydroxy-vitamin D3 receptors in space-flown vs. grounded control rat kidneys. The Physiologist, 28(4):379, 1985.

Morey, E.R., and Baylink, D.J. Inhibition of bone

formation during space flight. Science, 201:1138, 1978.

Novikov, V.E., and Il'in, E.A. Age-related reactions of rat bones to their unloading. Aviation, Space, and Environmental Medicine, 52(9):551–553, 1981.

Rambaut, P.C., and Johnston, R.S. Prolonged weightlessness and calcium loss in man. Acta Astronautica, 6:1113–1122, 1979.

Rambaut, P.C., Leach, C.S., and Whedon, G.D. A study of metabolic balance in crewmembers of Skylab IV. Acta Astronautica, 6:1313–1322, 1979.

Schneider, V.S. and McDonald, J. Skeletal calcium homeostasis and countermeasures to prevent disuse osteoporosis. Calcified Tissue International, 36:S151–S154, 1984.

Smith, M.C., Rambaut, P.C., Vogel, J.M., and Whittle, M.W. Bone mineral measurement—Experiment M078. In: Biomedical results from Skylab (NASA SP-377). Edited by R.S. Johnston and L.F. Dietlein. U.S. Government Printing Office, Washington, D.C., 1977.

Stupakov, G.P. Artificial gravity as a means of preventing atrophic skeletal changes. Space Biology and Aerospace Medicine, 15(4):88–90, 1981.

Stupakov, G.P., Kazeykin, V.S., Kozlovskiy, A.P., and Korolev, V.V. Evaluation of changes in human axial skeletal bone structures during long-term space flights. Kosmicheskaya Biologiya I Aviakosmicheskaya Meditsina, 18(2):33–37, 1984.

Vogel, J.M., and Whittle, M.W. Bone mineral changes: The second manned Skylab mission. Aviation, Space, and Environmental Medicine, 47:396–400, 1976.

Volozhin, A.I., Didenko, I.Ye., and Stupakov, G.P. Chemical composition of mineral component of human vertebrae and calcaneus after hypokinesia. Kosmicheskaya Biologiya I Aviakosmicheskaya Meditsina, 15(1):60–63, 1981.

Whedon, G.D., Lutwak, L., Rambaut, P.C., Whittle, M.W., Smith, M.C., Reid, J., Leach, C.S., Stadler, C.R., and Sanford, D.D. Mineral and nitrogen metabolic studies—Experiment M071. In: Biomedical results from Skylab (NASA SP-377). Edited by R.S. Johnston and L.F. Dietlein. U.S. Government Printing Office, Washington, D.C., 1977.

Wronski, T.J., Morey-Holton, E.R., Maeses, A.C., and Walsh, C.C. Spacelab 3: Histomorphometric analysis of the rat skeleton. The Physiologist, 28(4):376, 1985.

Yagodovsky, V.S., Trifaranidi, L.A., and Goroklova, G.P. Space flight effects on skeletal bones of rats. Aviation, Space, and Environmental Medicine, 47:734–738, 1976.

Young, D.R., Niklowitz, W.J., Brown, R.J., and Jee, W.S.S. Immobilization-associated osteoporosis in primates. Bone, 7:109–117, 1986.

13 Hematology, Immunology, Endocrinology, and Biochemistry

CAROLYN LEACH HUNTOON

PHILIP C. JOHNSON

NITZA M. CINTRON

Exposure to the space environment produces a wide range of effects on body tissues and fluids. Many of the changes observed in returning astronauts are thought to be caused by the cephalad shift of fluids accompanying weightlessness, or by removal of the load from weight-bearing tissues. However, some of these changes, particularly hormonal ones, may be related to stress and other variables associated with space flight.

Measurement of the variables discussed in this chapter requires analysis of blood, urine, and saliva samples. Usually, samples have not been acquired during space flight, but have been obtained and studied preflight, and as soon as possible (often within a few hours) after landing. However, inflight samples were obtained on one Gemini and one Apollo flight, the Skylab missions, and some Space Shuttle and Soyuz flights, for measurement of selected parameters.

HEMATOLOGY

The most significant hematological changes resulting from space flight are reductions in plasma volume and red blood cell mass.

CHANGES IN PLASMA VOLUME

Plasma volume changes have not yet been measured during weightlessness. With one exception, decreases in plasma volume have been observed in postflight studies following every United States space mission (Table 13-1; Johnson, 1983). Plasma volume is thought to decrease soon after onset of weightlessness, but recovery occurs within 8 days after landing (Leach and Johnson, 1984). Although central venous pressure (CVP) has not been measured during the first few hours in flight, bed rest studies have indicated that an early increase in CVP leads to decreases in venous pressure and plasma volume (Blomqvist et al., 1980; Leach, Johnson, and Suki, 1983). Venous pressure was found to have decreased by 4 hours after launch on the D-1 mission (Kirsch et al., 1986).

RED BLOOD CELL MASS

The loss of red blood cell mass recorded after U.S. missions and hemoglobin mass after Soviet missions is shown in Table 13-1. In the Soviet program, hemoglobin mass, rather than red cell mass, was measured by spectroscopic methods, thereby avoiding the injection of radioisotopes (Balakhovskiy, Legen'kov, and Kiselev, 1980). Results from both the U.S. and Soviet programs show considerable variation in the hematological responses of individual crewmembers. However, it appears that the decrease in red cell mass plateaus after about 60 days of exposure to weightlessness. Skylab data and hematological measurements on Spacelab 1 crewmembers (Leach and Johnson, 1984) indicate that the loss of red cell mass is not made up for at least 2 weeks, even after return to Earth.

Observed changes in red blood cell count have been even more variable than those noted in red cell mass and hemoglobin mass. Soviet scientists have reported that red cell count remains constant on flights of 3 days or less (Gazenko, Kakurin, and Kuznetsov, 1976). Erythrocyte counts have been variable after Soviet flights up to 18 days (Legen'kov et al., 1977). During the 10-day Spacelab 1 mission, erythrocyte count increased slightly, but on landing day it was slightly decreased (Leach and Johnson, 1984), decreasing further during the recovery period. Cosmonauts participating in missions of 18 days to 6 months have shown postflight decreases in erythrocyte counts (Legen'kov et al., 1977) which returned to baseline values within 6 weeks (Vorobyov et al., 1983). After the 28-day Skylab mission, erythrocyte count was decreased. After the 59-day and 84-day missions, red

TABLE 13-1

HEMATOLOGICAL CHANGES FOUND IN U.S. AND SOVIET MANNED MISSIONS (MEAN PERCENT CHANGE FROM PREFLIGHT BASELINE)

Program	Days in Space	Number of Subjects	Plasma Volume	RBC Mass	Hb Mass
Gemini	4–8	4	−8	−17	
Apollo	6–13	21	−4	−8	
Skylab	28–84	9	−13	−11	
Apollo-Soyuz	9	3	−11	−7	
Spacelab 1	10	4	−6	−9	
Soyuz 14	15	2			−12
Salyut 3–6	16–175	16			−20

cell count was increased, but began to decrease 1 day after landing (Kimzey, 1977).

Red Blood Cell Production and Destruction

Reticulocyte count, as a percentage of erythrocyte count, has usually shown a postflight decrease. Immediately after Skylab missions, reticulocyte count was as low as 44 percent of mean preflight value. After the 28-day mission, it had not attained preflight levels by 21 days after landing, but 3 weeks after the 59-day and 84-day missions reticulocyte counts were higher than preflight levels (Johnson, Driscoll, and LeBlanc, 1977). Although reticulocyte count decreased by more than 50 percent during and immediately after the 10-day Spacelab 1 mission, the change was not significant and on the day after landing only a 6 percent decrease was evident (Leach et al., 1985). Reticulocyte count decreased after flights of the Salyut-6 series, but increased later; this reticulocytosis persisted for over a month following the longest flights (Vorobyov et al., 1983).

Serum erythropoietin was measured in samples taken during and after the Spacelab 1 flight. By 24 hours after launch, erythropoietin had decreased by 50 percent, and continued to decrease during and after the flight, although the decrease was not statistically significant and preflight levels were relatively high (Leach et al., 1985). Soviet investigators, using a different assay for erythropoietin, reported increases in blood and urine levels in Salyut-6 cosmonauts after landing, especially after the shorter flights (16-30 days) (Legen'kov et al., 1977; Yegorov, 1980). Differences in flight duration or method may explain the discrepancy between these results and those from Spacelab. Soviet investigators have considered their findings to indicate that readaptation to normal gravity after long flights stimulates erythropoiesis (Yegorov, 1980).

Red Blood Cell Metabolism

A variety of enzymes and metabolites involved in red cell metabolism were assessed in postflight samples from the Skylab missions to evaluate the maintenance of erythrocyte integrity (Mengel, 1977). Levels of red cell components involved in peroxidation of lipids, enzymes of red cell metabolism, and 2,3-diphosphoglyceric acid (DPG) and adenosine triphosphate (ATP) were analyzed. This study was prompted by postflight findings of decreased red cell mass in U.S. missions which used a hyperoxic atmosphere. Although amounts of enzymes and metabolites changed, there was no consistent pattern and no evidence of lipid peroxidation, which is associated with irreversible damage to red blood cells. There was no change in amount of DPG or ATP during or after the Spacelab 1 flight (Leach et al., 1985), in which there was no hyperoxic exposure.

Soviet investigators found that changes in ATP content and activity of glycolytic enzymes of erythrocytes were a function of mission duration (Ushakov, 1981). A 1-week flight produced no alterations. During 30- and 63-day flights, glycolytic activity declined, while ATP content remained stable. Red cells of cosmonauts on 96- and 175-day flights displayed substantial decline in ATP content, with an elevated glycolysis rate (Yegorov, 1980). These changes were considered to be adaptive rather than results of changes in the basal metabolic processes of the cells.

Red Blood Cell Shape

Blood samples of Skylab and Spacelab 1 crewmembers (taken pre-, in-, and post-flight) were examined with light and scanning electron microscopy for alterations in the shape of red blood cells. Usually, 80 to 90 percent of erythrocytes have a biconcave discoid shape, and the rest have one of a number of more or less flattened shapes. Nondiscoid shapes can be caused by changes in plasma or in the cells themselves (Bessis et al., 1973). Inflight samples from Skylab showed a decline in the proportion of discocytes, accompanied by increases in the proportions of other cell types, particularly echinocytes (crenated cells) (Kimzey, 1977). While this was also observed in Spacelab samples, the inflight changes were not statistically significant, whereas a week after landing there was a significant increase of 210 percent in the proportion of echinocytes (Leach et al., 1985). Cosmonauts on Salyut-6 missions (96, 140, 175, and 185 days) also showed postflight decreases in discoid red blood cells, and increases in "mulberry" and spherical shapes (Vorobyov et al., 1983). Some crewmembers also had a few cells with shapes that are not normally seen. Although such changes were considered to be of potential clinical significance, the alterations in red cell shape distribution readily reversed after even the longest flight (Vorobyov et al., 1983), suggesting that space flight produced no permanent alteration of bone marrow function.

Possible Mechanisms Underlying Loss of Red Blood Cell Mass

The decrease in red cell mass associated with space flight has been observed since the early Gemini missions (Fischer, Johnson, and Berry, 1967). It was proposed initially that these losses were related to the 100 percent oxygen atmosphere in the spacecraft, which may have produced mild oxygen toxicity resulting in alterations in red cell integrity and premature intravascular hemolysis. However, subsequent hematological data from Skylab (Johnson, Driscoll, and LeBlanc, 1977) and the ground-based 59-day Skylab Medical Experiments Altitude Test (SMEAT) (Johnson, 1973) did not support this hypothesis. Skylab and the SMEAT simulation chamber had normobaric oxygen concentrations (70 percent oxygen and 30 percent nitrogen, at 258 torr), but only the Skylab astronauts showed decreases in red cell mass. Red cell mass also decreased in Spacelab crewmembers, who were not exposed to hyperoxia (Leach and Johnson, 1984).

Elimination of hyperoxia as a cause of red blood cell loss during space flight and the transient low postflight reticulocyte counts leaves several other possible causes: (1) increased destruction of red blood cells by the reticuloendothelial system or cell lysis, (2) permanent loss of erythrocytes by loss of blood or extravasation, (3) temporary sequestration of erythrocytes in the reticuloendothelial system, or (4) transient suppression of red blood cell production.

Studies of red cell metabolism in astronauts (Mengel, 1977) and cosmonauts (Yegorov, 1980) have revealed consistent abnormalities. If substantial hemolysis occurs, haptoglobin should be expected to decrease; and in Spacelab 1 astronauts, it did not (Leach et al., 1985). The first inflight and postflight measurements of serum ferritin were performed on samples from Spacelab 1, and ferritin increased significantly between 1 and 7 days after launch, returning to preflight levels between 1 and 8 days after landing (Leach et al., 1985). Although red cell survival times after space flight are normal (Johnson, 1983; Leach et al., 1985), the method of measurement used would not detect random loss (unrelated to age) of red cells.

The increase in ferritin may be an indication that the normal destruction of red blood cells by the spleen is accelerated in weightlessness. The spleen is the major site for efficient removal of red cells and reuse of their contents.

Ground-based simulations of space flight have shown that removal of blood for analysis does not result in red cell mass losses as great as those occurring after flight (Leach et al., 1985). There is no evidence that loss of blood occurs by extravasation.

Changes in the distribution of red cell shapes may contribute to premature sequestration of some cells by the spleen. However, measurement of spleen-liver ratios on the Apollo-Soyuz Test Project and in control subjects showed increases in controls, but not in astronauts (Kimzey and Johnson, 1977). These findings dispute an increase in reticuloendothelial trapping. Moreover, in the Spacelab 1 experiment, the percentage of echinocytes did not increase significantly until 1 week after landing (Leach et al., 1985).

Although measurements indicate that erythropoietin decreases during flight, further research is needed to obtain consistent results. Iron incorporation has been found to be normal after space flight (Johnson, 1983; Leach et al., 1985). Even if erythropoiesis is suppressed during space flight, the rapid onset of the decrease in red cell mass indicates that it is not caused solely by decreased erythrocyte production.

The evidence suggests that the decrease in red cell mass induced by space flight may be due mainly to a transient increase in destruction of red cells by the spleen, along with the failure of red cell production to compensate for the loss (Johnson et al., 1985). Losses in red cell and hemoglobin mass might result from a feedback mechanism triggered by the decrease in plasma volume (Cogoli, 1981). Simultaneous reduction of plasma volume and red cell mass would result in a nearly constant red cell count, along with stable inflight concentrations of hematocrit and hemoglobin.

IMMUNOLOGY

The most important effects of weightlessness on the immune system appear to be a decrease in the number of T lymphocytes and impairment in their function.

Increased white blood cell counts were noted on landing days in astronauts participating in Apollo (Kimzey et al., 1975), Skylab (Kimzey, 1977), and Shuttle test flights (Taylor and Dardano, 1983), but not in Spacelab 1 crewmembers (Leach et al., 1985). The increases in leukocytes were attributed to increases in neutrophils. The increased number of neutrophils, accompanied by decreases in lymphocyte and eosinophil numbers, indicates that increases in epinephrine and glucocorticoids caused the changes in white blood cells observed after these flights (Taylor and Dardano, 1983). Similar changes in neutrophils, lymphocytes, and eosinophils were reported for Salyut flights (Anonymous, 1974). An unusual finding from the Spacelab 1 mission was an inflight increase in neutrophil precursors (band neutrophils) (Leach et al., 1985).

Skylab astronauts showed reduced numbers of T cells postflight (Kimzey, 1977), while cosmonauts showed decreased numbers of natural killer T cells after the 185-day Salyut-6 flight (Vorobyov et al., 1983) and decreased activity of killer cells after the 150-day Salyut-7 flight (Vorobyev et al., 1986).

The function of the cellular component of the immune system has been evaluated in astronauts by measuring RNA and DNA synthesis in purified lymphocyte cultures in response to an *in vitro* mitogenic challenge with phytohemagglutinin (PHA). The PHA responsiveness to lymphocytes was markedly decreased on landing day for Skylab (Kimzey, 1977) and Space Shuttle (Taylor and Dardano, 1983) crewmembers. In Skylab crews, PHA responsiveness returned to preflight levels by 3 to 7 days postflight. The lymphocytes of Salyut-6 cosmonauts who participated in missions of 96 and 140 days also showed decreased nucleic acid synthesis in response to PHA challenge (Gazenko, 1979; Gazenko et al., 1981). These findings suggest that space flight can be accompanied by a transient impairment in the function of the cellular immune system, but the clinical significance of the observed changes is not yet clear.

Certain alterations in serum proteins, including a significant rise and subsequent decrease in alpha-2 macroglobulin, were consistently observed postflight during the Apollo program, suggesting that space flight is associated with changes in the humoral immune system (Kimzey et al., 1975). However, no significant changes were found in any of a number of plasma proteins during the Skylab missions (Kimzey, 1977), or in immunoglobulins G, M, A, D, and E during the Spacelab 1 flight (Voss, 1984). The effect of space flight on plasma proteins has also been examined by Soviet investigators (Guseva and Tashpulatov, 1980). The blood of cosmonauts after space flights lasting 2, 16, 18, 49 and 175 days was analyzed for protein composition. The 2-day flight was characterized by a decrease in gamma globulin (especially IgG and IgA) and beta-2 glycoprotein fractions. Increases in albumin and most globulins were seen after the 16- and 18-day space flights. Upon completion of the 49-day flight, changes were observed only in globulin fractions: levels of C_3 and C_4 complement factors and IgG, IgA, and IgM were higher than before

flight. After the 175-day flight, serum levels of IgG were significantly reduced (Yegorov, 1980). These varied changes in blood protein concentrations were considered to indicate that adaptive changes in blood protein levels occur gradually as flight duration increases. After 18 days of flight, preflight levels of some proteins are restored, but levels of others continue to change (Guseva and Tashpulatov, 1980).

ENDOCRINOLOGY

CHANGES IN FLUID AND ELECTROLYTE METABOLISM AND ASSOCIATED ENDOCRINOLOGY

With respect to fluid and electrolytes, the most significant changes accompanying space flight are reduction in total body fluid and loss of electrolytes.

Many endocrine and biochemical changes observed in conjunction with space missions fit a consistent picture of homeostatic adjustments of circulatory dynamics, renal function, and endocrine response, probably initiated by fluid shifts and associated environmental stresses. The cephalad shift of fluids is thought to produce a transient increase in central blood volume that is detected by stretch receptors in the heart and interpreted as an increase in total blood volume. A compensatory loss of water and sodium from the renal tubules is effected through a series of neural, humoral, and direct hydraulic mechanisms (Gauer and Henry, 1963; Leach, 1979, 1981).

It has been proposed (Leach, 1981) that certain key events initiate the redistribution of fluids and eventually promote the establishment of a new steady state of reduced extracellular fluid volume. These are:

- Suppression of the renin-angiotensin-aldosterone system
- Suppression of antidiuretic hormone (ADH)
- Increased secretion of humoral natriuretic substances
- Reduced thirst.

Suppression of aldosterone and ADH should cause diuresis, which has been observed in weightlessness simulation studies. Yet it has not usually been found to occur in space flight, probably for a number of reasons. Operational constraints have made it difficult to accurately document urine volumes in the early part of a mission. Usually water intake is markedly reduced during the first few days in flight, at least partly because of space adaptation syndrome and drugs taken to prevent or ameliorate it. Skylab data indicate that the nine crewmen decreased their water intake by approximately 700 ml/day during the first 6 days in flight (Leach and Rambaut, 1977). Since their urine volume decreased by only 400 ml/day during the same period, a net loss of water occurred. In an experiment performed on one Shuttle flight in which urine pools (less than 24 hours) were collected from one crewmember, an increased rate of urinary excretion of fluid did occur on the second day of the flight (Leach, 1987). Physiological mass measurements on Skylab documented rapid weight loss within the first few days in flight, indicating that it was due primarily to fluid loss. Most of this weight loss was rapidly regained postflight (Thornton and Ord, 1977).

Additional observations that lend support to the general fluid shift hypothesis include inflight increases in urinary output of sodium, potassium, and chloride during the Skylab flights (Leach and Rambaut, 1977), and increased rates of potassium and calcium excretion early in the Shuttle

mission on which urine was collected in flight (Leach, 1987).

The onset of reexposure to gravity induces many changes which must be distinguished from the remnants of effects of weightlessness. Results of analysis of postflight samples from Space Shuttle astronauts include increases in urine osmolality and decreases in urine volume, sodium, potassium, and chloride (Leach, 1983, 1984). It was concluded from these results and those of Skylab studies (Leach and Rambaut, 1977) that fluid and electrolyte conservation begins very soon after reentry into gravity (Leach, 1983). Fluid retention has also been a consistent finding in cosmonauts after Salyut flights, but excretion of potassium and calcium was found to increase (Vorobyov et al., 1983).

Inflight and postflight changes in levels of hormones that control fluid and electrolyte metabolism are summarized in Tables 13-2 and 13-3. Results for different flights have varied considerably for some hormones.

During the Spacelab flights, an increase in plasma ADH apparently was not effective in causing fluid retention (Leach et al., 1986). Urinary ADH decreased during Skylab (Leach and Rambaut, 1977) and Salyut-7 (Vorobyov et al., 1986) flights, but during the Space Shuttle flight in which urine was collected in samples representing less than 24 hours, the rate of ADH excretion increased during the first 24 hours of flight and then returned to preflight levels. Stimulation of the emetic reflex as a result of space adaptation syndrome may cause a centrally-induced increase in ADH secretion (Rowe et al., 1979), so that caution is necessary in interpreting this as a peripheral effect of fluid transfer. Plasma aldosterone decreased inflight in Spacelab astronauts (Leach et al., 1986) but did not change significantly during the Skylab flights (Leach and Rambaut, 1977). This can be explained by the dynamic changes which

TABLE 13-2

INFLIGHT CHANGES IN HORMONES INVOLVED IN REGULATION OF FLUID AND
ELECTROLYTE METABOLISM

Hormone	Skylab	Shuttle	Salyut-7
ADH			
Plasma	Not measured	Increase	Not measured
Urine	Decrease	Increase[a], then return to preflight level	Decrease[a]
Aldosterone			
Plasma	No change	Decrease	Not measured
Urine	Increase	Increase on 6th day[a]	Decrease, then increase
Angiotensin I			
Plasma	Increase, then return to preflight level	Decrease, then increase	Not measured
Cortisol			
Plasma	Increase	Decrease	Not measured
Urine	Increase	Increase, then return to preflight level[a]	Decrease, then increase[a]
ACTH			
Plasma	Decrease (at different times throughout flights)	Increase	Not measured
ANF			
Plasma	Not measured	Increase, then decrease	Not measured

[a] One subject.

occur within hours of onset of weight-lessness. Aldosterone first decreases and then increases as the system responds to sodium loss. Urinary aldosterone, on the other hand, increased in both Skylab and the Space Shuttle flight on which urine was collected, although in the latter the rate of aldosterone excretion did not increase until near the end of the 6-day mission. Plasma renin activity (angiotensin I) decreased for 48 hours and then increased (Leach et al., 1986), but during Skylab flights it increased early, then returned to preflight levels and continued to decrease for several weeks (Leach and Rambaut, 1977). During Skylab flights, plasma cortisol increased over preflight levels, but it decreased after several days during the Spacelab missions (Leach et al., 1986). Adrenocorticotropic hormone (ACTH) decreased at various times during Skylab

flights, but it increased in Spacelab. Urinary cortisol increased in both Skylab and the previously noted Shuttle flight, although in the latter flight the rate of cortisol excretion returned to preflight levels on the second day (Leach, 1987). Plasma atrial natriuretic factor (ANF) was recently found to increase early and decrease by 6 days on a Shuttle flight (Leach et al., 1987).

Postflight hormone levels generally differ from those measured during flight. ADH, measured only in urine, has been found not to change significantly, showing that the decrease in water clearance is a result of renal blood flow rather than a need for water conservation (Leach, 1977; Leach and Rambaut, 1977; Leach, 1983). Plasma levels of aldosterone have increased after Skylab, Space Shuttle, and short Salyut flights (Leach and Rambaut,

TABLE 13-3

POSTFLIGHT (LANDING DAY) CHANGES IN HORMONES INVOLVED IN REGULATION OF FLUID AND ELECTROLYTE METABOLISM

Hormone	ASTP[a]	Skylab	Shuttle	Soyuz	Salyut
ADH Urine	No change	No change	No change	Not measured	Increase
Aldosterone Plasma	No change	Increase (on next day)	Increase	Not measured	Increase (short flights); decrease (long flights)
Urine	Increase	Increase	Increase	Increase (short flights); no change (long flights)	Increase
Angiotensin I Plasma	Increase	No change	Increase	Not measured	Increase (short flights); decrease (long flights)
Cortisol Plasma	No change	No change	Increase	Increase	Increase (short flights); no change (long flights)
Urine	Increase	Increase	Increase	Increase	Increase
ACTH Plasma	Not measured	No change	Increase	Not measured	No charge
ANF Plasma	Not measured	Not measured	Increase (early); decrease (later)	Not measured	Not measured

[a] Apollo-Soyuz Test Project.

1977; Leach, 1983; Grigoriev et al., 1987), but after long Salyut flights plasma aldosterone has decreased (Kalita and Tigranyan, 1986). Postflight increases in urinary aldosterone have been consistent, indicating the need for sodium conservation (Leach, 1977; Leach and Rambaut, 1977; Leach, 1983; Gazenko, Kakurin, and Kuznetsov, 1976; Vorobyov et al., 1983). Postflight changes in plasma renin have varied considerably: angiotensin I was increased after the Apollo-Soyuz Test Project (ASTP) and Space Shuttle and short Salyut flights (Leach, 1977; Leach, 1983; Grigoriev et al., 1987), decreased after Salyut/Soyuz flights (Vorobyov et al., 1983), and remained stable after Skylab flights where G suits were worn to maintain blood pressure in the upright position. Plasma cortisol increased after Shuttle (Leach, 1984) and short Soyuz flights (Gazenko, Kakurin and Kuznetsov, 1978), but did not change after ASTP (Leach, 1977), Skylab (Leach and Rambaut, 1977), or long Salyut/Soyuz flights (Vorobyov et al., 1983). Urinary cortisol, like aldosterone, has been found to increase postflight in all programs, in response to the reimposition of gravity. Soviet investigators have found that blood levels of pressor prostaglandins decreased postflight, while those of depressor prostaglandins increased postflight (Gazenko et al., 1981).

Although the events depicted in the fluid redistribution model appear to reflect physiological adjustments to space flight reasonably well, the endocrinological findings are not yet completely understood. In particular, the predicted decrease in urinary levels of aldosterone soon after exposure to microgravity has not been observed, but plasma aldosterone did decrease during Spacelab flights (Leach et al., 1986) and after Soyuz flights (Vorobyov et al., 1983). Inflight increases in urinary aldosterone are consistent with observed losses of potassium, but not with losses of sodium, suggesting that aldosterone in-

crease compensates for another factor, such as the natriuretic factor or increased renal blood flow. Since space flight is also associated with events such as emotional stress, space adaptation syndrome, variable drug usage, gravity loads, and altered work/rest cycles, it is possible that the simultaneous adjustment of many physiological variables masks or negates certain predicted homeostatic responses to fluid shifts.

Water and electrolyte replenishment has been useful as a countermeasure against loss of fluid and electrolytes induced by space flight (Grigoriev, 1983; Bungo and Johnson, 1983). Although these countermeasures did not prevent the loss of red cell mass during the Spacelab 1 flight (Leach and Johnson, 1984), they may have partly alleviated the problem of reduced plasma volume upon landing, which is thought to be a cause of orthostatic intolerance postflight (Bungo and Johnson, 1983). Vigorous isotonic and isometric exercise regimens appear to offer multiple benefits as countermeasures, and may diminish the loss of electrolytes and metabolites associated with changes in mineral metabolism (Tipton, 1983). Lower body negative pressure has also been used successfully by cosmonauts prior to reentry, to relieve problems caused by fluid redistribution (Grigoriev, 1983).

STRESS

Plasma levels of human growth hormone (HGH), an indicator of stress, increased in Skylab crewmembers in the first few days of flight (Table 13-4). Urinary cortisol was increased throughout these flights (Leach and Rambaut, 1977). Increases in plasma HGH, cortisol, ACTH, and aldosterone; urinary aldosterone, cortisol, epinephrine, and norepinephrine (Table 13-5); and serum creatine phosphokinase, lactic acid

TABLE 13-4

INFLIGHT CHANGES IN VARIOUS HORMONES

Hormone	Skylab	Shuttle
Plasma		
HGH	Increase (first few days)	Not measured
Insulin	Decrease (after 2 weeks)	Not measured
PTH	No change	Not measured
Catecholamines	Decrease	Not measured
Urine		
Catecholamines	No change	No change[a]

[a] One subject.

dehydrogenase, and gamma-glutamyl transpeptidase have been observed after Space Shuttle flights, indicating that Shuttle crewmembers are subject to stress (Leach, 1983). These parameters usually returned to preflight levels within 2 weeks after landing. Soviet investigators have also reported increased catecholamine levels in blood and urine of cosmonauts, and increased excretion of cortisol and aldosterone after landing (Table 13-5) (Vorobyov et al., 1983). It was suggested that the sympathoadrenal and adrenal glucocorticoid systems are activated postflight for readaptation to gravity.

LOSS OF BODY MASS

It is important to understand the mechanism of weight loss during flight, in order to establish correct nutritional and exercise requirements. The average total body weight loss for Skylab crewmembers was 2.7 kg, 1.5 kg of which was attributed to loss of lean body mass (including 1.1 kg body water) (Leonard, Leach, and Rambaut, 1983). The remainder of the loss was calculated to be derived from fat stores. Most of the loss of lean body mass occurred during the first month of flight, while total body mass continued to decrease throughout flights as long as 84

days. This study suggested that appropriate diet and exercise should reduce weight loss, and that maintenance of a positive energy balance should minimize loss of body fat.

Thyroxine is thought to be an important regulator of cellular energy production. It has not been measured in inflight samples, but was found to increase after Skylab and Salyut (Kalita and Tigranyan, 1986) flights (Table 13-5). An increase in this hormone would cause increased oxygen consumption, heat production, and metabolism of protein, carbohydrates, and fats. Oxygen consumption did in fact increase significantly during Skylab flights (Michel et al., 1977). In the first few days of flight, blood glucose increased slightly, but soon decreased below preflight levels and remained low for the rest of the flight (Leach, Altchuler, and Cintron-Trevino, 1983). Decreased plasma cholesterol after flight (Alexander, Leach, and Fischer, 1975; Leach and Rambaut, 1977) is consistent with an inflight increase in thyroxine, which is also believed to increase the rate of metabolism of cholesterol to cholic acid (Williams and Glomset, 1968). Increases in thyroid-stimulating hormone have also been noted postflight (Table 13-5) (Leach and Rambaut, 1977; Leach, 1983).

Catecholamines are known to play an

important role in metabolic regulation by increasing the rate of energy utilization and mobilizing stored fuels in metabolizing tissues (Young and Landsberg, 1979). Plasma levels of epinephrine and norepinephrine decreased during the final Skylab flight (Leach, 1981), but urinary catecholamine levels did not change significantly during Skylab flights or in the Shuttle inflight urine collection experiment (Table 13-4). It is not clear whether changes in plasma catecholamines have significant effects on metabolism during flight.

Part of the loss of lean body mass is believed to result from muscle atrophy. Early in the history of manned space flight, significant decrements in muscle tone and strength and physical work capacity were observed during and immediately after missions (Thornton and Rummel, 1977). Biochemical measurements provided evidence that this deconditioning is caused largely by increased degradation of muscle tissue. The six crewmembers of the first two Skylab flights showed a negative inflight nitrogen balance (-4.5 grams per day) and decreases in total body potassium (Whedon et al., 1977). An increase in plasma amino acids has been observed in cosmonauts after flight (Ushakov and Vlasova, 1976). Excretion of creatinine, sar-

cosine, and 3-methylhistidine occurred during Skylab flights (Leach, Rambaut, and DiFerrante, 1979), an indication that the contractile proteins of skeletal muscle are degraded in weightlessness.

The rate of protein turnover in skeletal muscle is believed to be influenced by insulin, thyroxine, and growth hormone (Lemon and Nagle, 1981). Plasma insulin decreased during most Skylab flights (Table 13-4) (Leach, Altchuler, and Cintron-Trevino, 1983), and decreased insulin favors catabolism. (Changes in thyroxine and growth hormone concurrent with space flight are discussed above.)

A high correlation ($r=.79$) between methylhistidine and cortisol excretion during Skylab missions indicated that cortisol probably plays a role in muscle degradation during space flight (Leach, Rambaut, and DiFerrante, 1979). Increased plasma and urinary cortisol during Skylab flights were concurrent with decreases in plasma insulin (Table 13-4) (Leach, Altchuler, and Cintron-Trevino, 1983).

CHOLESTEROL BIOCHEMISTRY

Blood levels of cholesterol in Apollo and Skylab astronauts were significantly decreased after flight (Alexander, Leach, and

TABLE 13-5

POSTFLIGHT (LANDING DAY) CHANGES IN VARIOUS HORMONES

Hormone	ASTP[a]	Skylab	Shuttle	Salyut / Soyuz
Plasma				
HGH	Increase	Increase	No change	No change
Insulin	Increase	No change	Increase	Increase
PTH	Not measured	No change	Not measured	Not measured
T_3	Not measured	Decrease	No change	No change
T_4	Not measured	Increase	Increase	Increase
TSH	No change	Increase	Increase	No change
Urine				
Catecholamines	Decrease in norepinephrine	Increase	Increase	Increase

[a] Apollo-Soyuz Test Project.

Fischer, 1975; Leach and Rambaut, 1977). In the Space Shuttle Program, lipoprotein carriers of cholesterol were measured for the first time (Leach et al., 1988). Total cholesterol, triglycerides, high density lipoprotein (HDL) cholesterol, low density lipoprotein (LDL) cholesterol, and very low density lipoprotein (VLDL) cholesterol were measured before flight and immediately after landing. Of these, only HDL cholesterol changed significantly, decreasing by 13 percent. In blood samples drawn 3-23 days after landing, HDL cholesterol was still significantly different from preflight levels. These changes noted after Shuttle flights of several days are not thought to have clinical significance, but because of the association between cholesterol carriers and heart disease, these compounds should continue to be measured, especially after longer space flights.

in plasma albumin throughout Skylab flights indicate that ionized calcium is increased, but bound calcium is decreased in the blood during space flight (Leach, 1981).

The precise cause of bone mineral loss during weightlessness is not known. No change in plasma levels of parathyroid hormone (which stimulates calcium resorption) was found in Skylab crewmembers (Table 13-4) (Leach and Rambaut, 1977). High levels of cortisol, which was increased in plasma and urine during Skylab flights (Table 13-3), have been reported to cause bone mineral loss and negative calcium balance in humans (Kimberg, 1969); this may be the mechanism by which the calcium changes occur, since cortisol levels generally seem to be proportional to the rate of calcium loss.

CALCIUM METABOLISM

Loss of calcium in urine has been observed after most long space flights. Calcium balance studies showed that at least 200 mg of calcium were lost per day of flight by Skylab astronauts (Whedon et al., 1977). Mineral content of the calcaneus (heel bone) decreased by as much as 7.9 percent (Rambaut and Johnston, 1979), and urinary hydroxyproline increased 47 percent above preflight levels after 84 days of flight (Leach, 1981).

Bone is the body's main calcium reservoir, and it is in equilibrium with serum calcium. Since fecal and urinary calcium continued to increase during Skylab flights despite constant dietary intake of calcium, calcium losses are thought to result from losses of bone mineral (Rambaut and Johnston, 1979). Phosphorus balance was also consistent with increased bone resorption (Rambaut and Johnston, 1979). An increase in serum calcium and decrease

RENAL FUNCTION

Renal function has not yet been studied directly during or after space flight, but creatinine clearance has been used as an estimate of glomerular filtration rate (GFR). Inflight measurement of creatinine clearance in Skylab crewmembers indicated that GFR increased during flight (Leach, 1981). Free-water clearance, which indicates the responsiveness of the kidney collecting duct epithelium to ADH, was slightly decreased from preflight clearance (Leach, 1981). Together with decreased ADH excretion (observed in Skylab astronauts), this may reflect increased sensitivity of the renal tubule to ADH (Leach et al., 1983). Increased resorption of water might be related to increased GFR.

Serum uric acid decreased after Apollo, Skylab, and Shuttle flights (Alexander et al., 1975; Leach and Rambaut, 1977; Leach, 1983), while blood urea nitrogen increased after the same flights; these findings may indicate a change in renal function, as well as tissue changes.

Studies to determine renal artery pressure, blood flow, and glomerular filtration rate are planned to understand the effects of weightlessness on kidney function.

IN-FLIGHT PHARMACOKINETICS

The above observations that a wide range of physiological and biochemical changes occur during space flight suggest that these changes may alter the kinetics and dynamics of drugs administered to crewmembers during flight. While the need for elucidating such changes had been recognized, technical and operational constraints of the multiple blood sampling required for these studies limited their implementation during space flight. For this reason, the usefulness of salivary concentration profiles as an alternate noninvasive method for clinical monitoring of certain drugs was investigated. The feasibility of such an application of saliva drug levels depends upon the distribution of detectable levels into saliva and establishment of a consistent saliva/plasma (S/P) ratio over the entire disposition profile of the drug (Graham, 1982; Danohof and Breimer, 1978). In an attempt to determine the applicability of noninvasive salivary drug monitoring for pharmacokinetics and pharmacodynamic evaluation of therapeutic agents during Shuttle missions, three drugs that are frequently used by crewmembers were selected for inflight study: acetaminophen, a common pain relief medication whose disposition characteristics are well established; scopolamine, a drug currently used for the symptomatic relief of space adaptation syndrome; and dextroamphetamine, given in combination with scopolamine during missions.

Ground-based investigations to establish the S/P ratios of acetaminophen and scopolamine were conducted in normal subjects. Following oral administration, both acetaminophen and scopolamine were shown to distribute into saliva with consistent S/P ratios (Cintron et al., 1985; Putcha et al., 1986). Pharmacokinetic evaluation and bioavailability estimations of these drugs using saliva and plasma concentration data were in good agreement. Based on these results, salivary pharmacokinetics of acetaminophen (650 mg) and scopolamine/dextroamphetamine (0.4/5 mg) during space flight were evaluated following oral administration to crewmembers before and during missions.

Significant changes in the concentration profiles were observed during space flight (Cintron et al., 1987a; Cintron et al., 1987b). These changes were more pronounced during the absorption phase of the profile than during the elimination phase. Rate of absorption and time to reach peak saliva concentration calculated from preflight and inflight data indicate that there is a significant decrease in the absorption rate of acetaminophen during flight. There is a resultant twofold increase in the time to reach peak concentration during flight. Elimination rate of the drug, however, did not change significantly. Scopolamine analysis of a limited number of samples from inflight studies also suggests that detectable changes in saliva concentration-time profiles of scopolamine occur during missions. Collectively these results support predictions that changes in drug dynamics may occur during flight as a result of the physiologic condition of crewmembers. Such changes in the pharmacokinetics of drugs administered to crewmembers during a mission may result in ineffective therapeutic responses or unexpected side effects.

The limited inflight data accumulated thus far are inadequate for characterization of the degree and magnitude of and the mechanisms underlying space flight-induced pharmacokinetic changes because of a number of interfering variables influencing the disposition profiles and kinetic parameter estimates of drugs. While information about some of these variables (e.g., mission day) is available, information about such factors as the incidence of motion sickness, ingestion of other medications during the flight, and the overall physical and physiological responses of each participating crewmember to microgravity are unavailable. A thorough and comprehensive evaluation of inflight pharmacokinetics of drugs under controlled experimental conditions is planned for future Spacelab missions, where some of the factors contributing to the variability in data can be monitored, if not controlled. The information thus obtained can be applied not only to predict the therapeutic consequences of operationally critical drugs administered to crewmembers during flight, but also to identify and describe alterations in key processes within the body that are relevant to overall metabolic homeostasis in man.

SUMMARY

Weightlessness produces a number of changes in blood, and in fluid and electrolyte balance. The cephalad shift of fluids and the resulting transient increase in central blood volume initiate a series of compensatory mechanisms. A decrease in red cell mass appears to be caused by random removal of red cells by the reticuloendothelial system. After a 30- to 60-day delay, the red cell mass begins a partial recovery, even if exposure to weightlessness continues. Recovery appears to be incomplete even after 6 months of continuous exposure. Reduction of plasma volume is probably accomplished by decreased fluid intake and loss of fluid through the urine. Loss of electrolytes persists throughout flight, but conservation of fluid and electrolytes seems to begin immediately upon return to Earth's gravity. Changes in the levels of hormones involved in control of fluid and electrolyte metabolism have sometimes been inconsistent with the effects of weightlessness on serum electrolyte levels and fluid excretion. Some of these hormones are also affected by physical and emotional stresses present during space flight, and it is possible that the effects of these factors mask predicted homeostatic responses. Body weight reduction in flight results from loss of fluid, lean body mass, and fat stores. Weightlessness-induced changes in levels of hormones such as thyroxine, insulin, catecholamines, and cortisol may affect metabolism of protein, carbohydrates, and fats, thus helping to bring about body mass loss. Cortisol also plays a role in bone mineral loss. Indirect studies of renal function during space flight indicate that glomerular filtration rate may increase during weightless conditions, and more direct studies are in progress. Changes in the rate of absorption of acetaminophen and scopolamine during Space Shuttle flights suggest that physiological and biochemical changes may affect pharmacodynamics of drugs administered to crewmembers.

REFERENCES

Alexander, W.C., Leach, C.S., and Fischer, C.L. Clinical biochemistry. In: Biomedical results of Apollo (NASA SP-368). Edited by R.S. Johnston, L.F. Dietlein, and C.A. Berry. U.S. Government Printing Office, Washington, D.C., 1975.

Anonymous. Basic medical results of the flights of the Soyuz-13, Soyuz-14 (Salyut-3) and Soyuz-15 spacecraft. Translated into English from Osnovnyye meditsinskiye rezultaty poletov kosmicheskikh korabley Soyuz-13, Soyuz-14 (Salyut-3) and

Soyuz-15. Moscow, Academy of Sciences, USSR, 1974. NASA TT F-16,054, 1974.

Balakhovskiy, I.S., Legen'kov, V.I., and Kiselev, R.K. Changes in hemoglobin mass during real and simulated space flights. Space Biology and Aerospace Medicine, 14(6):14–20, 1980.

Bessis, M., Weed, R., and LeBlond, P. Red cell shape. New York: Springer-Verlag, Inc., 1973.

Blomqvist, C.G., Nixon, J.V., Johnson, R.L., Jr., and Mitchell, J.H. Early cardiovascular adaptation to zero gravity simulated by head-down tilt. Acta Astronautica, 7:543–553, 1980.

Bungo, M.W., and Johnson, P.C., Jr. Cardiovascular examinations and observations of deconditioning during the Space Shuttle orbital flight test program. Aviation, Space, and Environmental Medicine, 54:1001–1004, 1983.

Cintron, N.M., Putcha, L., and Vanderploeg, J.M. Salivary concentrations for clinical drug monitoring of scopolamine. Annual Meeting of Aerospace Medical Association, 1985.

Cintron, N.M., Putcha, L., and Vanderploeg, J.M. Inflight pharmacokinetics of acetaminophen in saliva. In: Results of the Life Sciences DSOs Conducted Aboard the Space Shuttle 1981-1986. Edited by M.W. Bungo, T. Bagian, M.A. Bowman, and B.M. Levitan. Space Biomedical Research Institute, Johnson Space Center, Houston, Texas, 1987a.

Cintron, N.M., Putcha, L., and Vanderploeg, J.M. Inflight salivary pharmacokinetics of scopolamine and dextroamphetamine. In: Results of the Life Sciences DSOs Conducted Aboard the Space Shuttle 1981-1986. Edited by M.W. Bungo, T. Bagian, M.A. Bowman, and B.M. Levitan. Space Biomedical Research Institute, Johnson Space Center, Houston, Texas, 1987b.

Cogoli, A. Hematological and immunological changes during space flight. Acta Astronautica, 1981, 8:995–1002.

Danohof, M., and Breimer, D.D. Therapeutic drug monitoring in saliva. Clin. Pharmacokinet. 3:39–57, 1978.

Fischer, C.L., Johnson, P.C., and Berry, C.A. Red blood cell mass and plasma volume changes in manned space flight. Journal of the American Medical Association, 200:579–583, 1967.

Gauer, O.H. and Henry, J.P. Circulatory basis of fluid volume control. Physiological Reviews, 43:423–481, 1963.

Gazenko, O.G. (Ed.) Summaries of reports of the Sixth All Soviet Union Conference on Space Biology and Medicine. Vol. I and II. Kaluga, USSR, 5–7 June, 1979.

Gazenko, O.G., Genin, A.M., and Egorov, A.D. Major medical results of the Salyut-6/Soyuz 185-day space flight (NASA NDB 2747). Proceedings of the XXXII Congress of the International Astronautical Federation, Volume II, Rome, Italy, 6–12 September, 1981.

Gazenko, O.G., Kakurin, L.I., and Kuznetsov, A.G. (Eds.) Space flights in the Soyuz spacecraft. Biomedical research. Translated into English from Kosmicheskiye polety na korablyakh "Soyuz." Biomeditsinskiye issledovaniya. Moscow, Nauka Press, 1976. NASA TT F-17524, 1977.

Graham, G.C. Non-invasive clinical methods of estimating pharmacokinetic parameters. Pharma. Ther. 18:333–349, 1982.

Grigoriev, A.I. Correction of changes in fluid-electrolyte metabolism in manned space flights. Aviation, Space, and Environmental Medicine, 54:318–323, 1983.

Grigoriev, A.I., Popova, I.A., and Ushakov, A.S. Metabolic and hormonal status of crewmembers in short-term space flights. Aviation, Space, and Environmental Medicine, 58 (Suppl.):A121–125, 1987.

Guseva, Ye.V., and Tashpulatov, R.Yu. Effects of flights differing in duration on protein composition of cosmonauts' blood. Space Biology and Aerospace Medicine, 14(1):15–20, 1980.

Johnson, P.C. Hematology/immunology (M110 series). Part C: Blood volume and red cell life span (M113). In: Skylab medical experiments altitude test (SMEAT) (NASA TM X-58115). Johnson Space Center, Houston, Texas, 1973.

Johnson, P.C. The erythropoietic effects of weightlessness. In: Current concepts in erythropoiesis. Edited by C.D.R. Dunn. New York, John Wiley and Sons Ltd., 1983.

Johnson, P.C., Driscoll, T.B., and Huntoon, C.L. Iron kinetics during exposure to microgravity. Aviation, Space, and Environmental Medicine, 56:482, 1985.

Johnson, P.C., Driscoll, T.B., and LeBlanc, A.D. Blood volume changes. In: Biomedical results from Skylab (NASA SP-377). Edited by R.S. Johnston and L.F. Dietlein. U.S. Government Printing Office, Washington, D.C., 1977.

Kalita, N.F., and Tigranyan, R.A. Endocrine status of cosmonauts following long-term space missions. Space Biology and Aerospace Medicine, 20(4):84–86, 1986.

Kimberg, D.V. Effects of vitamin D and steroid hormones on the active transport of calcium by the intestine. New England Journal of Medicine, 280:1396–1405, 1969.

Kimzey, S.L. Hematology and immunology studies. In: Biomedical results from Skylab (NASA SP-377). Edited by R.S. Johnston and L.F. Dietlein. U.S. Government Printing Office, Washington, D.C., 1977.

Kimzey, S. L., Fischer, C.L., Johnson, P.C., Ritzmann, S.E., and Mengel, C.E. Hematology and immunology studies. In: Biomedical results of Apollo (NASA SP-368). Edited by R.S. Johnston, L.F.

Dietlein, and C.A. Berry, U.S. Government Printing Office, Washington, D.C., 1975.

Kimzey, S.L., and Johnson, P.C. Hematological and immunological studies. In: The Apollo-Soyuz Test Project medical report (NASA SP-411). Edited by A.E. Nicogossian. U.S. Government Printing Office, Washington, D.C., 1977.

Kirsch, K.A., Haenel, F., and Rocker, L. Venous pressure in microgravity. Naturwissenschaften, 73:447–449, 1986.

Leach, C.S. Biochemistry and endocrinology results. In: The Apollo-Soyuz Test Project medical report (NASA SP-411). Edited by A.E. Nicogossian. U.S. Government Printing Office, Washington, D.C., 1977.

Leach, C.S. A review of the consequences of fluid and electrolyte shifts in weightlessness. Acta Astronautica, 6:1123–1135, 1979.

Leach, C.S. An overview of the endocrine and metabolic changes in manned space flight. Acta Astronautica, 8:977–986, 1981.

Leach, C.S. Medical results from STS 1–4: Analysis of body fluids. Aviation, Space, and Environmental Medicine, 54 (Supp. 1):S50–S54, 1983.

Leach, C.S. Biochemical and endocrine changes. 55th Annual Scientific Meeting, Aerospace Medical Association, San Diego, CA, May 6–10, 1984.

Leach, C.S. Fluid control mechanisms in weightlessness. Aviation, Space, and Environmental Medicine, 58 (Suppl):A74–A79, 1987.

Leach, C.S., Altchuler, S.I., and Cintron-Trevino, N.M. The endocrine and metabolic responses to space flight. Medicine and Science in Sports and Exercise, 15:432–440, 1983.

Leach, C.S., Chen, J.P., Crosby, W., Dunn, C.D.R., Johnson, P.C., Lange, R.D., Larkin, E., and Tavassoli, M. Spacelab 1 hematology experiment (1NS103): Influence of space flight on erythrokinetics in man (NASA TM-58268). Johnson Space Center, Houston, TX, 1985.

Leach, C.S., and Johnson, P.C. Influence of space flight on erythrokinetics in man. Science, 225:216–218, 1984.

Leach, C.S., Johnson, P.C., and Cintron, N.M. The regulation of fluid and electrolyte metabolism in weightlessness. Proceedings of the 2nd International Conference on Space Physiology, Toulouse, France, November 20–22, 1985 (ESA SP-237), Paris: European Space Agency, pp. 31–36, 1986.

Leach, C.S., Johnson, P.C., and Cintron, N.M. The endocrine system in space flight. Acta Astronautica 17:161–166, December, 1987.

Leach, C.S., Johnson, P.C., Krauhs, J.M. and Cintron, N.M. Cholesterol in Serum Lipoprotein Fractions after Space Flight. Aviation, Space, and Environmental Medicine, 59:1034–1037, 1988.

Leach, C.S., Johnson, P.C., and Suki, W.N. Current concepts of space flight induced changes in hor-

monal control of fluid and electrolyte metabolism. The Physiologist, 26 (Supp.):S-24-S-27, 1983.

Leach, C.S., and Rambaut, P.C. Biochemical responses of the Skylab crewmen: An overview. In: Biomedical results from Skylab (NASA SP-377). Edited by R.S. Johnston and L.F. Dietlein. U.S. Government Printing Office, Washington, D.C., 1977.

Leach, C.S., Rambaut, P.C., and DiFerrante, N. Amino aciduria in weightlessness. Acta Astronautica, 6:1323–1333, 1979.

Legen'kov, V.I., Kiselev, R.K., Gudim, V.I., and Moskaleva, G.P. Changes in peripheral blood of crewmembers of the Salyut-4 orbital station. Space Biology and Aerospace Medicine, 11(6):1–12, 1977.

Lemon, P.W.R., and Nagle, F.J. Effects of exercise on protein and amino acid metabolism. Medicine and Science in Sports and Exercise, 13:141–149, 1981.

Leonard, J.I., Leach, C.S., and Rambaut, P.C. Quantitation of tissue loss during prolonged space flight. American Journal of Clinical Nutrition, 38:667–679, 1983.

Mengel, C.E. Red cell metabolism studies on Skylab. In: Biomedical results from Skylab (NASA SP-377). Edited by R.S. Johnston and L.F. Dietlein. U.S. Government Printing Office, Washington, D.C., 1977.

Michel, E.L., Rummel, J.A., Sawin, C.F., Buderer, M.C., and Lem, J.D. Results of Skylab medical experiment M171—metabolic activity. In: Biomedical results from Skylab (NASA SP-377). Edited by R.S. Johnston and L.F. Dietlein. U.S. Government Printing Office, Washington, D.C., 1977.

Putcha, L., Cintron, N.M., Vanderploeg, J.M., Chen, Y., and Dardano, J.R. Comparative concentration profiles of acetaminophen in plasma and saliva of normal subjects. World Conference Clinical Pharmacology and Therapeutics, Stockholm, Sweden, August, 1986.

Rambaut, P.C., and Johnston, R.S. Prolonged weightlessness and calcium loss in man. Acta Astronautica, 6:1113–1122, 1979.

Rowe, J.W., Shelton, R.L., Helderman, J.H., Vestal, R.E., and Robertson, G.L. Influence of the emetic reflex on vasopressin release in man. Kidney International, 16:729–735, 1979.

Taylor, G.R. and Dardano, J.R. Human cellular immune responsiveness following space flight. Aviation, Space, and Environmental Medicine, 54 (Supp. 1):S55–S59, 1983.

Thornton, W.E., and Ord, J. Physiological mass measurements in Skylab. In: Biomedical results from Skylab (NASA SP-377). Edited by R.S. Johnston and L.F. Dietlein. U.S. Government Printing Office, Washington, D.C., 1977.

Thornton, W.E., and Rummel, J.A. Muscular deconditioning and its prevention in space flight. In:

Biomedical results from Skylab (NASA SP-377). Edited by R.S. Johnston and L.F. Dietlein. U.S. Government Printing Office, Washington, D.C., 1977.

Tipton, C.M. Considerations for exercise prescriptions in future space flights. Medicine and Science in Sports and Exercise, 15:441–444, 1983.

Ushakov, A.S. Nutrition during long flight. Translated into English from Zdorov'ye, 4(304):4–5, 1980, NASA TM-76436, 1981.

Ushakov, A.S., and Vlasova, T.F. Free amino acids in human blood plasma during space flights. Aviation, Space, and Environmental Medicine, 47:1061–1064, 1976.

Vorobyov, E.I., Gazenko, O.G., Shulzenko, Ye.B., Grigoriev, A.I., Barer, A.S., Yegorov, A.D., and Skiba, I.A. Preliminary results of medical investigations during 5-month space flight aboard Salyut-7 Soyuz-T orbital complex. Space Biology and Aerospace Medicine, 20 (2):27–34, 1986.

Vorobyov, E.I., Gazenko, O.G., Genin, A.M., and Egorov, A.D. Medical results of Salyut-6 manned space flights. Aviation, Space, and Environmental Medicine, 54 (Supp. 1):S31–S40, 1983.

Voss, E.W., Jr. Prolonged weightlessness and humoral immunity. Science, 225:214–215, 1984.

Whedon, G.D., Lutwak, L., Rambaut, P.C., Whittle, M.W., Smith, M.C., Reid, J., Leach, C., Stadler, C.R., and Sanford, D.D. Mineral and nitrogen metabolic studies, experiment M071. In: Biomedical results from Skylab (NASA SP-377). Edited by R.S. Johnston and L.F. Dietlein. U.S. Government Printing Office, Washington, D.C., 1977.

Williams, R.H., and Glomset, J.A. Lipid metabolism and lipopathies. In: Textbook of Endocrinology, 4th ed. Edited by R.H. Williams, Philadelphia: W.B. Saunders Co., 1968.

Yegorov, A.D. Results of medical research during the 175-day flight of the third main crew on the Salyut-6-Soyuz orbital complex. Translated into English from Rezultaty meditsinskikh issledovaniy vo vremya 175-sutochnogo poleta tretyego osnovnogo ekipazha na orbitalnom komplekse Salyut-6-Soyuz. Moscow: USSR Academy of Sciences, 1980. NASA TM-76450, 1981.

Young, J.B., and Landsberg, L. Catecholamines and the sympathoadrenal system: The regulation of metabolism. In: Contemporary Endocrinology, Vol. 1, Edited by S.H. Ingbar. New York, Plenum Medical Book Co., 1979.

14 Microgravity: Simulations and Analogs

ARNAULD E. NICOGOSSIAN
LAWRENCE F. DIETLEIN

In Earth's gravity, it is only possible to duplicate the microgravity of space for brief periods (30 to 40 seconds) during Keplerian aircraft maneuvers. Despite this handicap, ground-based simulations and analogs have yielded a great deal of information concerning the acclimation of humans to microgravity, providing much insight into the expected responses of various human body systems to extended space flight. One commonly utilized analog is hypokinesia, induced by prolonged confinement to bed or chair, water immersion, or immobilization. Additional ground-based techniques such as dehydration and *in vitro* rotation of cells have been utilized to investigate certain physiological alterations associated with microgravity. This chapter describes a number of these analogs or techniques, and summarizes the advantages and disadvantages of each.

BED REST

The most widely used analog for microgravity is bed rest. The technique has been in use for decades, in hundreds of studies performed to determine the physiological effects of prolonged horizontal posture (Nicogossian et al., 1979). U.S. and international research (up to 1980) on the effects of bed rest on major body systems has been critically reviewed by Nicogossian (1980). Although prolonged bed rest cannot be considered a true simulation of microgravity since the influence of gravity is obviously still present (only parabolic flight is a true simulation), it does induce many physiological changes that are remarkably similar to those observed in space: muscle atrophy, bone demineralization, redistribution of fluids and body mass, and decreases in plasma volume and red blood cell (RBC) mass (Genin, 1977; Sandler, 1976). Cardiovascular changes include decreases in cardiac output, stroke volume, heart size, and end diastolic volume. Following bed rest, subjects exhibit decreased orthostatic tolerance similar to that typically demonstrated by returning astronauts Sandler and Vernikos, 1986.

Although the physiological effects of bed rest are in most respects qualitatively similar to those of microgravity, there are some notable differences. For example, bone mineral losses appear to be more severe during space flight (Rambaut and Johnston, 1979), and while diuresis is common during the early days of bed rest, it has not yet been clearly demonstrated in space flight (Greenleaf, Shvartz, and Keil, 1981). In addition, bed rest does not produce the full range of aberrant vestibular signs and symptoms characteristic of space flight, although vestibular disturbances that could be attributable to "deconditioning" are observed (Kotovskaya, Gavrilova, and Galle, 1981).

BED REST WITH HEAD-DOWN TILT

Soviet scientists have demonstrated that bed rest with head-down tilt (antiorthostatic position) elicits some of the early physiological effects of microgravity with greater fidelity than horizontal bed rest (Kakurin, et al., 1976). In particular, head-down tilt results in more rapid and pronounced fluid shifts, along with related symptoms of facial puffiness, nasal congestion, fullness of the head, and "sensory realignments" similar to those experienced by cosmonauts. Table 14-1 compares clinical symptomatology experienced by subjects during the recumbent posture and various degrees of head-down tilt. Although the head-down position results in more pronounced fluid shifts, selective catheterization studies indicate that the shifts are not accompanied by a persistent increase in central venous pressure (Katkov, et al., 1979; Nixon, et al., 1979).

In a joint 7-day bed rest study American and Soviet scientists compared the effects

TABLE 14–1

CLINICAL SYMPTOMS DURING HORIZONTAL POSTURE AND HEAD-DOWN TILT

Symptoms	Bed Rest Position			
	0°	−4°	−8°	−12°
Lowered taste and olfactory sensitivity threshold	−	+	+	+ +
Sensation of blood rushing to and heaviness in the head	−	+	+	+ +
Nasal congestion	−	+	+ +	+ + +
Uncomfortable feeling in the nose and throat, hoarse voice	−	+	+	+ +
Increase in intranasal resistance	+	+	+ +	+ + +
Vertigo and nausea	−	−	+	+
Spatial illusions	−	−	+	+ +
Nystagmus of eyes	−	−	+	+ +
Facial puffiness and overfilling of sclera and conjunctiva vessels	−	+	+ +	+ +
Sensation of fullness in the eyes, fatigue in the eyes in reading, drop in central sight acuity	−	+	+ +	+ +

Kakurin et al., 1976.
− = Symptoms absent
+ = Symptoms present (+ +, + + + = pronounced symptoms)

of the horizontal and −6° head-down positions (Gazenko and Grigor'yev, 1980; Joint U.S./U.S.S.R. Hypokinesia Program, 1979). Results of this study indicated that the two treatments have similar physiological effects, but that the head-down position results in more pronounced cardiac deconditioning as measured by post-bed rest lower body negative pressure (LBNP) and exercise tolerance tests.

SHUTTLE FLIGHT SIMULATIONS

A number of studies conducted in preparation for the first Space Shuttle flights exposed subjects to 10 to 15 days of bed rest followed by centrifuge runs of up to +3 Gz. These simulations provided valuable data concerning physiological changes in men and women of varying ages and their tolerance to post-bed rest acceleration (Goldwater, et al., 1978; Jacobson, et al., 1974; Leverett, et al., 1971; Miller and Leverett, 1965; Montgomery, et al., 1979; Newsom, et al., 1977; Sandler, 1980; Sandler, et al., 1978, 1979). The investigators concluded that tolerance to +Gz acceleration degrades after bed rest, primarily because of the reduction in plasma volume. Male subjects, especially in the older groups, appear to tolerate postbed rest centrifugation runs up to +3 Gz with fewer adverse effects than females or younger subjects.

Studies utilizing Shuttle flight simulations have helped to identify population risk factors in men and women of various age groups, and test the efficacy of such countermeasures as electrolyte and fluid replenishments, antigravity suits, exercise, and periodic application of acceleration and LBNP during bed rest. Such simulations can also be used to investigate the cumulative effects of repeated short-term space flights.

CHAIR REST

Although few studies have utilized prolonged chair rest as an analog for microgravity, it appears that this treatment modality results in many of the same physiological decrements as bed rest, namely, loss of plasma volume, decreased RBC mass, and cardiovascular deconditioning (Lamb, et al., 1964; Lamb, 1965). Although not so pronounced as with bed rest, the changes are nonetheless puzzling, since headward fluid shifts are absent. It is possible that decreased metabolic loads secondary to inactivity may be a factor in the etiology of cardiovascular deconditioning in both bed rest and space.

WATER IMMERSION

Water immersion has been used as an analog for microgravity by a number of investigators interested primarily in acute renal and circulatory changes associated with space flight (Gauer, 1975, Epstein, 1978). Immersion results in rapid fluid shifts secondary to changes in hydrostatic forces and negative pressure breathing. Immersion is followed rapidly by a pronounced involuntary diuresis, with loss of electrolytes and decrease in plasma volume. These events may be triggered by activation of cardiac stretch receptors and suppression of antidiuretic hormone (the Gauer-Henry reflex); there is also evidence that early hemodilution and suppression of vasopressin play a role (Greenleaf, Shvartz and Keil, 1981). Studies on immersed animals, however, suggest that other pathways may be involved (Gilmore and Zucker, 1978).

Characteristics of the diuretic response are influenced by, and exquisitely sensitive to, the subject's state of hydration

(Gauer, 1975; Leach, 1981). Normally, hydrated subjects exhibit an increase in free-water clearance, whereas dehydrated subjects show increased osmolar clearance.

Decreased orthostatic tolerance typically follows water immersion; however, the magnitude of the change depends upon the physical condition of the subject. Although diuresis occurs earlier and is more pronounced in nonathletes during water immersion, they demonstrate less degradation in orthostatic tolerance than athletes (Boening, et al., 1972; Stegemann, et al., 1975). Stegemann et al. (1975) suggest that this discrepancy can be explained by a reduction in the effectiveness of the blood pressure control system in endurance-trained subjects.

Although fluid shifts and many additional physiological responses occur rapidly during water immersion, other methods of simulating microgravity are usually preferred due to problems associated with maintaining hygiene and precise thermal control (Sandler, 1979). The problem of skin maceration makes immersion for periods in excess of 24 hours impractical; long-term studies using water immersion are therefore not feasible. To address these limitations, Soviet scientists have employed a "dry immersion" technique (Figure 14-1) in which subjects are protected from water contact by a thin plastic sheet, enabling long-term studies. Indeed, this may represent the ideal analog of microgravity, since it has been demonstrated that the physiological changes related to fluid redistribution endure longer when induced by this immersion technique (Gogolev, et al., 1980).

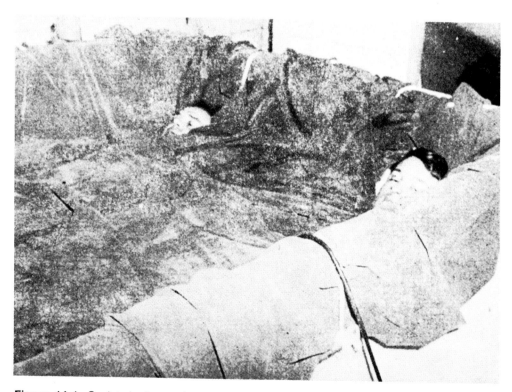

Figure 14-1. Soviet dry immersion technique for simulation of zero-gravity effects.

IMMOBILIZATION

Animal studies constitute a significant portion of the research on hypokinesia. Investigators employ partial- or whole-body casts as well as confinement in small cages to produce hypokinesia, particularly for studies of circulatory dynamics and the musculoskeletal system. For example, Dickey et al. (1979) found that primates maintained in horizontal body casts for 2 to 4 weeks exhibit many changes similar to those observed in bed-rested humans and individuals exposed to space flight: slightly increased heart rate, slightly decreased RBC mass, as well as decreased orthostatic tolerance, plasma volume, and responsiveness to vasoactive drugs. In a later study (Dickey et al., 1982), the resulting cardiovascular deconditioning was shown to be secondary to diminished effective circulating blood volume during orthostatic stress.

Some investigators, particularly in the U.S.S.R., confine animals in small cages for prolonged periods to simulate weightlessness. Although confinement does not result in fluid shifts, it does produce a number of physiological effects similar to those observed in space—particularly in the musculoskeletal system. Animal studies offer the advantage of direct observation of physiological changes. Rats confined for up to 2 months demonstrate weight loss; decreases in the size of the gastrocnemius muscle; and decreased protein content in muscle, cardiac, renal, and liver tissue (Fedorov and Shurova, 1973). Degenerative and atrophic changes are observed in mixed (soleus) and red muscle fibers (Kurash, et al., 1981). Bone demineralization is also noted in confined animals, and studies of rats suggest that excessive dietary phosphorus aggravates demineralization during hypokinesia (Ushakov, et al., 1980). Dogs confined for 6 months demonstrate a number of circulatory and skeletal abnormalities, particularly in the caudal extremities. The animals exhibit morphological alterations in the vascular network of the fascia, increased blood stasis in the bone marrow vessels, and changes in the femur and tibia indicative of dystrophic processes (Novikov and Vlasov, 1976). In rabbits, 3 to 4 weeks of confinement result in extensive enlargement and deformation of intra-organ veins (Muratikova, 1980).

PARTIAL BODY SUPPORT SYSTEMS

In order to minimize problems associated with immobilization and more accurately reproduce events occurring in space, some investigators have adopted a system of partial body support. In a typical system, the animal is attached to a harness and suspended in a head-down position, with complete unloading of the hind limbs. The front limbs do not bear weight, but can be used by the animal to maneuver itself in a circular pattern.

Studies on rats suspended in harnesses suggest that the resulting physiological changes are similar to those in space. Compared to controls, suspended rats exhibit less weight gain per gram of food consumed (Morey, 1979); decreased metabolic rate (Jordan, et al., 1980); inhibition of periosteal bone formation, particularly in older rats (Morey, 1979; Morey, et al., 1979; Novikov and Il'in, 1981); and decreased thymus size with no accompanying decrease in immunocompetence (Caren, et al., 1980). With the exception of calcium balance, most changes in fluid and electrolyte balance during the first few days of suspension appear to be similar to those observed in rats and humans in space (Meininger, et al., 1978). Preliminary cardiovascular studies suggest increased right atrial pressure, absence of diurnal variation in heart rate and mean arterial blood pressure, and increased cardiac output, all of which indicate a cephalad shift of body fluids (Popovic, cited by Morey, 1979).

Partial body support systems which align subjects at a 9.5° angle from the horizontal have been developed both by NASA (Hewes, et al., 1966) and Soviet scientists. These systems attempt to simulate the physiological changes experienced in the one-sixth gravity of the lunar surface. Studies with primates reveal alterations in motor activity, early diuresis, decreased erythropoiesis, EEG abnormalities, weight loss, and post-treatment orthostatic intolerance. Information gleaned from these simulations may be useful for planning longer-duration space flights in which some degree of artificial gravity is available, and for long-term lunar operations.

DEHYDRATION

One model primarily designed to investigate the erythropoietic effects of space flight involves dehydration (Dunn, 1978; Dunn and Lange, 1979; Dunn, Leonard, and Kimzey, 1981). Mice deprived of water for days demonstrate weight loss, reduced plasma volume, and elevated hematocrit, and decreased RBC production as estimated by ^{59}Fe incorporation into erythron. Although the suppression of erythropoiesis in hydrated animals with absolute increases in RBC volume is related to decreased production of a humoral regulator, serum titers of this substance do not change after dehydration. This indicates that the mechanisms underlying suppression of erythropoiesis differ, depending upon whether the elevated hematocrit results from an absolute or relative increase in RBC volume. Dunn

and Lange (1979) suggest that changes in RBC formation associated with dehydration, and possibly space flight, may also be related to factors such as negative energy balance. Using computer simulations, Dunn et al. (1981) conclude that the primary cause of erythropoiesis suppression in dehydrated mice is reduced food intake.

Although the mechanisms resulting in human dehydration are clearly different from those operant in laboratory mice, similar factors may mediate suppression of erythropoiesis, once dehydration occurs and plasma volume declines. For this reason, studies of dehydrated mice may yield important information about hematological changes in space.

IN VITRO SIMULATION

Several investigators have simulated reduced gravity for the *in vitro* study of cells by means of rotation. When the axis of rotation is perpendicular to the gravity vector and intersects the cell at its center, the viscosity of the cytoplasm prevents the immediate adjustment of particle distribution in response to the changing direction of gravity. At an appropriate rotation rate, a stationary distribution similar to that observed in microgravity is attained (Schatz and Teuchert, 1972). Cogoli et al. (1980) used a clinostat to produce this low-gravity environment and study its effects on lymphocytes. They found that low-gravity simulation depresses lymphocyte activation by the mitogen concanavalin A, as measured by DNA synthesis and ultrastructure changes. Compared to controls, lymphocyte activation was reduced by 50 percent in cells incubated for 3 days with the mitogen. In contrast, ultrastructural alterations in lymphocytes exposed to 4-g and 16-g indicated accelerated activation and aging. Since transient depressions of mitrogen-induced lymphocyte activation have been observed in returning astronauts and cosmonauts, this model promises to elucidate the mechanisms involved.

MATHEMATICAL MODELS AND COMPUTER SIMULATION

Another tool that biomedical researchers use to understand the function of body mechanisms and control systems in microgravity is the mathematical model. Such models represent each portion of the physiological feedback system by a mathematical expression. These expressions are combined to describe the entire physiological system of interest. The resulting model can be programmed into a computer and simulations obtained. Computer simulation output is often quite realistic, and contributes to a unique representation of real body systems. For example, a number of physiological models can be developed for the cardiovascular, respiratory, ther-

moregulatory, calcium, red blood cell production, and other systems. These models can be combined and integrated into a larger, more comprehensive whole-body model. Such whole-body models have been used to investigate the processes of adaptation to weightlessness, and in a similar fashion, help scientists understand the importance of gravity in shaping physiological function on Earth. The models have also been used to design environmental control systems for spacecraft and space suits.

While no ground-based simulation technique can precisely duplicate microgravity, studies utilizing these techniques provide important information about the acclimation process. They permit investigators to verify and extend inflight biomedical observations, develop new hypotheses for further inflight testing, and validate the efficacy of countermeasures. Since an increasingly heterogeneous population will be exposed to space flight in the Shuttle era and beyond, simulation studies allow investigators to define individual differences in response characteristics and detect potential problems in various subgroups.

REFERENCES

Boening, D., Ulmer, H.V., Meier, U., Skipka, W., and Stegemann, J. Effects of a multi-hour immersion on trained and untrained subjects: 1. Renal function and plasma volume. Aerospace Medicine, 43:300–305, 1972.

Caren, L.D., Mandel, A.D., and Nunes, J.A. Effect of simulated weightlessness on the immune system in rats. Aviat., Space, and Envir. Med., 51(3):251–255, 1980.

Chernov, I.P. The stress reaction of hypokinesia and its effect on general resistance. Space Biology and Aerospace Medicine, 14(3):86–90, 1980.

Cogoli, A., Valluchi-Morf, M., Mueller, M., and Briegler, W. Effect of hypogravity on human lymphocyte activation. Aviat., Space, and Envir. Med., 51(1):29–34, 1980.

Dickey, D.T., Billman, G.E., Teoh, K., Sandler, H., and Stone, H.L. The effects of horizontal body casting on blood volume, drug responsiveness and +Gz tolerance in the rhesus monkey. Aviat., Space, and Envir. Med., 53(2):142–146, 1982.

Dickey, D.T., Teoh, K.K., Sandler, H., and Stone, H.L. Changes in blood volume and response to vasoactive drugs in horizontally casted primates. The Physiologist, 22(6)(supplement):S27–S28, 1979.

Dunn, C.D.R. Effect of dehydration on erythropoiesis in mice: Relevance to the "anemia" of space flight. Aviat., Space, and Envir. Med., 49:990–993, 1978.

Dunn, C.D.R. and Lange, R.D. Erythropoietic effect of space flight. Acta Astronautica, 6:725–732, 1979.

Dunn, C.D.R., Leonard, J.I., and Kimzey, S.L. Interactions of animal and computer models in investigations of the "anemia" of space flight. Aviat., Space, and Envir. Med., 52(11):683–690, 1981.

Epstein, M. Renal effects on head-out water immersion in man; implications for understanding of volume homeostasis. Physiology Review, 58:529–581, 1978.

Fedorov, I.V., and Shurova, I.F. Content of protein and nucleic acids in the tissues of animals during hypokinesia. Space Biology and Medicine, 2:22–28, 1973.

Gauer, O.H. Recent advances in the study of whole body immersion. Acta Astronautica, 2:39–39, 1975.

Gazenko, O.G., and Grigor'yev, A.I. Modeling the physiological effects of weightlessness: Soviet-American Experiment. NDB 92 (NASA TM-76317). Translated into English from Vestnik Akademii nauk U.S.S.R., 2:71–75, 1980.

Genin, A.M. Laboratory simulation of the action of weightlessness on the human organism. NASA TM-75072. Translated into English from Laboratornoye modelirovaniye deystviya nevesomosti na organism cheloveka. Interkosmos Council, Academy of Sciences U.S.S.R. Report, 1–17, 1977.

Gilmore, J.P., and Zucker, I.L.H. Contribution of vagal pathways to the renal responses to head-out immersion in the nonhuman primate. Circulation Research, 42(2):263–267, 1978.

Gogolev, K.I., Aleksandrova, Ye.A., and Shul'zhenko, Ye.B. Comparative evaluation of changes in the human body during orthostatic (head-down) hypokinesia and immersion. NDB 311. Translated into English from Fiziologiya Cheloveka, 6(6):978–983, 1980.

Goldwater, D., Sandler, H., Popp, R., Danellis, J., and Montgomery, L. Exercise capacity, body composition, and hemoglobin levels of females during bed rest Shuttle flight simulation. Preprints of the Annual Scientific Meeting, Aerospace Medical Association, New Orleans LA, 1978.

Greenleaf, J.E., Shvartz, E., and Keil, L.C. Hemodilution, vasopressin suppression, and diuresis during water immersion in man. Aviat., Space, and Envir. Med., 52(6):329–336, 1981.

Hewes, D.E., Spady, A.A., and Harris, R.L. Comparative measurements of man's walking and running gaits in Earth and simulated lunar gravity (NASA TM D-3363). National Aeronautics and Space Administration, Washington, D.C., 1966.

Jacobson, L.H., Hyatt, K.H., and Sandler, H. Effects of simulated weightlessness on responses of untrained men to Gx and Gz acceleration. Journal of Applied Physiology, 36:745–762, 1974.

Joint U.S./U.S.S.R. Hypokinesia Program (NASA TM-76013). National Aeronautics and Space Administration, Washington, D.C., 1979.

Jordan, J.P., Sykes, H.A., Crownover, J.C., Schatte, C.L., Simmons, J.B., and Jordan, D.P. Simulated weightlessness: Effects of bioenergetic balance. Aviat., Space, and Envir. Med., 51(5):132–136, 1980.

Kakurin, L.I., Lobachik, V.I., Mikhailov, V.M., and Senkevich, Yu.A. Antiorthostatic hypokinesia as a method of weightlessness simulation. Aviat., Space, and Envir. Med., 47:1083–1086, 1976.

Kaplanskiy, A.S., and Durnova, G.N. Role of dynamic space flight factors in the pathogenesis of involution of lymphatic organs (experimental morphological study). Space Biology and Aerospace Medicine, 14(2):45–52, 1980.

Katkov, V.Y., Chestukhin, V.V., Zybin, O.Kh., Mikhaylov, V.M., Troshin, A.Z., and Utkin, V.N. Effect of brief head-down hypokinesia on pressure in various parts of the healthy man's cardiovascular system. Space Biology and Medicine, 13(3):86–93, 1979.

Kotovskaya, A.R., Gavrilova, L.N., and Galle, R.R. Effect of hypokinesia in head-down position on man's equilibrium function. Space Biology and Aerospace Medicine, 15(4):34–38, 1981.

Kovalev, O.A., Lysak, V.F., Severovostokova, V.I., and Sheremetevskaya, S.K. Local redistribution of blood under the effect of fixation stress against a background of hypokinesia, NDB 57 (NASA TM-76322). Translated into English from Fiziologii Zhurnal, 26(1):120–124, 1980.

Kurash, S., Andzheyevska, A., and Gurski, Ya. Morphological changes in different types of rat muscle fibers during long-term hypokinesia. Space Biology and Aerospace Medicine, 14(6):45–52, 4 February 1981.

Lamb, L.E. Hypoxia—An anti-deconditioning factor for manned space flight. Aerospace Medicine, 36(2):97–100, 1965.

Lamb, L.E., Johnson, R.L., and Stevens, P.M. Cardiovascular deconditioning during chair rest. Aerospace Medicine, 35:646, 1964.

Leach, C.A. A review of the consequences of fluid and electrolyte shifts in weightlessness. Acta Astronautica, 6:1123–1135, 1981.

Leverett, S.D., Shubrooks, S.J., and Shumate, W. Some effects of Space Shuttle reentry profiles on human subjects. Preprints of the Annual Scientific Meeting, Aerospace Medical Association, Washington, D.C., 1971.

Meininger, G.A., Deavers, D.R., and Musacchia, X.J. Electrolyte and metabolic imbalances induced by hypokinesia in the rat. Federal Proceedings, 37:633, 1978.

Miller, P.B., and Leverett, S.D. Tolerance to transverse (+Gx) and headward (+Gz) acceleration after prolonged bed rest. Aerospace Medicine, 36:13–15, 1965.

Montgomery, L.D., Goldwater, D., and Sandler, H. Hemodynamic response of men 45–55 years to

+Gz acceleration before and after bed rest. Preprints of the Annual Scientific Meeting, Aerospace Medical Association, Washington, D.C., 1979.

Morey, E.R. Space flight and bone turnover: Correlation with a new rat model of weightlessness. BioScience, 29:168–172, 1979.

Morey, E.R., Sabelman, E.E., Turner, R.T., and Baylink, D.J. A new rat model simulating some aspects of space flight. The Physiologist, 22(6) (supplement):S23–S24, 1979.

Muratikova, V.A. Effect of hypokinesia on blood vessels of the rabbit sympathetic trunk. NDB 60 (NASA TM-76328). Translated into English from Arkhiv Anatomii, Gistologii i Embriologii, 78(5):40–45, 1980.

Newsom, B.D., Goldenrath, W.L., Winter, W.L., and Sandler, H. Tolerance of females to +Gz centrifugation before and after bed rest. Aviat., Space, and Envir. Med., 48:327–331, 1977.

Nixon, J.U., Murray, R.G., Bryant, C., Johnson, Jr., R.L., Mitchel, J.H., Holland, O.B., Gomes-Sanchez, C., Vergne-Marini, P. and C.G. Blomqvist. Early cardiovascular adaptation to simulated zero gravity. J. Appl. Physiol.: Respirat. Environ. Exercise Physiol., 46(3):541–548, 1979.

Novikov, I.I. and Vlasov, V.B. Morphology of the circulatory bed of elements of the soft stroma and bones of the rear extremities of the dog upon extended hypodynamia. Biomedical and Behavioral Science, 59:9, 1976.

Novikov, V.E., and Il'in, E.A. Age-related reactions of rat bones to their unloading. Aviat., Space, and Envir. Med., 52(9):551–553, 1981.

Rambaut, P.C., and Johnston, R.S. Prolonged weightlessness and calcium loss in man. Acta Astronautica, 6:1113–1122, 1979.

Sandler, H. Cardiovascular effects of weightlessness. In: Progress in cardiology. Volume 6. Edited by P.N. Yu and R.R. Goodwin. Philadelphia, Lea and Febiger, 1976.

Sandler, H. Low-g simulation in mammalian research. The Physiologist, 22(6) (supplement):S19–S22, 1979.

Sandler, H. Effects of bed rest and weightlessness on the heart. In: Hearts and heart-like organs. Vol. II—Physiology. Edited by G.H. Bourne. New York, Academic Press, 1980.

Sandler, H., Goldwater, D.J., and Rositano, S.A. Physiologic responses of female subjects during bed rest Shuttle flight simulation. Preprints of the Annual Scientific Meeting, Aerospace Medical Association. New Orleans, LA, 1978.

Sandler, H., Goldwater, D., Rositano, S.A., Sawin, C.F., and Booher, C.R. Physiologic response of male subjects ages 46–55 years to Shuttle flight simulation. Preprints of the Annual Scientific Meeting, Aerospace Medical Association, Washington, D.C., 1979.

Sandler, H., and Vernikos, J. Inactivity: Physiological Effects. New York, Academic Press, 1986.

Schatz, A., and Teuchert, G. Effects of combined 0 g simulation and hypergravity on eggs of the nematode, Ascaris suum. Aerospace Medicine, 43(6):614–619, 1972.

Stegemann, J., Meier, U., and Skipka, W., et al. Effects of a multi-hour immersion with intermittent exercise on urinary excretion and tilt table tolerance in athletes and nonathletes. Aviat., Space, and Envir. Med., 46(1):26–29, 1975.

Ushakov, A.S., Smirnova, T.A., Pitts, G.C., Pace, N., Smith, A.H., and Rahlmann, D.F. Body composition of rats flown aboard Cosmos 1129. The Physiologist, Supplement, 23(6):S41–S44, December, 1980.

Zagorskaya, Ye.A. Corticosteroid content of rat adrenals in the presence of hypokinesia combined with graded physical exercise. Space Biology and Aerospace Medicine, 14(6):53–56, 4 February 1981.

HEALTH MAINTENANCE OF SPACE CREWMEMBERS

section V

15 Medical Evaluation for Astronaut Selection and Longitudinal Studies

SAM L. POOL

EDWARD C. MOSELEY

Candidates for astronaut selection are medically evaluated, using principles and techniques of preventive medicine to rule out serious medical risk factors and identify those individuals with maximum career potential. The system for medical evaluation employs modern diagnostic and evaluation procedures; the process is designed to assist the astronaut selection board in selecting candidates whose current state of health indicates exceptional promise in terms of the rigors of astronaut training and performance, and whose long-term health prospects are excellent.

Since NASA—and the nation—have a great investment in the training of an astronaut, the medical evaluation process is designed to ensure that this investment is not jeopardized during a normal career because of identifiable medical problems. Aside from flight medical examinations, annual medical evaluations are conducted for clinical purposes and to evaluate any long-term effects that may be associated with differential exposure to microgravity.

HISTORY OF ASTRONAUT SELECTION

DEVELOPMENT OF THE SELECTION PROCESS: 1958–1969

In November 1957, President Dwight D. Eisenhower established the President's Scientific Advisory Committee. One of the first recommendations of this committee was that the nation establish a civilian agency to pursue an aggressive program of space exploration. The White House released a paper in March 1958 listing key reasons for supporting the exploration of space. These included man's compelling drive to explore and discover, defense considerations, and national prestige. However, the committee's primary focus was on the new opportunities for scientific observation and experimentation that would broaden knowledge and understanding of the Earth, the solar system, and, ultimately, the universe.

After lengthy deliberations on Capitol Hill, the National Aeronautics and Space Act of 1958 was enacted by Congress in July of that year. Based on the work of a Space Task Group established at Langley Field, Virginia, the highest national priority for personnel selection was granted to the first manned spacecraft project, Project Mercury. Considerable effort was expended by members of the Space Task Group to determine which types of individual would function most effectively as an astronaut. Since no data were available at that time on physiological changes in space, most of the qualifications for such individuals were necessarily based on a combination of conjecture and experience with high-performance aircraft operations.

The Space Task Group, together with a Special Committee on the Life Sciences, developed a selection procedure based on what they believed the duties of an astronaut would be (Link, 1965). Simply stated, these were:

1. To survive; i.e., to demonstrate the ability of man to fly in space and to return safely
2. To perform; i.e., to demonstrate man's capacity to perform effectively under conditions of space flight
3. To serve as a backup for automatic controls and instrumentation; i.e., to increase the reliability of space systems
4. To serve as a scientific observer; i.e., to go beyond what the instruments and satellites can observe and report

5. To serve as an engineering observer and, acting as a true test pilot, to improve the flight system and its components.

The Space Task Group explored various categories of professionals to determine which vocations might furnish individuals best qualified for training and duty as astronauts. Categories considered were pilots, balloonists, submariners, deep-sea divers, mountain climbers, explorers, flight surgeons, and scientists.

By December, 1958, a set of proposed civil service standards had been drafted. It was expected that representatives from the Department of Defense and industry would nominate approximately 150 men by the end of January, 1959. Of these, 39 candidates would be selected for further testing. Subsequently, the White House stipulated that only active military test pilots would be considered for selection as astronauts. It was also decided that it would be inappropriate to jeopardize candidates' military careers should medical anomalies be discovered in the course of the stringent medical examinations intrinsic to the selection process. Therefore, such information was not to be entered on candidates' permanent medical records. Additionally, candidates were required to be graduates of test pilot school and to have at least 1,500 hours of flying time in high-performance jet aircraft.

This decision simplified the selection process considerably since it provided a known pool of applicants, each with a complete medical file at the time of application, and a medical history spanning his service career. The records of 500 individuals were subsequently reviewed, including candidates from the Air Force, Navy, Marine Corps, and Army. NASA announced in January, 1959, that 110 candidates met the basic requirements, and 69 candidates from this prescreened group reported to Washington under special military orders.

In Washington, these individuals were further screened through interviews with NASA project officials, psychiatric evaluations by two Air Force medical officers, reviews of their medical records and background, and a battery of written tests. On the basis of this initial evaluation 32 pilots were selected to undergo the second phase of evaluation.

The 32 finalists were screened with an extensive battery of medical and psychological tests, some of which were devised specifically for this purpose on the basis of the best medical judgment and state-of-the-art medical practice. Some of the most up-to-date procedures were included in the test battery; for example, exercise capacity was determined using a bicycle ergometer.

The first phase of the medical evaluation program was conducted for NASA by the Lovelace Clinic in Albuquerque, New Mexico. Each candidate spent 7.5 days undergoing detailed medical examinations at the Lovelace facility. These examinations were followed by a series of provocative physiological stress tests administered at the USAF Aerospace Medical Laboratory at Wright-Patterson Air Force Base, Ohio. Stress tests were designed to simulate, as far as could be anticipated, the combination of stresses an astronaut might encounter during a Mercury mission. Tolerance was tested through use of a centrifuge, low pressure chambers, an anechoic chamber, thermal exposure units, and aircraft modified to fly "Keplerian" trajectories producing a brief period of weightlessness. As a final step, peer ratings were obtained.

On April 2, 1959, NASA announced that seven astronauts had been chosen for Project Mercury. According to the Lovelace report, the seven were ultimately selected because of their exceptional resistance to physical and psychological stresses and

their particular scientific discipline or specialty. The average age was 35.2 years.

Subsequently, eight additional groups were selected to join the astronaut corps, for a total (as of 1986) of 157 individuals, including 13 women. From 1962 through 1969, medical evaluations for astronaut selection were conducted at Brooks Air Force Base, San Antonio, Texas, using the protocol shown in Table 15-1. Since 1977, medical evaluations using NASA-developed standards have been conducted at the L.B. Johnson Space Center (JSC), Houston, Texas. Table 15-2 shows the nine selection groups and statistics relating to each group.

It is interesting to note that all the astronaut selections through 1969 were conducted without a specific set of "pass-fail" medical standards. Instead, individuals in each selection group were ranked in terms of health and physical fitness against other individuals in the same group. Since these examinations were conducted by experts in the field of aerospace medicine, it is clear that individuals who were unqualified for duty as high-performance test pilots had a lower probability of receiving a high ranking. However, since all candidates had been repeatedly screened during their careers as pilots of high-performance aircraft, there was little likelihood that such medical defects would be found. As a result, there were uncertainties as to which medical criteria should be considered disqualifying.

INTRODUCTION OF FORMAL MEDICAL STANDARDS

Medical evaluations of the first seven astronauts were exhaustive and included sperm counts, total body radiation counts, and physiological tests which took several pages to list. In 1962, when the second astronaut selection was made, the examination process had been streamlined somewhat, although many elements from the

TABLE 15-1

MEDICAL AND PSYCHOLOGICAL TESTS ADMINISTERED TO ASTRONAUT CANDIDATES[a]

1. Medical history and review of systems
2. Physical examination
3. Electrocardiographic examinations, including routine electrocardiographic studies at rest, during hyperventilation, carotid massage, and breath holding, a double Master exercise tolerance test, a cold pressure test, and a precordial map
4. Treadmill exercise tolerance test
5. Vectorcardiographic study
6. Phonocardiographic study
7. Tilt table studies
8. Pulmonary function studies
9. Radiographic studies, including cholecystograms, upper GI series, lumbrosacral spine, chest, cervical spine, and skull films
10. Body composition study, using tritium dilution
11. Laboratory examinations, including complete hematology workup, urinalysis, serologic test, glucose tolerance test, acid alkaline phosphatase, BUN, sodium potassium, bicarbonate, chloride, calcium, phosphorus, magnesium, uric acid, bilirubin (direct and indirect), thymol turbidity, cephalin flocculation, SGOT, SGPT, total protein with albumin and globulin, separate determination of Alpha 1 and Alpha 2, Beta and Gamma globulins, protein-bound iodine, creatinine, cholesterol, total lipids and phospholipids, hydroxyproline, and red blood cell intracellular sodium and potassium. Stool specimens were examined for occult blood and microscopically for ova and parasites. A urine culture for bacterial growth was done, and a 24-hour specimen analyzed for 17-ketosteroids and 17-hydroxycorticosteroids
12. Detailed examination of the sinuses, larynx, and Eustachian tubes
13. Vestibular studies
14. Diagnostic hearing tests
15. Visual fields and special eye examinations
16. General surgical evaluation
17. Procto-sigmoidoscopy
18. Dental examination
19. Neurological examination
20. Psychological summary, including Wechsler Adult Intelligence Test, Bender Visual-Motor Gestalt Test, Rorschach Test, Thematic Apperception Test, Draw-A-Person Test, Gordon Personal Profile, Edwards' Personal Preference Schedule, Miller Analogies Test, and Performance Testing
21. Electroencephalographic studies
22. Centrifuge testing

[a] 1962 through 1969, Brooks Air Force Base, San Antonio, Texas. From Hawkins and Zieglschmid, 1975.

TABLE 15-2

MEDICAL EVALUATION FOR ASTRONAUT SELECTION PILOT AND MISSION SPECIALIST[a]

1. Medical history
2. Physical examination
3. Laboratory
    A. Hematology
    B. Blood chemistry
    C. Urine
    D. Feces
    E. Endocrine
    F. Radiological
       Chest, PA, and lateral abdominal (KUB)
4. Dental
5. Otorhinolaryngological
6. Ophthalmological
7. Neurological
8. Genito-Urological
9. Cardiopulmonary
10. Psychiatric
11. Radiation exposure
12. Musculoskeletal

[a] 1980 through 1984, Medical Sciences Division of Lyndon B. Johnson Space Center, Houston, Texas.

previous examinations were retained, such as psychological testing (Table 15-1). It is interesting to note that even though medical evaluation and psychological testing were stressed in the early astronaut selection evaluations, there were no established guidelines, and no clear patterns emerged. Apparently, physicians relied on their flight surgery experiences and based their judgments of mental fitness on whether the candidate would have been qualified for aviation.

NASA's formulation of medical evaluation standards for candidate Shuttle astronauts represented a departure from tradition. In developing a set of space flight medical evaluation standards, NASA thoroughly reviewed medical standards used by the Air Force, Navy, Department of Defense (DoD), and the Federal Aviation Authority (FAA). The new standards were based on 18 years of manned space flight experience and the emergence for the first time of two categories of astronauts: pilot and mission specialist. Since duties for these designations were different, it was decided that the standards for mission specialist could be somewhat more relaxed than those for pilot. Closely related to this were requirements for visual acuity. The selection process was being geared for people in their 30's who were primarily test pilots. Whereas a standard of 20/20 vision for younger pilots would have been appropriate, it was not necessarily correct for older pilots who had begun to experience minor degradations in vision due to the normal aging process. The result was a 20/50 standard, a higher upper limit than that used in a typical DoD selection of younger aviators. For the mission specialist, the visual acuity standard was set at 20/100. Ultimately there was agreement upon a set of standards which established an official basis for making the process fair, repeatable, and reliable. Medical evaluation components are listed in Table 15-2. Table 15-3 shows the chronology of selection of astronauts for the U.S. space program.

In January 1977, NASA published the Medical Evaluation and Standards for Astronaut Selection: NASA Class I—Pilot Astronaut, and NASA Class II—Mission Specialist (NASA, 1977a, 1977b). These were augmented in April of that year by corresponding standards for the category NASA Class III—Payload Specialist (NASA, 1977c). These standards served as a basis for selections in 1978 and 1980, when 54 candidates were approved for ratings of pilot or mission specialist. Among those selected were eight women. These standards were revised in 1983, and in 1984 a new category was added (NASA Class IV) for space flight participants.

Tables 15-4 and 15-5 compare values for some physiological health indices for those astronauts selected prior to 1970 and those chosen in the two most recent selections.

Table 15-6 shows the principal differences in medical standards for Class I, II, III, and IV crewmembers. Medical risk factors for acute and chronic diseases are weighed equally for all four classes.

The medical evaluation procedures and standards for astronaut selection established in 1977 (revised in 1983) parallel requirements developed by DoD for high-performance aircraft pilots. They have been augmented with tests to evaluate ability to withstand space flight stresses. Certain stress and endurance tests, initially used as part of the selection process for astronauts, are now included in the training curriculum. These tests include Keplerian parabolic flights, altitude chamber indoctrination, water tank immersion training, survival training, and workload tolerance evaluations. These tests were moved from the selection process to the training phase, since pass/fail selection criteria cannot readily be applied. They are

TABLE 15-3

CHRONOLOGY OF SELECTION OF SPACE PERSONNEL IN U.S. PROGRAM TO 1985

Year	Number Category	Selected	Average Age (yrs) at Selection
1959	Mercury Pilots	7	35
1962	Pilots/Astronauts	9	32
1963	Pilots/Astronauts	14	31
1965	Scientist/Astronauts	6	30
1966	Pilots/Astronauts	19	32
1967	Scientist/Astronauts	11	31
1969	Pilots/Astronauts	7	29
1978	Pilots	15	32
	Mission Specialists	20	
1980	Pilots	8	34
	Mission Specialists	11	
1984	Pilots	7	32
	Mission Specialists	10	
1985	Pilots	6	33
	Mission Specialists	7	
	Total:	157	

TABLE 15-4

MEDICAL PARAMETERS FROM ASTRONAUTS SELECTED BEFORE 1970

Selection Group	Selection Year	Weight (Mean)	(SD)	Sys BP (Mean)	(SD)	Dia BP (Mean)	(SD)	Chol (Mean)	(SD)	Trig (Mean)	(SD)	Glucose (Mean)	(SD)	O₂ (max) (Mean)	(SD)
Males (73)															
1	1959	166	13	121	8.3	77	1.1	194	26.8	—		103	4.6	35.0	3.2
2	1962	162	13	122	11.8	75	8.4	177	33.8	—		93	7.1	—	
3	1963	161	13	127	12.9	79	11.8	174	16.7	116	36.3	102	9.3	42.2	5.9
4	1965	158	13	123	15.3	77	11.6	151	42.5	117	24.7	84	14.0	46.3	5.5
5	1966	166	15	124	13.4	76	7.6	197	45.7	99	18.5	109	12.3	43.8	4.6
6	1967	164	23	128	10.5	76	9.0	194	72.0	73	28.7	99	8.9	44.4	5.4
7	1969	162	15	127	10.0	68	7.7	194	44.4	93	36.2	112	7.9	43.7	2.7

TABLE 15-5

MEDICAL PARAMETERS FROM CREWS SELECTED FOR SHUTTLE PROGRAMS

Selection Group	Selection Year	Weight (Mean)	(SD)	Sys BP (Mean)	(SD)	Dia BP (Mean)	(SD)	Chol (Mean)	(SD)	Trig (Mean)	(SD)	Glucose (Mean)	(SD)	O₂ (max) (Mean)	(SD)
Males (71)															
8	1977	164	20	122	10.3	78	7.3	192	43.8	82	37.9	95	8.9	46.4	7.7
9	1980	160	14	118	8.8	79	5.1	167	30.6	74	21.0	94	4.5	49.4	5.8
10	1984	165	23	122	8.3	75	7.1	203	48.5	55	26.3	90	5.2	48.6	5.5
11	1985	120	19	114	10.4	73	9.3	180	24.3	58	12.3	89	5.2	51.3	4.2
Females (13)															
8	1977	131	22	107	11.3	76	3.8	191	47.2	67	24.3	84	6.9	35.0	5.9
9	1980	113	13	118	0.0	75	9.5	150	36.8	54	0.7	86	1.4	40.8	2.6
10	1984	121	16	95	3.4	62	5.9	214	30.1	80	16.2	80	4.3	39	6.1
11	1985	133	4	92	8.0	60	0.0	158	1.0	65	12.5	89	0.5	39	1.3

TABLE 15-6

DIFFERENCES IN STANDARDS BETWEEN NASA MEDICAL CLASS I, II, III, AND IV SPACE FLIGHT EVALUATIONS[a]

Item	Astronauts	
	Pilots (Class I)	Mission Specialist (Class II)
Distant vision	20/50 or better uncorrected; correctable to 20/20 each eye	20/100 or better uncorrected; correctable to 20/20 each eye
Near vision	Uncorrected <20/20 each eye	Uncorrected <20/20 each eye
Hearing loss (db) per 150, 1964 Standard	500 Hz 1000 Hz 2000 Hz each ear 30 25 25	500 Hz 1000 Hz 2000 Hz better ear 30 25 25 worse ear 35 30 30
Height (in)	64–76 in	60–76 in
Refraction/Astigmatism	Specified	Specified
Contraction visual field	15°	15°
Phorias	ESO >15 EXO >8 Hyper >2	ESO >15 EXO >8 Hyper >2
Depth perception	Verhoeff—no errors in 8 presentations	Verhoeff—any error in 8 presentations
Color vision	Pass Farnsworth Lantern	Pass Farnsworth Lantern
Blood pressure	140/90	140/90
Radiation exposure	<5 rem/year	<5 rem/year
	Payload Specialists (Class III)	Space Flight Participants (Class IV)
Distant vision	Corrected less than 20/40, better eye	Correctable to 20/40, better eye
Near vision	Corrected < 20/40, better eye	Correctable to 20/40, better eye
Hearing loss (db) per 150, 1964 Standard	500 Hz 1000 Hz 2000 Hz better ear 35 30 30	Must hear whispered voice 3 ft. (hearing aid permitted)
Height (in)	Not specified	Not specified
Refraction/Astigmatism	Not specified	Not specified
Contraction visual field	30°	Not specified
Phorias	Not specified	Not specified
Depth perception	Not specified	Not specified
Color vision	Not specified	Not specified
Blood pressure	150/90 R_x permitted	160/100 R_x permitted
Radiation exposure	Not specified	Not specified

[a] Medical standards, NASA Class I pilot astronaut—selection and annual medical certification, Revision: December 1983, JSC 11569 NASA; Class II mission specialist—selection and annual medical certification, Revision: December 1983, JSC 11570; NASA Class III payload specialist—selection and annual medical certification, Revision: December 1983 JSC 11571; NASA Class IV—medical certification criteria, space flight participant program, Issued: December 1984.

retained in training under the philosophy that physiological stress testing enhances endurance for the environmental factors of space flight. It is believed that these tests, given during the 1-year indoctrination period prior to formal acceptance into the astronaut corps, help to prepare candidates for space flight stresses.

MEDICAL ISSUES IN SPACE CREW SELECTION

With the formulation of medical standards, NASA established individual medical evaluation programs for pilot and mission specialist astronauts, as well as for the nonastronaut payload specialist. Of the 519 applicants examined since 1977, 25 percent were disqualified for medical reasons. Of those, 75 percent of the rejections were due to visual, psychiatric, and cardiovascular problems. Vision problems alone accounted for 54 percent of those rejected, with visual acuity accounting for 60 percent of all ophthalmological problems. Other diagnoses showed a wide degree of variability. Table 15-7 shows the disqualifying medical conditions encoun-

tered during selections dating back to 1959. Results from selections prior to 1969 have been pooled, since no standardized evaluation process was used during that period.

The relevance of selection standards is demonstrated by the fact that, to date, all of the selected astronaut candidates have completed their prescribed 1-year training period successfully. Another important consequence of the publication of NASA medical standards is that, in combination with the unique operational aspects of the STS, they provide the field of space medicine with the long-awaited opportunity to establish longitudinal health trend studies which were difficult to conduct in the past.

LONGITUDINAL MEDICAL DATA

Biomedical results from Mercury, Gemini, and Apollo were based largely on comparisons of pre- and postflight physiological status and on observation of postflight

TABLE 15-7

DISQUALIFYING MEDICAL CONDITIONS FOUND FOR ASTRONAUTS AT SELECTION

Standard	1959–67	1977	1980	1984	1985
Visual	49	28	9	5	3
Surgical	13	4	7	0	0
Neurological	13	3	7	1	0
Cardiovascular	14	13	5	1	1
Hematological	3	1	3	0	0
Otolaryngological	17	1	3	2	0
Metabolic / Endocrine	9	4	3	2	0
Gastrointestinal	11	1	0	1	0
Genito-Urinary	12	2	1	0	0
Pulmonary	2	1	0	0	2
Dental	1	0	0	0	0
Psychiatric	6	1	13	4	0

physiological readaptation. Inflight medical monitoring focused only on certain functions essential to the assessment of crew health and safety, and the evaluation of basic physiological response to activities such as EVA. It was not until the advent of Skylab that provisions were made for extensive experimentation in space to determine the rate and time course of adaptation to space flight conditions, based on scheduled analyses of metabolic, cardiovascular, and biochemical parameters under a variety of stressed and nonstressed conditions (Johnston, 1977).

Results of all Skylab experiments, as well as the operational adjustments of crewmembers to microgravity, are summarized in other chapters and will not be reiterated here. The bottom line is that significant physiological changes occurred on all space flights of all durations; however, all changes appeared reversible, returning to preflight baselines with no apparent long-range deficits.

In 1976, a retrospective survey was conducted concerning aging and the development of coronary artery disease among U.S. astronauts selected prior to 1970 (Degioanni et al., 1976). The conclusion was that the incidence of coronary artery disease among U.S. astronauts was not significantly different from that of the general population. In the context of the length of observation (15 years) and the rate of occurrence of the disease under investigation (N=1 out of a sample size of 73), this conclusion was probably premature. The pre-1977 astronaut population is a relatively homogeneous, prescreened group of men with a low index for cardiovascular risk factors. This description is supported by a review of trend data for weight, recumbent blood pressure, fasting blood sugar, and triglycerides for this group (Figure 15-1). All of these health indices remained remarkably stable during the period of observation (1969 through 1979). The small variations in

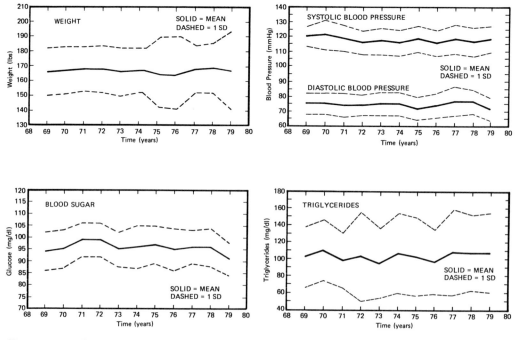

Figure 15-1. Ten-year review of four health indices for astronauts selected before 1970.

weight recorded in the years 1975 and 1976 probably represent fluctuations in the number of astronauts examined, and changes in lifestyle (decreased activity) due to the absence of space missions and associated training during this period of time. Changes in blood cholesterol levels are presented in Figure 15-2. A steady and significant increase in blood cholesterol values over time is noted, which is comparable to trends observed in the general population. However, values for high density lipoprotein (HDL) and the persistently high maximum oxygen consumption levels ($VO_2 = 42 + 8$ ml/kg/body), as well as a lower-than-expected percent fat for age (15.7), all indicate that cardiovascular risk profiles of astronauts were well below the national average.

Objectives in this area are to conduct longitudinal retrospective and prospective studies of medical data from astronauts and controls. The studies to be covered involve individuals in a relatively closed population in an attempt to correlate physiological changes and occupational exposure. Areas of particular interest consist of acute responses and long-term adaptive mechanisms to weightlessness, changes noted in annual physical examinations, and effects of aging and disease. The approach includes: (a) entering and storing all astronaut medical exams (annual, flight, and illness) in computer databases; (b) collecting and storing similar information on a control group of civil servants (matched on age, sex, body size, and smoking history); (c) analyzing longitudinal information comparing these groups; (d) cumulatively evaluating pre/postflight physiological changes across missions; and (e) periodic reviews to define and include new parameters.

LONGITUDINAL STUDIES METHODOLOGY

When the Skylab Program ended in 1970, it was clear that humans could survive and function effectively on a mission of up to 83 days; all inflight physiological changes were apparently transitory. (Since that time, Soviet programs have extended exposure time to orbital flight to almost 1 year.) However, because of the small num-

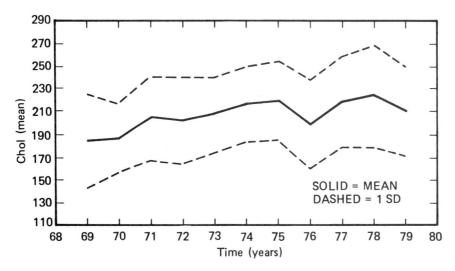

Figure 15-2. Changes in blood cholesterol levels of astronauts selected before 1970 (N=57).

ber of subjects, the variable characteristics of the few missions flown, and the recency of the missions, results of studies concerning the long-term effects of space flight exposure are not known.

Some of the problems associated with implementing longitudinal studies are shown in Table 15-8. For obvious reasons, longitudinal studies in the traditional epidemiological sense of using large populations and statistically controlling a variable are currently impossible as far as the astronaut corps is concerned. Furthermore, with this relatively small population, a random medical problem may be overweighted. A carefully matched control group may experimentally verify what could not be shown statistically. Because of the limited number of cases, selection of an appropriate control group is crucial and will be discussed in detail later. The formulation of certain critical tests in the absence of any real knowledge about long-term effects of space flight is particularly difficult. Further, there are ethical, practical, and political implications in obtaining certain otherwise desirable measurements, e.g., bone biopsy.

Because of changes in personnel and testing procedures, addition of new tests, and introduction of new equipment, maintaining quality control over a long period of time is very difficult. NASA has committed to a program for "decades" of medical studies for astronauts; however, this may not be sufficient, since follow-up examinations are voluntary for individual astronauts. Although over 90 percent of astronauts return periodically for follow-up exams, some, for various reasons, do not. Follow-up of the peer group is even more difficult, since their return expenses are not paid (as they are for astronauts). This may be compensated by selecting a larger number of peers than minimally required.

While these difficulties are substantial, they can frequently be overcome if they

TABLE 15-8

SOME PROBLEMS ASSOCIATED WITH LONGITUDINAL STUDIES

Small size of study population
Stable commitment of resources
Selecting appropriate control groups
Selection of critical tests
Stable testing and quality control
Commitment to decades of follow-up
Difficulty of follow-up
Attrition of peer group

---

are realistically faced, and if practical compromises are made. Some progress is evident in the methods ultimately used in the NASA longitudinal studies described below.

Recognizing the limited evidence and realizing that the Space Shuttle Program would ultimately raise questions concerning possible effects of multiple space flight exposure, questions and methodology needed to formally evaluate long-range effects of space flights were carefully defined (Kannel, 1982).

Since long-range physiological and anatomical changes occur as a function of age, it was clearly important to find a suitable peer group that had not been exposed to microgravity. In general, military pilots were considered by most symposium participants as the best peer group controls; however, a subsequent, careful examination suggested that JSC civil servants might be almost as good a choice as military pilots, and certainly more practical from an implementation viewpoint.

First, all JSC employees are offered an annual medical examination by a medical group under contract to the Center. Almost 100 percent of the employees avail themselves of this opportunity each year. While this exam is not as comprehensive as astronaut examinations, it is generally similar in content, and the same technicians and equipment are used for both astronauts and employees, providing equivalent procedures, instruments, and quality control. Second, as the space program matures, and includes additional non-pilot, scientist astronauts, civil servants may prove to be more medically representative of astronauts than pilots. Ideally, prospective longitudinal studies should include a pilot control group, since NASA policy is to use military pilots.

A final reason for selecting a subset of JSC civil servants for a peer group is practicality. In 1978, all previous SF 88 medical examination records for each of about 3,000 JSC employees were entered in a database. Since the average employee had been at the Center for 10 years, the purpose of this activity was to develop an annual cumulative trend chart on selected variables for each individual. In addition, all astronaut medical and operational examinations were entered in a computer database for possible use for medical operations decision-making.

With these considerations in mind, a decision was made to use JSC employees as the primary control group for evaluating general health changes possibly attributable to space flight. The next step was to identify matching peers for each astronaut from a dispensary database of over 40,000 records. First, a body size index commonly used by epidemiologists was calculated for each annual examination and an average was computed for each JSC employee and astronaut. Next, astronaut data were entered into the JSC dispensary database, sorted by age, body size, smoking history, sex, number of annual exams available, and physical activity code (where available).

From this list, each astronaut was matched with five equivalent civil servants according to the parameters identified.

Five controls for each astronaut were chosen to reduce attrition and problems associated with missing data. This same process has been used to identify five matching subjects for all astronauts, including the 13 selected in 1985.

LONGITUDINAL STUDY RESULTS FOR PRE-SHUTTLE ASTRONAUTS

The astronaut corps consists of two groups with respect to age—those selected before 1970 and those selected from 1977 to 1985. The former group flew in programs from Mercury through Skylab and are referred to in this paper as "pre-Shuttle astronauts," even though several have flown on the Shuttle. Currently, this pre-Shuttle group ranges in age from about 43 to 59, with a mean age of 51 and a standard deviation of 3.77. In contrast, the Shuttle group has a mean age of 39 with a standard deviation of 3.34, thereby ranging in age from about 31 to 43. Relatively few Shuttle astronauts have flown, while virtually all members of the pre-Shuttle group have flown. In short, the pre-Shuttle astronauts have had time to manifest any long-term health decrements that may have resulted from their space flight experience. For this reason, a retrospective longitudinal study was completed using annual medical evaluations over the last 15 years for both pre-Shuttle astronauts and controls. Of the 73 astronauts selected from 1959 through 1969, 3 were killed in the Apollo fire, 4 were killed in aircraft accidents, 1 in an automobile accident, and 9 resigned early in the program. This left a total of 56 astronauts that were included in the study.

Table 15-9 shows the results of body size and age matching for pre-Shuttle astronauts. As can be seen, weight, height, and body size show no significant difference between astronauts and their matching control group of civil servants. The

TABLE 15-9

RESULTS OF BODY SIZE AND AGE MATCHING

Parameter Measured	Astronauts	Peer Group
Weight		
Mean	166.5	166.0
Standard Deviation	14.5	16.2
Height		
Mean	69.8	70.2
Standard Deviation	1.7	1.8
Age		
Mean	38.3	38.0
Standard Deviation	4.0	4.4
Number of subjects	110.0	474.0

number of cases are 56 and 280 for astronauts and peers, respectively. In 1970, 84 percent of the astronauts ranged between ages 33 and 41. The average astronaut in the study aged from 38 in 1970 to 52 by the end of the study in 1984. The youngest and oldest astronauts in 1970 were 31 and 47, respectively. Naturally, the peer group has aged at an equivalent rate.

Table 15-10 lists the health screening variables measured annually at JSC for astronauts and nonastronaut employees. To better understand the relationship between these 42 variables, a factor analysis was completed using 8,600 SF88 records of JSC employees (see Table 15-11). From the intercorrelations of all 42 variables, the analysis identified 11 independent dimensions or factors. The variables most highly correlated with these factors were as expected. Of some interest was the fact that age did not appear as an independent di-

TABLE 15-10

VARIABLES AVAILABLE FOR STUDY

Age	OD	FEV1
Height	OS	FVC
Weight	Hearing (R500)	Glucose
Sitting BP (Sys)	Hearing (R1000)	BUN
Sitting BP (Dia)	Hearing (R2000)	SGOT
Recumbent BP (Sys)	Hearing (R3000)	Cholesterol
Recumbent BP (Dia)	Hearing (R4000)	Triglycerides
Sitting (Pulse)	Hearing (R6000)	Uric Acid
After exercise (Pulse)	Hearing (L500)	Specific Gravity
After 2 min. (Pulse)	Hearing (L1000)	pH
Recumbent pulse	Hearing (L2000)	HGB
Distant vision (R)	Hearing (L3000)	HCT
Distant vision (L)	Hearing (L4000)	WBC
Near vision (R)	Hearing (L6000)	
Near vision (L)		

TABLE 15-11

FACTOR ANALYSIS (42 CLINICAL VARIABLES, N=8, 628)

Factor Number	Factor	% Variance
I	Audition (3K–6K)	19
II	Biochemical	13
III	Blood pressure	11
IV	Heart rate	10
V	Respiration	8
VI	Audition (1K–2K)	7
VII	Distant vision	7
VIII	Interocular pressure	7
IX	Near vision	7
X	Audition (.5K)	6
XI	Body size	5
	TOTAL	100

mension, but was related primarily to Factors I, VIII, and IX (audition, interocular pressure, and near vision), and to a lesser extent to Factors II, III, and VI (biochemical, blood pressure, and audition [1K-2K]). This was seen in later analyses as increasing slopes over time. The analysis shows that one or two variables from each factor would be sufficient to describe the overall changes in these health screening variables, since those associated with a single factor are highly correlated.

The primary descriptive and inferential analysis for this study was to calculate mean and standard deviation for each variable in each group, for each year. Regression lines were then calculated for each group, statistically compared, and tested to determine if they were significantly different in direction or level. The variables selected for analysis were those suggested by the factor analysis.

Three parameters were selected to represent the cardiovascular dimension. These were sitting systolic blood pressure, sitting diastolic blood pressure, and heart rate 3 minutes after exercise.

Figure 15-3 shows the means for astronauts and peer groups for sitting systolic blood pressure for each year from 1970 to 1984. A regression line fitted to the astronauts' means over the 15 years shows the trend is significantly upward, while the regression line for the peer group shows the trend to be significantly sharper, rising from 116 to almost 130. The difference between the two regression lines is significant ($P < .0001$). Standard deviations ranged from 7 to 10 for the astronauts and 8 to 11 for the peer group.

Figure 15-4 shows sitting diastolic blood pressure with the astronaut and the peer group trend rising almost in parallel. Again, the difference between the two regression lines is significant, with astronauts consistently exhibiting lower pressures. While not shown, sitting pulse was consistently lower for astronauts and decreased significantly over the years.

Figure 15-5 shows the mean pulse after 2 minutes of exercise for pre-Shuttle astronauts and peer group over 15 years. The 15-year trend shows that pulse rates for astronauts tended to decrease, while those of controls remained constant or showed some average increase. Recumbent blood pressure (systolic and diastolic) and pulse showed no differences in trends between

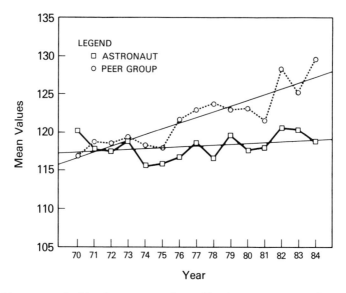

Figure 15-3. Mean systolic blood pressure of pre-Shuttle astronauts and peer group over 15 years. Significantly different regression lines are also shown.

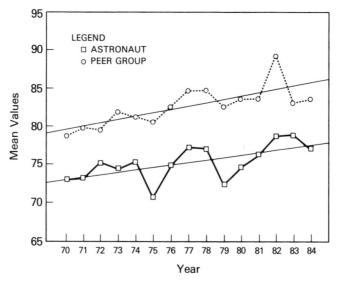

Figure 15-4. Mean diastolic blood pressure of pre-Shuttle astronauts and peer group over 15 years. Significantly different regression lines are also shown.

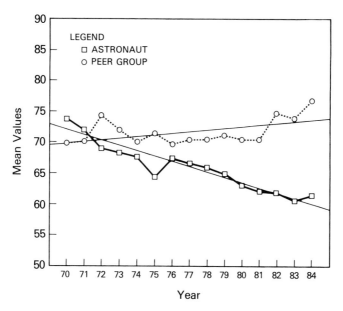

Figure 15-5. Mean pulse after 2 minutes of exercise for pre-Shuttle astronauts and peer group over 15 years. Regression lines shown are significantly different.

the two groups. Standing blood pressure and standing pulse also showed no differences in trends between the two groups.

To summarize, the overall 15-year trend for pre-Shuttle astronauts was improved cardiovascular responsiveness (which was initially better than that of the peer group), which could be a result of more physical activity on the part of astronauts. As more astronauts retire, it will be interesting to see if this trend continues, and if the incidence of heart attacks is lower. In any event, there is no evidence of any long-range occupational hazards to the cardiovascular system for the variables considered.

Results of visual trends are shown by near vision, distant vision, and interocular pressure. Figure 15-6 shows the mean visual acuity for near-vision of pre-Shuttle astronauts as compared to the control group across the 15-year period. Because of selection, astronaut visual acuity was significantly greater than the peer groups, with virtually all having uncorrected 20/

20 vision as compared to wide variability of the peer group. They remained significantly more visually acute throughout the last 15 years.

The upward trend for both groups was significant (P < .0001) when regression lines were tested; this is consistent with the significant correlation with age noted in the factor analysis for the general population.

Measures of pre-Shuttle astronaut variability on visual acuity markedly increased in 1975, and increased consistently across the remaining 10-year period, showing increasing need for glasses which peaked in 1976 when the average age was 44. The 1983–84 mean rise in acuity variability corresponds to a time period when the youngest of these astronauts reached age 44–45. In fact, a search was made of the databases of both pre-Shuttle astronauts and peer groups for the age when vision first degraded from 20/20. This search indicated that pre-Shuttle astronauts were significantly older than mem-

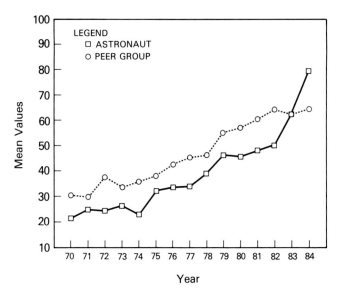

Figure 15-6. Mean near-vision measurements for pre-Shuttle astronauts and peer group over 15 years. Both upward trend and difference between the groups are significant.

bers of the peer group when their vision degraded: age 44 for astronauts and 40 for the 256 peers.

The effect of selection on vision was also evident in distant vision, as shown in Figure 15-7. For pre-Shuttle astronauts, distant-vision acuity rises insignificantly. However, for the peer group (between 189 and 243 people), a very high number (about 35 percent) showed poor distant vision, with no improvement throughout the 15-year period. The remaining individuals show a significant upward trend—again, consistent with the factor analysis showing significant but modest correlation of distant vision with age.

Finally, interocular pressure (OD and OS) showed no difference between the groups. In summary, there is no evidence of visual loss beyond what is age related.

Figure 15-8 shows mean comparisons for the two groups on hearing of the left ear at 4000 Hz. Average decibel loss for pre-shuttle astronauts may appear to be significant, but the variability of about 20

decibels for both groups shows the difference to be insignificant. Hearing at 2,000 Hz and 3,000 Hz is very similar, while hearing above and below that range shows considerable overlap between the two groups.

The upward trend for both groups was significant for virtually all frequencies, reinforcing the high correlation with age noted in the factor analysis. Given the flying record of this group of pre-Shuttle astronauts, a greater loss was in fact expected.

Figure 15-9 shows glucose means for each group over the 15-year period. Standard deviations average about 8 and the difference between the two groups is significant. Unlike the other measures presented, biochemistries are analyzed in the clinical laboratory for astronauts and in the dispensary for the peer group. From 1975 to 1979 a different procedure was used, which undoubtedly accounts for the differences seen during that period.

Significant differences were also seen in

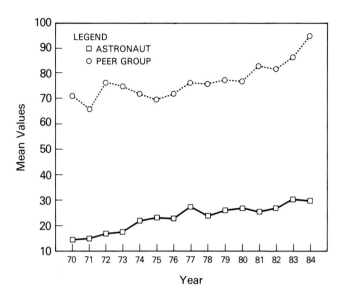

Figure 15-7. Mean distant-vision measurements for pre-Shuttle astronauts and peer group over 15 years. Both upward trend and difference between groups are significant. About 35% of the peer group had poor initial distant vision.

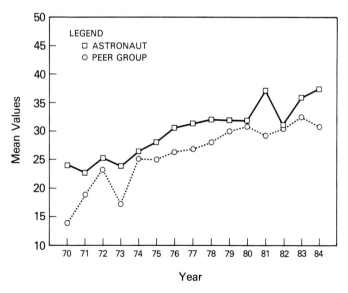

Figure 15-8. Mean hearing loss at 4,000 Hz for pre-Shuttle astronauts and peer groups over 15 years. Difference between the groups is not significant, although the upward trend of hearing loss is significant.

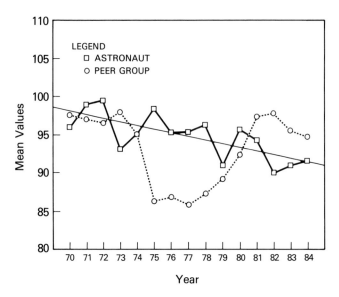

Figure 15-9. Mean glucose for pre-Shuttle astronauts and peer group over 15 years.

triglycerides, and BUN appeared to be the result of changes in instruments, procedures, or both, at the two laboratories. To enhance control in the future, changes will involve an overlap period so all data can be scaled to equivalence. No differences were found between the groups on total cholesterol, PH, HCT, HGB, and WBC. In summary, none of the biochemistry data suggested readings outside normal clinical limits.

Finally, with respect to the respiratory system, instrument and procedure differences also prevented full comparison between astronauts and their peer group. Astronauts' respiratory functions were evaluated by a flow meter during treadmill testing, while the peer group was given forced vital capacity and forced expiratory capacity measures. Fortunately, in recent years some peer groups have been evaluated by the treadmill, using the same instrumentation and protocol as for astronauts.

FUTURE STUDIES AND MEDICAL PROGRAMS IN THE SPACE STATION ERA

Results of the study of pre-Shuttle astronauts revealed no impairment in any of the variables examined, but were generally the same or better than a matched peer group. This does not necessarily mean that no differences would be found in parameters which were not measured. Of perhaps equal importance is the development of a method to identify control groups for the retrospective and prospective studies being planned.

From a retrospective point of view, studies are underway to evaluate treadmill results from both astronauts and controls, in order to develop and validate a general health index, and to determine the frequency and types of illness events reported by astronauts and controls. With respect to prospective longitudinal studies, efforts are underway to better document bone and muscle parameters, establish a radiation registry, and collect questionnaire responses on lifestyle variables which can dramatically influence medical evaluation.

In order to assess systematically the effects of space flight on humans, several types of studies are planned by NASA, differing primarily in the length of time devoted to data collection:

1. Short-term studies based on analyses of data from single flights. These will add to the information collected describing physiological changes during space flight. The ongoing STS space motion sickness study is an example. This study involves routine collection of pre-, in-, and postflight space motion sickness-related data from Space Shuttle crewmembers and passengers through at least the mid-1980's. The goals are to (1) validate ground-based predictive tests of susceptibility to space motion sickness, and (2) define operationally acceptable countermeasures.

2. Mid-term longitudinal studies spanning several missions. These studies will measure the effects, if any, of repeated exposures to the space flight environment. Attention will be given to issues such as cumulative effect of radiation exposure and rate of bone mineral loss.

3. Long-term longitudinal studies aimed at collecting career data through a medical surveillance program to develop occupational information based on diseases or injuries incurred during or following space flight.

Much of the data in NASA longitudinal studies will be obtained from standardized annual medical evaluations. The resulting biomedical database will be divided into astronaut-pilot, astronaut-mission specialist, and payload specialist categories. This will allow studies concerning the effects of different work requirements in space, as well as differential length and frequency of exposure to space flight. These longitudinal studies will help to validate medical standards, better define medical risk factors associated with space flight, characterize the "health profile in zero gravity," and, as appropriate, define new problems associated with space flight which might result from exposure of population groups other than astronauts.

MEDICAL PROGRAMS IN THE STS AND SPACE STATION ERA

The Space Transportation System (STS) has opened new opportunities for gathering flight-related biomedical data. To support the increased number of flight crew personnel, an efficient biomedical system must be established for the orderly and timely collection of standardized biomedical data from selection, retention, and flight medical evaluations. An essential requirement here is the initiation of longitudinal studies of large groups of space travelers. The publication of NASA Medical Standards in 1977, along with the novel operational features of the Space Shuttle, allow the establishment of longitudinal follow-up studies, bringing space biomedical research into accord with standard public health practices. Although these studies will be of limited pathophysiological and etiological value in the foreseeable future, they will provide valuable feedback mechanisms for (1) designing high-quality experiments addressing specific hypotheses and (2) developing more accurate modeling capabilities. Over the years, longitudinal studies of astronaut health trends may serve as a basis for many operational decisions.

As the nation's research and development organization for aeronautics and space, NASA must look continuously to the future. New goals emerge as extant goals are reached; each advance toward a new program objective in turn serves as a building block for future programs. In view of future manned space exploration, it may be necessary to consider using the Space Station as a test bed for qualifying humans for missions of increasingly longer durations.

Tours of duty on Space Station will re-quire exposure of humans to microgravity for long periods of time; advanced missions will likely extend exposure times. In addition, critical questions persist regarding the physiological adaptation of humans to long-term stays in microgravity. For these reasons, investigations are required to further define the processes of adaptation to microgravity and readaptation to gravity, and to initiate development of appropriate countermeasures.

REFERENCES

Colton, T. Statistics in medicine. Boston, Little, Brown & Co., 1974.

Degioanni, J., Nicogossian, A., Karstews, A.I., Burchard, E.C., and Zieglschmid, J.F. A survey of fifteen years of medical experience with astronauts. In: Preprints of the 48th ASMA Annual Scientific Meeting, Bal Harbour, FL., 1976.

Hawkins, W.R., and Zieglschmid, J.F. Clinical aspects of crew health. In: Biomedical results of Apollo (NASA SP-368). Edited by R.S. Johnston, L.F. Dietlein, and C.A. Berry. National Aeronautics and Space Administration, U.S. Government Printing Office, Washington, D.C., 1975.

Johnston, R.S. Skylab Medical Program Overview. In: Biomedical results from Skylab (NASA SP-377). Edited by R.S. Johnston and L.F. Dietlein, National Aeronautics and Space Administration, U.S. Government Printing Office, Washington, D.C., 1977.

Kannel, W.B. (Chairman), American Institute of Biological Sciences. Ad Hoc Working Groups to NASA on Longitudinal Studies, 1982.

Link, M.M. Space medicine in Project Mercury (NASA SP-4003). U.S. Government Printing Office, Washington, D.C., 1965.

NASA. Medical evaluation and standards for astronaut selection: NASA class I—Pilot Astronaut (JSC-11569). Prepared by Space and Life Sciences Directorate, NASA Lyndon B. Johnson Space Center, Houston, TX, January 1977a.

NASA. Medical evaluation and standards for astronaut selection: NASA class II—Mission Specialist (JSC-11570). Prepared by Space and Life Sciences Directorate, NASA, Lyndon B. Johnson Space Center, Houston, TX, January 1977b.

NASA. Medical evaluation and standards: NASA class III-Payload Specialist (JSC-11571). Prepared by Space and Life Sciences Directorate, NASA Lyndon B. Johnson Space Center, Houston, TX, April 1977c.

NASA. Summary Report, Johnson Space Center, Houston, TX, August 1982.

Nicogossian, A., Pool, S., and Rambaut, P. The Shuttle and its importance to space medicine. Presented at the 31st IAF Congress, Tokyo, Japan, 22–25 September, 1980.

16 Biomedical Training of Space Crews

JEFFREY R. DAVIS

ARNAULD E. NICOGOSSIAN

Biomedical training, which has always been part of the total training program for space crews, is designed for two purposes. The first is to familiarize crewmembers with the unique features of the space environment, especially weightlessness, as these features produce physiological changes and affect performance. The second is to prepare crewmembers to manage unforeseen medical events, such as illness or injury during a mission.

Physiology training in space medicine is a direct outgrowth of training used in military aviation medicine. Aviation programs are concerned with traditional problems of high-speed, high-altitude flight. Physiological stresses include low pressure and temperature, lack of oxygen, vibration, high linear and angular acceleration forces, and many other variables. Altitude chambers and human centrifuges are used extensively in aviation physiology training programs. In the early stages of manned space flight, much of this training technology was applied, with some modification, to the demands of space flight.

Astronauts were trained in high-altitude physiology, human response to thermal extremes, survival in varying recovery environments, tolerance to different acceleration forces, and the effects of psychological stressors such as confinement and isolation. To the extent possible, an introduction to the physiology of weightlessness was added.

Extravehicular tasks attempted in the Gemini 9 and 11 missions were not particularly successful prior to the development of zero-gravity simulations for training purposes. In Gemini 9, the task was to check out and don the Astronaut Maneuvering Unit to be used as an assist during EVA. Foot restraints proved to be inadequate, requiring the pilot to exert a continuous high workload to maintain body position. Heat and perspiration were produced at rates exceeding the removal capacity of the life support system, and fog accumulated on the space suit visor until the astronaut's vision was almost totally blocked (Schultz et al., 1967).

Shortly after Gemini 9, the pilot used

an underwater zero-gravity simulation to test various restraint systems. It was concluded at the time that this type of simulation very nearly duplicated the actual weightless condition and could be used profitably to study problems inherent to extravehicular operations. As a result of these tests, it was decided that the Gemini 12 flight crew would use an underwater zero-gravity simulator in their EVA training. During the two periods of intensive underwater simulation and training subsequently added to the program, the pilot followed scheduled flight procedures and systematically duplicated the planned EVA. Among other benefits, he was able to condition himself to relax completely within the suit. All movements were slow and deliberate, using only those muscles required for task performance. This technique was then applied to the actual EVA of Gemini 12.

Results of the Gemini 12 EVA showed that all tasks attempted were feasible using the techniques perfected in the zero-gravity simulator, as well as improved body restraints. EVA workload could be controlled within desired limits through proper procedures and indoctrination. It was concluded that any task that could be accomplished readily in a valid underwater simulation would have a high probability of success during actual EVA (Machell et al., 1967). Underwater simulation training for performance in weightlessness was included in all subsequent training programs.

A second training issue results from problems encountered in returning a spacecraft to Earth. When a spacecraft cannot be recovered quickly, emergency medical services (except in the unusual presence of a physician crewmember) must be provided by trained crewmembers using onboard medical supplies. While medical advice can be provided by Mission Control in the event of a serious illness or injury, direct treatment must be provided by another crewmember.

During orbital flight, a spacecraft can make an emergency return to Earth within a matter of hours, given prior preparations, but this is desirable neither in terms of mission objectives nor economy. In certain cases, an emergency return simply may not be possible, however pressing the circumstances. This was amply demonstrated during the Apollo 13 mission. After insertion into a lunar trajectory, an oxygen tank ruptured and exploded, with serious damage to other spacecraft components. Oxygen required for breathing and for the fuel cells was rapidly depleted. It was initially calculated that only about 38 hours of power, water, and oxygen were available: about one-half the amount needed to circumnavigate the moon and return to Earth. By transferring to the Lunar Module, greatly reducing power consumption, and improvising onboard carbon dioxide removal systems, the crew was able to accomplish a successful return. While the lowered cabin temperature made it uncomfortably cold, the only serious medical problem that arose was a urinary tract infection developed by one crewmember. Apollo 13 served to demonstrate the need for meticulous planning and training for inflight emergencies. Medical training for crewmembers, supported by simulator practice, is an important part of this emergency planning.

During the Space Station era, requirements for medical training will be driven by the nature of the crew escape/rescue capability present on orbit. Current planning for Space Station includes the concept of a "safe haven"—an isolatable volume within the station which contains all necessary supplies (food, water, clothing, medical supplies, etc.) as well as life support systems to sustain life until the crew can be rescued. Current estimates of the time required to effect a rescue (assuming that the Shuttle is not present on orbit) range from 28 to 45 days.

HEALTH MAINTENANCE FACILITY

The Health Maintenance Facility (HMF) will permit preventive, diagnostic, and therapeutic care on board the Space Station. Design of the HMF applies state-of-the-art medical capabilities and hardware to the specialized and self-contained spacecraft environment (see Chapter 21).

TRAINING FOR THE STRESSES OF SPACE

An astronaut may encounter any number of stresses, including weightlessness, noise and vibration, unusual acceleration forces, temperature extremes, and isolation. Every effort is made to minimize these stresses through appropriate spacecraft design and attention to mission parameters. However, the possibility always remains that through an unusual combination of circumstances, one or more of these stresses might suddenly increase, exceeding safe levels. The Apollo 13 inflight emergency provides an excellent example. In this mission, the crew operated under very low thermal conditions, with suit inlet temperatures dropping to as low as 5°C (41°F).

The philosophy of environmental stress training is that repeated exposure to a stress factor results in a better understanding of its effects and an enhanced ability to cope with it. This type of training, which in one sense might better be termed "conditioning," was given considerable emphasis by the United States and the So-viet Union in the early preparations for manned space flight. Since then, emphasis has abated somewhat in the American program, while continuing at much the same level in the Soviet Union.

Training for Project Mercury emphasized exposure to environmental conditions such as high acceleration forces, zero gravity, heat, noise, and spacecraft tumbling motion (Link and Gurovskiy, 1975). Particular attention was given to manual control of the spacecraft during the high acceleration loads imposed during launch and reentry. In order to examine this capability and provide training for dealing with acceleration, a number of simulations were undertaken in the centrifuge at the Naval Air Development Center, Johnsville, Pennsylvania. These training programs were considered quite valuable in providing practice in operating spacecraft systems and allowing astronauts to develop their adaptive capabilities to accelerative forces.

Centrifuge training has continued throughout the Soviet program, but was discontinued in the U.S. prior to the Apollo missions. As experience in manned space flight increased, more attention was given to enhancing performance in weightlessness and less to environmental stress factors per se. While indoctrination concerning the consequences of hypoxia and exposure to reduced pressure is still a practice through the use of altitude chambers, greater use is made of the NASA KC-135 aircraft which can provide brief periods of weightlessness when flying a Keplerian trajectory. Figures 16-1 and 16-2 show the use of this aircraft to train astronauts in tasks that become challenging in weightlessness, such as handling food and maneuvering in space suits. Even though the trainee has only a few seconds of zero gravity in which to experiment with such tasks, this practice is judged useful for later mission performance.

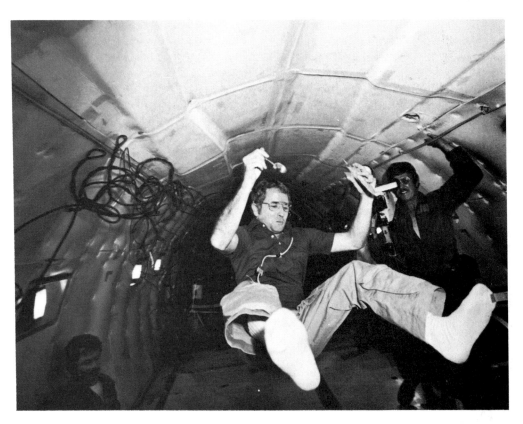

Figure 16-1. Astronaut Richard Truly practicing use of the Space Shuttle food system while in weightlessness in the KC-135 aircraft.

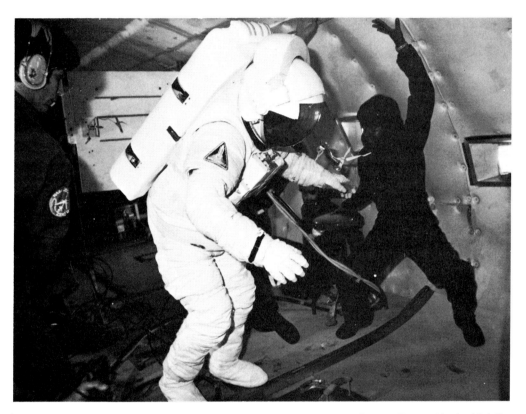

Figure 16-2. Astronaut Gordon Fullerton practicing with the Space Shuttle Extravehicular Mobility Unit in the KC-135 aircraft.

Water immersion techniques to simulate zero gravity have distinct advantages over aircraft flying a zero-gravity profile, since there are no time constraints. Under conditions of neutral buoyancy in a water tank, astronauts can practice tasks required during EVA until the desired proficiency is achieved. Since the Gemini 12 flight, all astronauts have been trained in this manner. Figures 16-3 and 16-4 show training operations at the two NASA facilities used for this purpose.

MEDICAL TRAINING

All spacecraft carry a medical kit tailored to mission duration, availability of physicians, and training level of crewmembers. The purpose of medical training is to provide crewmembers with the knowledge and skills necessary to respond to inflight illnesses and injuries in an appropriate and timely manner. This objective is met through both the general medical training included in each astronaut's initial training, and mission-specific training over 6 months prior to a mission (Vanderploeg and Hadley, 1982).

The initial medical training involves 16 hours of instruction during the first year after selection. The program covers altitude physiology and includes training in composition of the atmosphere; gas laws; signs, symptoms, and treatment of hypoxia; operation of life-support equipment; effects of increased gravity; antigravity maneuvers (Valsalva maneuver, etc.); use of the anti-gravity suit; and a demonstration of hypoxia.

Medical training for management of inflight episodes involves the entire crew and typically begins 6 months prior to a Shuttle flight. Briefing topics include com-

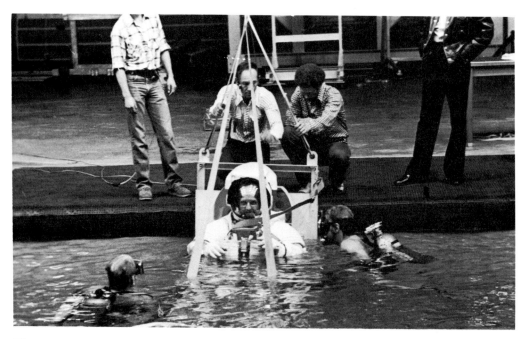

Figure 16-3. Astronaut Richard Truly entering the water immersion training facility at the Johnson Space Center.

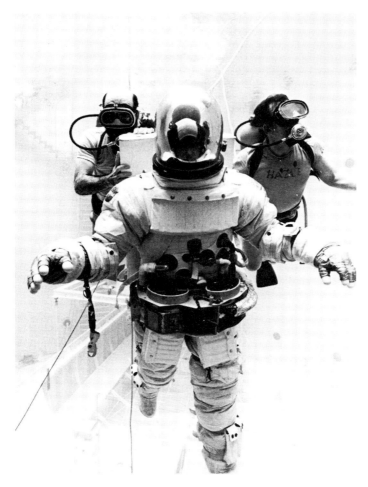

Figure 16-4. Astronaut Shannon Lucid using the Neutral Buoyancy Simulator at the Marshall Space Flight Center.

mon medical problems of space flight, such as motion sickness, lower back pain, cardiovascular adaptation, and use of (1) the Shuttle Orbiter Medical System (SOMS), (2) the Operational Bioinstrumentation System, (3) the anti-gravity suit, and (4) radiation monitoring equipment. The commander then designates two crewmembers to serve as medical officers for that flight. They are given additional training in one-gravity and zero-gravity performance of CPR, and diagnostic and therapeutic techniques. In addition, they are briefed on common ambulatory illnesses anticipated during a short flight, and the use of the medical checklist, part of the onboard flight data file. A final summary briefing is given for the entire crew at launch minus 10 days.

EMERGENCY MEDICAL SUPPORT

Launch and landing operations of the Space Shuttle are supported by an Emergency Medical Services System (EMSS) designed to provide an ill or injured crewman with rapid access to the appropriate level of medical care. The success of this system depends on availability of medical personnel and facilities, rapid transportation procedures, trained rescue personnel, and knowledgeable space crewmen. Training for space crewmen is directed principally toward use of the system. Eight major egress modes have been identified for launch and landing emergencies of the Space Shuttle (Pool, 1981). Figure 16-5 shows rescue operations being practiced. Figure 16-6 shows one of the NASA rescue vehicles.

TRAINING SYSTEM DEVELOPMENT

Training of space crews is a team effort that evolves in consonance with advances in medical knowledge. The physician, as one member of the team, provides inputs concerning environmental stress effects and medical requirements. Lessons learned from previous missions, combined with prospective activities for future missions, are analyzed in terms of the feasibility of coping with inflight medical episodes through a combination of medical training and onboard equipment. Proposed im-

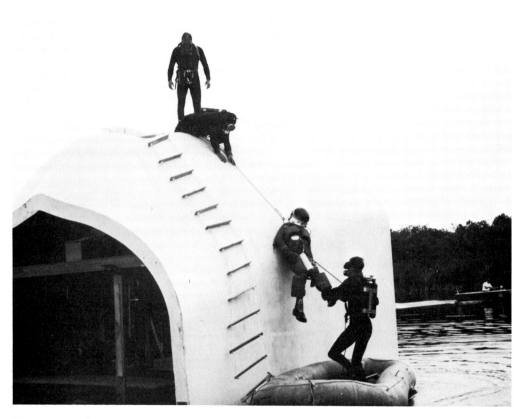

Figure 16-5. Rescue swimmers assisting an ''astronaut'' during recovery from an orbiter mockup which supposedly has landed in water.

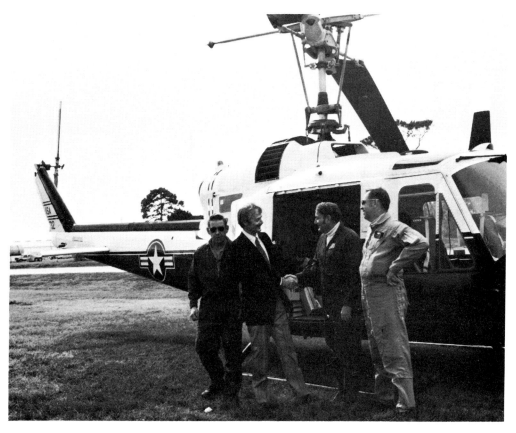

Figure 16-6. Rescue helicopter used by NASA for transport of injured crewmembers to medical facilities.

provements in procedures and equipment are verified under laboratory conditions, in spacecraft simulators, and during parabolic aircraft flights. Experienced astronauts review the procedures and provide invaluable feedback as to their feasibility for inflight use. At the completion of this process, new training procedures and new onboard medical equipment are incorporated into the space program. At some future time, as the Space Station becomes operational and as physician-astronauts are included in crew complements, more advanced biomedical training procedures will use the actual space platform as a training base, rather than relying heavily on ground-based simulations, as is now the case.

REFERENCES

Degioanni, J., Smart, R.C., and Snyder, R.D. Shuttle operational medical system (SOMS): Medical checklist, Preliminary, Rev. A (JSC-14798; LA-B-11110-5Q). Lyndon B. Johnson Space Center, Houston, TX, July 13, 1979.

Link, M.M. and Gurovskiy, N.N. Training of cosmonauts and astronauts. In: Foundations of space biology and medicine (Vol. III) (NASA SP-374). Edited by M. Calvin and O.G. Gazenko. U.S. Government Printing Office, Washington, D.C., 1975.

Machell, R.M., Bell, L.E., Khyken, N.P., and Prim, J.W., III. Summary of Gemini extravehicular activity. In: Gemini summary conference (NASA SP-138). U.S. Government Printing Office, Washington, D.C., 1967.

Pool, S.L. Emergency medical services system (EMSS). In: STS-1 medical report (NASA TM-58240). Edited by S.L. Pool, P.C. Johnson, Jr., and J.A. Mason. National Aeronautics and Space Administration, Scientific and Technical Information Branch, Washington, D.C., December 1981.

Schultz, D.C., Ray, H.A., Jr., Cernan, E.A., and Smith, A.F. Body positioning and restraints during extravehicular activity. In Gemini summary conference (NASA SP-138). U.S. Government Printing Office, Washington, D.C., 1967.

Vanderploeg, J.M. Crew medical training. In: STS-1 medical report (NASA TM-58240). Edited by S.L. Pool, P.C. Johnson, Jr., and J.A. Mason. National Aeronautics and Space Administration, Scientific and Technical Information Branch, Washington, D.C., December 1981.

Vanderploeg, J.M. and Hadley, A.T., III. Crew medical training and Shuttle Orbiter medical system. In: STS-2 medical report (NASA TM-58245). Edited by S.L. Pool, P.C. Johnson, Jr., and J.A. Mason. Lyndon B. Johnson Space Center, Houston, TX, May 1982.

17 Ground-Based Medical Programs

ARNAULD E. NICOGOSSIAN

SAM L. POOL

The principal goal of the ground-based medical program is to ensure the health and well-being of the astronauts and their families. A wide variety of programs have been implemented to support this goal, including: preflight health care, medical training, and support programs; inflight monitoring and observation; and postflight care and biomedical data collection. The health care record of the astronaut begins with medical selection and continues through his or her career into retirement, when annual physical exams are encouraged. The biomedical data collected through this program will enhance health care planning for the Space Station, and will be of value in designing new spacecraft and human habitats on such distant worlds as the moon or Mars.

PREFLIGHT PROGRAMS

Health care for the astronaut begins with the medical selection exam at the NASA Johnson Space Center (JSC) during an astronaut selection year. Astronaut candidate finalists spend 5 days at JSC and receive a thorough physical and laboratory exam, including treadmill, sigmoidoscopic, and X-ray examinations. They also receive subspecialist exams in ophthalmology, neurology, psychiatry, dentistry, and otolaryngology. Each candidate's results are compiled and presented to the Space Medicine Board at JSC, measured against NASA medical standards, and reported to the Medicine Policy Board at NASA Headquarters.

After selection, astronauts and their families receive outpatient medical and dental care at the JSC Flight Medicine Clinic. Astronauts also undergo a yearly medical examination certifying them for ongoing flight status. Problems which cannot be managed within the Flight Medicine Clinic are referred to a network of subspecialists within the Houston medical community. Astronauts and their families are encouraged to participate in a preventive medicine program with risk factor

283

analysis and follow-up counseling and intervention. Dietary and other information is available in the form of pamphlets and video tapes in the clinic, while quarterly newsletters on health care are mailed to the families. This program is designed to reduce chronic health problems (especially cardiovascular) as well as acute illnesses and injuries.

As crewmembers are assigned to specific flights, they enter into a rigorous training schedule. The manned test area of the Medical Operations Branch at JSC provides medical monitoring and care during EVA training in the Weightless Environment Training Facility (Figure 17-1), EVA suit qualification training in hypobaric chambers, and KC-135 aircraft parabolic flights for the simulation of microgravity. The medical personnel in the manned test area also provide classroom and hypobaric chamber training to pilots and all other personnel on flight status through a program with the Federal Aviation Administration. Hyperbaric treatment for decompression sickness is available at JSC and treatment protocols are conducted by experts in the manned test area.

Crewmembers also receive medical training for space flight from the Crew Surgeon assigned to the flight, who is typically one of the Flight Surgeons in the Medical Operations Branch. General training sessions cover medical and physiolog-

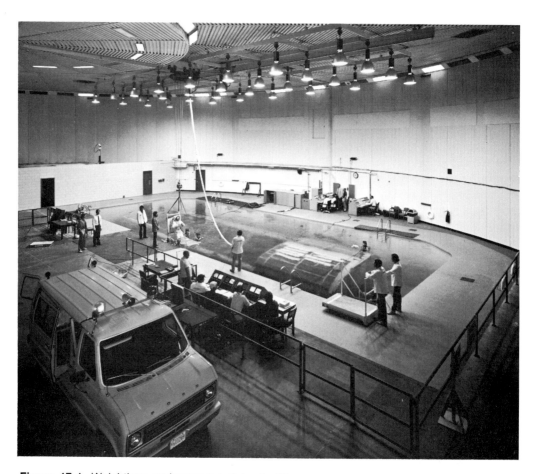

Figure 17-1. Weightless environment training facility.

ical problems encountered in microgravity, including space motion sickness, cardio-vascular deconditioning, reduced pressure environments, decompression sickness, radiation hazards, habitability, and the inflight medical care capability. Two crewmembers are selected as Crew Medical Officers (CMO) if no astronaut-physician is assigned to the flight. The CMOs receive additional training in the diagnostic and therapeutic capabilities of the Shuttle Orbiter Medical System (SOMS) and the Medical Checklist. The checklist is an onboard quick reference to common ambulatory and emergency medical problems and a complete description of the medications in the SOMS and their side effects. CMOs are trained to diagnose and treat common medical problems, give intramuscular and intravenous medications, and start intravenous lines, etc. They are also taught the use of the Contaminant Clean-up Kit (CCK) for protection against toxic or irritant materials that may contaminate the Shuttle atmosphere. Protection is available for crewmembers in the event of toxic spill, provided by 100 percent oxygen supplied by special crew helmets, or by goggles and masks for less toxic compounds.

Early Mercury and Gemini flights were sufficiently brief that there was little concern over the development of infectious disease in flight. As Gemini flights increased in duration, medical personnel acknowledged the possibility of disease and obtained a reduction in the number of personal contacts by crewmembers prior to launch. While there were no serious inflight episodes, Gemini crews did experience minor illnesses such as colds and influenza during prelaunch preparation.

During the Apollo Program, concern increased over the possibility and consequences of infectious disease, particularly with regard to the difficulty of completing a lunar landing should a crewmember become seriously ill during the early stages of the mission. All crewmembers on

Apollo 8 suffered viral gastroenteritis during the preflight period. Treatment was successful, and the spacecraft was launched on schedule. However, the recurrence of the infection in one crewmember in flight (Wooley and McCollum, 1975) greatly increased the awareness of the need for more stringent preflight measures to ensure astronaut health during a mission.

The Apollo 14 mission was the first to be conducted under a formalized Flight Crew Health Stabilization Program. The goal of the program was to eliminate inflight health problems by minimizing or eliminating adverse alterations in the health of flight crews during the immediate preflight period. The program combined four key elements: (1) clinical medicine, (2) immunology, (3) exposure prevention, and (4) epidemiological surveillance. The essence of the program was to institute, prior to launch, a 3-week period of strict control over locations to which flight crewmembers had access and number of personal contacts. Individuals required to be in contact with flight crewmembers were also carefully monitored for health status (Wooley and McCollum, 1975). The program was successful, immediately lowering the number of crewmembers experiencing illness during all mission periods.

The Health Stabilization Program, first instituted during Apollo, became a formal part of the Skylab mission sequence for two reasons. First, greatly extended periods of orbital flight increased the probability of inflight illness. Second, an inflight illness would have compromised the results of a number of biomedical experiments designed to examine in detail human physiological responses to the space environment. A 7-day postflight isolation period was added to allow extensive medical observation, examinations, and documentation of recovery from the physiological changes noted in flight.

A summary of the illnesses occurring in

the Apollo and Skylab Programs is presented in Table 17-1 (Ferguson, et al., 1977). Before the initiation of the Health Stabilization Program, 57 percent of prime crewmembers experienced some illness during the 21 days prior to launch, as well as illness events both in- and postflight. Illnesses included a number of upper respiratory infections, viral gastroenteritis, and one rubella exposure. These problems were notably absent under the administration of the Health Stabilization Program. (On Apollo 17 and Skylabs 3 and 4, crewmembers developed minor skin infections, or rashes, but medical personnel concluded that these occurred for reasons other than preflight exposure.)

The Space Transportation System (STS) presents new problems for health stabili-zation. Greater numbers of personnel are involved in launch preparation and, as missions become more frequent, more flight crewmembers will be under medical surveillance than in any previous program. Astronauts will also have more personal contacts prior to flight as preparations are completed for a variety of payloads.

The STS Health Stabilization Program identified three levels of health care coverage (NASA, 1981). Level I is the least stringent. This is a voluntary program based on health education and increased health awareness by flight crewmembers and contact personnel. It involves no special medical surveillance or examination beyond the initial health screening program usually completed 2 to 3 weeks before flight. Level II requires limited

TABLE 17-1

EFFECT OF THE FLIGHT CREW HEALTH STABILIZATION PROGRAM ON THE OCCURRENCE OF ILLNESS IN PRIME CREWMEMBERS

| Mission | Health Stabilization Program Absent | | | |
	Illness Type[a]	No. of Crewmen	Time Period[b]
Apollo 7	URI	3	M
8	VG	3	P,M
9	URI	3	P
10	URI	2	P
11			
12	SI	2	M
13	R	1	P
	Health Stabilization Program Operational		
Apollo 14			
14			
16			
17	SI	1	P
Skylab 2			
3	SI	2	M
4	SI	2	M

[a] Illness type: URI—upper respiratory infection; VG—viral gastroenteritis; SI—skin infection; R—rubella exposure.
[b] Time period: M—during mission; P—premission.
From Ferguson et al., 1977.

personal contact with flight crewmembers, and medical examination and surveillance of contact personnel. This is essentially the Health Stabilization Program used during previous space programs, but with reduced isolation time. Level III is a true isolation (quarantine) program which provides the maximum amount of health protection.

The appropriate level of health stabilization is decided for each STS mission by a Health Stabilization Board established at JSC. For the STS-1 mission, a Level II program was used. Personnel required to be in work areas were identified and given medical examinations. Those considered medically qualified were identified as primary contacts. The training facility and principal work areas for crewmembers were secured; only primary contacts were allowed entry, and they were instructed to wear surgical masks when within six feet of crewmembers. Each contact voluntarily reported any illness to the NASA Clinic. Table 17-2 shows the number, type, and location of personnel given medical examinations and approved as primary contacts for STS-1. The rate of illness for this population during the program was 28 illnesses per 1,000 persons per week (Ferguson, 1981). A summary of these illnesses is presented in Table 17-3. The STS-1 Program effectively excluded 38 known ill persons from crew work areas, thereby preventing exposure and possible illness.

The Health Stabilization Program for the STS-2 mission was reduced from a Level II to a Level I effort (Ferguson, 1982). This level, as noted, focuses on health awareness education for personnel entering crew work areas. Posters and signs were placed in these areas and information sheets were distributed to contacts. Special routes were established for crewmembers, to prevent accidental exposures. Only three illness reports were received from the 164 primary contacts during the 14 days of program operation. Crewmembers experienced no illness from infectious disease.

Illnesses were noted on missions 51-B, 51-F, 61-C, and preflight on D-1. These were thought to arise from increased crew contact with multiple personnel preflight, as well as from reduced surveillance. The Health Stabilization Program proposed for subsequent Shuttle missions is more stringent than the original Level I and II designations.

In addition to the Health Stabilization Program, a variety of other preflight medical programs have been developed to assure the safety and health of crews during flight. Middeck and/or Spacelab payloads are evaluated by the Payload Safety Review Board (PSRB) for hazards such as electric shock, fire potential, sharp edges, and broken glass. One of the primary medical hazards evaluated is the possible toxic contamination of the Shuttle atmosphere

TABLE 17-2

NUMBER, TYPE, AND LOCATION OF PERSONNEL GIVEN MEDICAL EXAMINATIONS AND APPROVED AS PRIMARY CONTACTS FOR STS-1

Type	Location					Subtotal
	(JSC)	(KSC)	(DFRC)	(ARC)	(Headquarters)	
NASA	216	35	7	1	5	264
Contractor	643	42	12	0	0	697
Others	10	1	0	0	0	11
Subtotal	869	78	19	1	5	Total: 972

From Ferguson, 1981.

TABLE 17-3

SUMMARY OF ILLNESSES IN STS-1 PRIMARY CONTACT POPULATION

Illness	Location (JSC)	(KSC)	(DFRC)	% of Total[a]
Upper respiratory function	24	3	3	81
Bronchitis	1	0	0	3
Pneumonia	0	0	0	0
Upper enteric illness	3	0	0	8
Lower enteric illness	2	0	0	5
Fever present	4	0	0	11
Headache present	1	0	0	3
Skin infection present	0	0	0	0
Other infectious illness	1	1	0	5

[a] Percentages total more than 100% because one illness may contain more than one symptom complex.
From Ferguson, 1981.

from a particular payload. Payloads that contain toxic material must have double or triple containment. Compounds are evaluated for toxic potential by the Biomedical Laboratories Branch and antidotes or other specific treatments are identified and flown in the Medical Accessory Kit, a companion kit to the SOMS. Toxic analysis and treatment procedures are written into the Shuttle toxicology database, which is available on computer to the Flight Surgeon in the Mission Control Center (MCC).

Middeck or Spacelab payload experiments that involve crewmembers as subjects are reviewed by the Human Research Policy and Procedures Committee (HRPPC) to ensure the safety and health of the crewmember. Preflight training procedures are reviewed for any pre- or postflight data collection, both on the ground and in the KC-135 aircraft, and JSC Flight Surgeons may be assigned to monitor training and data collection sessions at sites remote to JSC. International cooperation between medical boards of foreign payload customers and the NASA HRPPC has been very successful on previous Shuttle flights.

Flight Rules are developed for the Aeromedical section of the Flight Rule Book that governs all Shuttle flights. They are written to provide guidelines for an adequate atmosphere in terms of pressure and composition, to provide EVA prebreathe guidelines for prevention of decompression sickness in reduced pressure environments, and to detail effective countermeasures for inflight problems (such as fluid loading to counter cardiovascular deconditioning).

Planning for inflight medical contingencies is effected through NASA's Emergency Medical Services (EMS) and the Department of Defense (DoD). These two programs and contractor resources are committed to a Shuttle launch and landing to provide rescue and medical evacuation of injured crewmembers, if necessary. The EMS system consists of a worldwide network of medical and rescue specialists stationed at specified Shuttle launch and landing sites. Resources are prepositioned to ensure a timely response, preclude loss of life, and reduce the severity of injuries that do occur. NASA obtains DoD support through the DoD Manager for Shuttle Contingency Operations, based at Patrick AFB in Florida. The DoD provides helicopters, fixed-wing aircraft such as C-130s and C-9s, and rescue and medical personnel at the designated Shuttle launch and landing sites. Preflight simulations are conducted to coordinate the many professionals involved in providing EMS and to ensure that communications work smoothly throughout the exercise.

Flight Surgeons at JSC may be called upon to help investigate accidents involving NASA aircraft. All physicians who serve as Medical Officers of the Day (MOD) receive specific training in aircraft accident investigation and use of the medical equipment available at Ellington field. Simulations are conducted to ensure that the communications and investigations proceed smoothly for all personnel involved.

Flight Surgeons at JSC also undergo a detailed training program in all aspects of Shuttle medical support, and participate in the MCC simulations for all inflight phases of a mission. In essence, preflight training programs lead to certification of the Flight Surgeon as an MCC flight controller capable of working all phases of a Shuttle flight.

Occupational Health Services at many NASA centers support the Shuttle Program in a variety of ways. Occupational Health Clinics medically certify all personnel (other than crewmembers) who are essential for Shuttle missions. Through the Health Stabilization Program, the Clinics conduct the physical exams which permit support personnel to be "primary contacts" and Clinic personnel work with the crew for the 7 days prior to launch. Other essential mission support programs train employees who work with hazardous chemical or physical agents, to ensure the safety of such tasks as handling the fuels and testing the rocket engines.

PRE- AND POSTFLIGHT MEDICAL EXAMINATIONS

All space missions have included a schedule of detailed medical examinations of flight crewmembers prior to launch and following recovery. Preflight physical examinations, typically scheduled 10 days before launch, are conducted to detect any medical problems which might require remedial or preventive intervention, and to provide baselines for postflight comparison (Figure 17-2). The final examination immediately prior to launch medically certifies crewmembers for flight and documents their physical status at the beginning of the mission.

In the Orbital Flight Test (OFT) Program for the Space Shuttle, comprised of four orbital missions, there were four medical examinations preflight and three postflight. In addition, all crewmembers underwent vestibular testing beginning 180 days prior to the mission to establish personal treatment regimens.

After the OFT missions, two preflight and two postflight medical evaluations were performed as experience and a larger medical database led to a streamlining of medical operations to support an increased flight schedule. The schedule and contents of pre- and postflight evaluations for OFT missions are shown in Table 17-4. The duration listed for each examination is that used for the STS-1 mission. A formal medical debriefing accompanied the physical examination given immediately following recovery. Crewmembers were debriefed

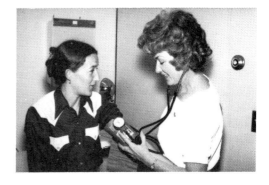

Figure 17-2. STS crewmember undergoing preflight medical examination at the Lyndon B. Johnson Space Center.

TABLE 17-4

SCHEDULE AND CONTENTS OF PRE- AND POSTFLIGHT EVALUATIONS USED FOR OFT MISSIONS[a]

Examination Date	Location	Duration	Examination Components
F − 30	JSC	1:05	LM, PX, D, V, T
F − 10	JSC	1:55	LM, ST, PX, A
F − 2	JSC	0:15	LM
F − 0	JSC	0:10	PX
L + 0	DFRC	0:30	LM, STW, PX
L + 3	JSC	1:45	ST, D, V, T, A, PX
L + 3–L + 7	JSC		T-38, check out

[a] Table key: A—audiometry; D—dental examination; LM—laboratory-microbiology; PX—physical examination; ST—(cardiovascular) stress tests, including 80 percent treadmill; STW—stand test - weight; T—tonometry; V—visual examination; F − 30—30 days before flight; L + 3—3 days after landing.
From Fischer and Degoianni, 1981.

using a standardized protocol to ensure accurate data collection and produce timely mission summaries. The STS-1 recovery medical examination revealed few physiological effects of space flight, as was anticipated for a mission lasting only 2 days and 6 hours. The crew did exhibit the expected hyperreflexia and dependent venous stasis (Fischer and Degoianni, 1981). The STS-2 mission, abbreviated to 2 days because of fuel cell problems, also involved only nominal change. In this case, the most notable finding was that both crewmembers were fatigued and underhydrated (LaPinta and Fischer, 1982). No residual space flight effects were observed during the next medical examination, conducted 3 days later.

INFLIGHT PROGRAMS

An important feature of medical surveillance during space missions is inflight monitoring of telemetered biomedical data. Sophisticated and highly reliable biotelemetry devices have been developed during the course of the U.S. and Soviet space programs. These allow real-time, comprehensive monitoring of biomedical status and provide critical data for medical personnel in the MCC. Table 17-5 shows the medical data collected and the techniques used to obtain this information.

The value of telemetered biomedical data as an aid in evaluating crewmember health status was demonstrated vividly during the Apollo 15 mission. Arrhythmias were noted while astronauts were on the lunar surface and, again, during return to Earth. Bigeminies and premature auricular and ventricular contractions were seen. These arrhythmias have been linked to potassium deficits and excessive workloads (Johnston and Hull, 1975). These unexpected cardiac events led to a comprehensive review of nutritional requirements and work schedules for subsequent lunar exploration missions.

Shuttle crews in flight are monitored indirectly for medical status by television and voice monitoring by the Flight Surgeon in the MCC, and directly through telemetry of biomedical data and Private Medical Communications (PMC). Heart rate was monitored for each crewmember through the first 12 flights of the Shuttle during prelaunch, launch, reentry, and landing. No significant findings were obtained, and the ECG monitoring was discontinued. ECG and other biomedical data (oxygen consumption, etc.) are obtained by telemetry during EVA maneuvers. These measurements allow the calculation of metabolic rates during EVA, which provided very useful data during flight 61-B when potential space construction techniques were evaluated by the EVA crewmembers. This flight demonstrated that acceptable construction techniques did not require large expenditures of energy.

PMCs between the crew and the Flight Surgeon in the MCC were conducted for STS 1-6. Crewmembers were able to discuss symptoms of space motion sickness (SMS) with a physician and receive treatment recommendations. As knowledge about SMS and its treatment increased, allowing greater preflight preparation, the daily inflight PMC was discontinued after STS-6. It is currently required only when an EVA is being considered prior to flight day 4 (approximately 72 hours mission elapsed time), the peak symptom period for SMS. A PMC may be requested at any other time by the Commander of the mission or the Flight Surgeon in the MCC.

Preflight education and inflight treatment of SMS will continue to be important for the Shuttle Program, particularly since incidence of SMS is now 67 percent in first-flight crewmembers. Because a majority of the cases (54 percent) are graded moderate to severe, SMS remains the major operational medical problem of short-duration space flight. Inflight treatment capability consists of oral, rectal, and IM/IV medications to reduce the nausea and vomiting associated with this syndrome. The operational impact of SMS is signif-

TABLE 17-5

SPACE FLIGHT MEDICAL DATA COLLECTED AND THE TECHNIQUES USED

Parameter Measured	American Missions	Soviet Missions
Cardiac activity and circulation	2-lead ECG with synchronous phonocardiography, vector-cardiography, blood pressure cuffs and automatic measurement of tonus, leg plethysmography during LBNP tests, venous compliance	Continuous 1-lead ECG, periodic 12-lead ECG, seismocardiography (myocardial contractility, kinetocardiography, blood pressure-pressure cuffs, tachooscillography and other measurements, sphygmography, rheoencephalography, and cardiac output (Bremser-Ranke)
Hematology	Hemoglobinometry, venous collection with separation and preservation	
Respiration	Impedance pneumography, spirometry, gas exchange	Perimetric pneumography, pulmonary volumes, gas exchange
CNS, sensory function, and performance	EEG, sleep analysis with EOG, voice communication, vestibular tests in rotating chair, overall task performance, otolith test-goggles, rod and sphere (for spatial orientation)	EEG, EOG, voice communication, vestibular tests, psychophysiological tests, overall task performance
Metabolism	Body mass measurement, biosampling, bicycle ergometry, metabolic analyzer (O_2 consumption, CO_2 production), body temperature (ear probe)	Biosampling

From Berry, 1975.

icant because EVAs cannot be scheduled until flight day 4 and minimum duration flights are defined as 96 hours mission elapsed time to ensure that a healthy crew is available for EVA or landing.

Finally, two computerized databases are available to assist the MCC Flight Surgeon: the aeromedical database and the Shuttle toxicology database. The aeromedical database provides essential data in the event of an onboard illness or Shuttle landing contingency and, to guide initial therapy, provides data on each crewmember for blood type, allergies, past medical history, and any unusual sensitivity to medications. The toxicology database provides a detailed description of any potential toxic hazard on the Shuttle and gives treatment recommendations, both supportive and specific.

acquired is then entered into the STS Medical Database, a computerized database that allows further stratification and analysis of the data. Subjective data related to symptoms of orthostatic intolerance are used by physicians in the Space Biomedical Research Institute for correlation with the blood pressure and ECG data obtained during postflight testing.

The NASA medical program continues beyond the active career of the astronaut. Retired astronauts are encouraged to participate in annual medical examinations at JSC to obtain data for analysis in a longitudinal study of this unique population exposed to microgravity. It is hoped that analysis of this longitudinal data will facilitate a greater understanding of the biological responses to microgravity.

POSTFLIGHT PROGRAMS

As noted above, postflight medical examinations are designed to recertify a crewmember for flight status after satisfactory recovery from the effects of microgravity. Postflight, crewmembers may demonstrate some disequilibrium, which has been described as a readaptation syndrome. This disequilibrium may persist up to 36 hours, but is usually gone by the time of the second postflight exam 3-7 days after landing.

During the two postflight exams, a detailed medical debriefing is conducted by the NASA Crew Physician using a standardized questionnaire to ensure the accuracy of the debriefing material. This technique has allowed the detailed characterization of SMS and has permitted the stratification of the syndrome into mild, moderate, and severe categories. Information from earlier flights is used to further refine the questionnaire. The data

FUTURE DIRECTIONS

As NASA plans longer-duration space flights on the Space Station, lunar colonies, or exploration of Mars, the need to study humans in microgravity will become more compelling. The limits of human tolerance to microgravity will need to be defined and effective countermeasures identified, where possible. Both preflight and inflight medical monitoring programs will increase in profile and importance, as necessary to ensure the health of crewmembers for longer periods in increasingly remote locations. Onboard medical diagnostic and therapeutic capabilities will be further refined to meet the challenges of providing health care under these conditions. New techniques for surgical procedures and an expanded understanding of pharmacodynamics are but two of the many challenges awaiting the health care provider on future space flights.

The information obtained from previous

manned space flights will be the foundation for future developments in providing health care on Space Station and beyond. Greater advances in preventive medicine, both in detection and intervention with risk factors, will become increasingly important as humans journey into remote microgravity environments.

REFERENCES

Berry, C.A. Medical care of space crews (Medical care, equipment, and prophylaxis). In: Foundations of space biology and medicine (Vol.III) (NASA SP-374). Edited by M. Calvin and O.G. Gazenko. U.S. Government Printing Office, Washington, D.C., 1975.

Ferguson, J.K. Health stabilization program. In: STS-1 medical report (NASA TM-58240). Edited by S.L. Pool, P.C. Johnson, and J.A. Mason. National Aeronautics and Space Administration, Scientific and Technical Information Branch, Washington, D.C., December 1981.

Ferguson, J.K. Health stabilization program. In: STS-2 medical report (NASA TM-58245). Edited by S.L. Pool, P.C. Johnson, and J.A. Mason. Lyndon B. Johnson Space Center, Houston, TX, May 1982.

Ferguson, J.K., McCollum, G.W. and Portnoy, B.L. Analysis of the Skylab flight crew health stabilization program. In: Biomedical results from Skylab (NASA SP-377). Edited by R.S. Johnston and L.F. Dietlein. U.S. Government Printing Office, Washington, D.C., 1977.

Fischer, C.L. and Degioanni, J. Evaluation of crew health. In: STS-1 medical report (NASA TM-58240). Edited by S.L. Pool, P.C. Johnson, and J.A. Mason. National Aeronautics and Space Administration, Scientific and Technical Information Branch, Washington, D.C., December 1981.

Hawkins, W.R. and Zieglschmid, J.F. Clinical aspects of crew health. In: Biomedical results of Apollo (NASA SP-368). Edited by R.S. Johnston, L.F. Dietlein, and C.A. Berry. U.S. Government Printing Office, Washington, D.C., 1975.

Johnston, R.S. and Hull, W.E. Apollo missions. In: Biomedical results of Apollo (NASA SP-368). Edited by R.S. Johnston, L.F. Dietlein, and C.A. Berry, U.S. Government Printing Office, Washington, D.C., 1975.

LaPinta, C.K. and Fischer, C.L. Evaluation of crew health. In: STS-2 medical report (NASA TM-58245). Edited by S.L. Pool, P.C. Johnson, and J.A. Mason. Lyndon B. Johnson Space Center, Houston, TX, May 1982.

National Aeronautics and Space Administration, Health stabilization program for the Space Transportation System (JSC 14899). Lyndon B. Johnson Space Center, Houston, TX, May 1981.

Wooley, B.C. and McCollum, G.W. Flight crew health stabilization program. In: Biomedical results of Apollo (NASA SP-368). Edited by R.S. Johnston, L.F. Dietlein, and C.A. Berry. U.S. Government Printing Office, Washington, D.C., 1975.

18 Countermeasures to Space Deconditioning

ARNAULD E. NICOGOSSIAN

Previous chapters have described physiological changes associated with short- and long-duration space missions. Some of these changes and adaptive processes, such as motion sickness, are self-limiting; others produce progressive changes in different body systems. These changes occasionally affect crew performance in flight. However, with continuing technological advances in space systems design, concerns have increased regarding the physiological implications of adaptation to weightlessness, and the ability of crewmembers to cope with complex and demanding tasks while physiologically stressed. Therefore, the search for countermeasures is considered to be of high priority in order to enhance performance in flight and upon return to a gravitational field, especially in light of the potential 2- to 3-year manned space missions for exploration of Mars or other planets.

MAINTENANCE OF PHYSICAL CONDITION

Two of the most immediate and significant effects of weightlessness are the headward shift of body fluids, and the removal of gravitational loading from bone and muscle. These changes lead to a progressive deconditioning (by Earth's standards) of the cardiovascular and musculoskeletal systems. Cardiovascular deconditioning is manifested by postflight orthostatic intolerance, decreased cardiac output, and reduced exercise capacity. Musculoskeletal system changes, brought about by hypodynamia and the absence of gravitational loading, are mostly reversible, but like cardiovascular changes they contribute substantially to weakness and poor gravitational tolerance in the postflight period. Both forms of deconditioning may also severely impair the ability of the weight-lessness-adapted individual to function adequately during the critical phases of reentry and landing, and to exit unassisted from the spacecraft.

Because the underlying factor producing the changes leading to cardiovascular and musculoskeletal deconditioning is the absence of gravity, efforts to reduce these deconditioning effects have focused primarily on restoring weight forces on the body and simulating Earth-normal physical movements, stresses and system interactions to the greatest extent possible. The most direct approach would be the generation of artificial gravity inside the spacecraft. Thus far, this has not been deemed practical, for technical and economic reasons. On a smaller scale, onboard centrifugation has been considered (Vil'-Vil'yams and Shul'zhenko, 1980), but this requires significant technological and engineering modification to current spacecraft systems.

Artificial gravity, in concept, has been proposed as a primary means to counteract bone and muscle mass loss in extended space missions of 1 year and longer. However, artificially-induced accelerative forces will produce coriolis acceleration on the vestibular system of individuals who will work and move about such environments (Graybiel, 1960; Lackner, 1986). This in turn will produce debilitating effects, especially when one moves from rotating to non-rotating environments. It has been established experimentally that a given rotation rate will determine the minimum space vehicle radius. For example, a rotation of 2 revolutions per minute will correspond to a radius of approximately 75 meters to produce an equivalent of 9.81 meters/sec^2 force. More rapid rotation rates will be associated with shorter radii; however, the incidence of coriolis forces under rapid head and body movements will be greater (Nicogossian and McCormack, 1987).

The single approach which has received wide operational acceptance to date in the U.S. and U.S.S.R. space programs is exercise, particularly when combined with the periodic application of low-level lower body negative pressure (LBNP) (up to -30 torr), as in the U.S.S.R. program. The provision of adequate daily dietary caloric and nutrient content constitutes another significant countermeasure, particularly for counteracting the losses of muscle mass and electrolytes that are important for the general metabolic regulation. Occasionally, electrical muscle stimulation has been utilized in flight to prevent changes in the muscular system. In recent years, in order to minimize the time devoted to physical training during flight, a search has begun for newer and more efficient countermeasures, including drugs. In general, these efforts have not produced ideal measures of protection and, in many instances, have raised additional questions regarding their potential effect on the time course of underlying mechanisms of "space deconditioning."

EXERCISE

Exercise Techniques

A variety of exercise techniques and devices have been employed in the Soviet and American space programs. An ideal exercise countermeasure represents the best possible compromise among efficacy, equipment size, ease of performance, and operational time requirements (Nicogossian et al., 1988). Since complete maintenance of one-gravity physical condition is not possible, the identification of functional capabilities that are compatible with different missions is also an important factor. It has been suggested that different types of exercise offer different degrees of protection and efficacy (Thornton, 1977; Nicogossian et al., 1988). Isotonic and isokinetic exercises work well in preventing mass and strength losses in certain muscle groups, while quiet standing under gravitational loading (by means of straps) may afford some protection against loss of bone mass. Walking under the same applied force appears to slow down muscle atrophy and improve coordination. Endurance exercises such as pedaling a bicycle ergometer minimize reductions in work capacity, as well as respiratory capacity, and may also increase circulating blood volume. However, the latter approach (which has been used whenever possible on long-term flights since the early 1970's) does not significantly affect the rate of mineral or muscle mass losses, which seem to level off after 6 months in space.

Thornton (1977) has suggested that combining exercise techniques and devices with application of one-gravity equivalent forces (e.g., on a passive treadmill) is the most effective way to reduce muscle, joint, and bone atrophy; minimize reductions in heart size/mass; and maintain coordination and exercise capacity.

Although the types of exercise best suited to the maintenance of different physiological functions can be fairly spec-ified, the optimum amount of daily exercise is uncertain. Table 18-1 gives an estimate of time required to maintain average nonathletic performance upon return to Earth.

Experience Gained From Inflight Exercise Programs

Exercise regimens prescribed for space missions have required gradually longer and more frequent periods of exercise—particularly as the length of missions has increased. On the first prolonged (18-day) Soviet manned flight, Soyuz-9, physical exercises were performed by the cosmonauts for two 1-hour periods each day. In a subsequent 24-day flight, 2.5 hours of exercise were employed daily, including walking/running on a treadmill. By 1975, a standard exercise regimen had begun to emerge, involving three exercise periods per day and a variety of equipment, for a total of 2.5 hours, with selection of exercises on the fourth day being optional (Dodge, 1976). On more recent Salyut and Mir flights, cosmonauts have been required to exercise 3 hours per day (divided

TABLE 18-1

EXERCISE TIME REQUIRED TO MAINTAIN ONE-GRAVITY CAPACITIES

Physical Parameter	Exercise Modality	
	(Walk)	(Jog)
Leg Strength	15–20 min/day	5 min/day
Leg Endurance	25–30 min/day	15–20 min/day
Cardiorespiratory Endurance	30 min/day	15–20 min/day
Bone Strength	1–2 hours/day	30–90 min/day
Coordination	10 min/day	5 min/day
	1-g Equivalent Hydrostatic Forces on Leg Vessels	
Blood & Fluid Redistribution & Loss	1–3 hrs/day in addition to above exercises. This should be a static exercise which would not interfere with other duties.	

Thornton (personal communications, 1981).

into two sessions) for 6 days per week. Also, the type of exercise, intensity, and equipment is rotated on a 4-day cycle. Some of these exercises were performed with a bicycle ergometer rated for increasing physical loads (Hooke et al., 1986). On the treadmill, cosmonauts were monitored for workloads, distance covered, and vital signs during exercise. A similar increase in exercise level was imposed during the three Skylab missions (0.5, 1.0, and 1.5 hours/day), although the total amounts were less than those used by the Soviets. Throughout the Skylab missions, successive improvements were seen in postflight leg strength and volume changes, orthostatic tolerance and recovery time, and cardiac output and stroke volume, even though each mission lasted 4 weeks longer than the last (Henry et al., 1977; Thornton and Rummel, 1977). During the first manned Skylab mission, only the bicycle ergometer was used. During the second mission, isokinetic devices MKI and II were added, and during the last and longest mission the treadmill was included in the overall daily exercise regimen. No significant change was observed in postflight leg muscle strength between the first and second missions, while significant improvements were noted in all crewmembers after the last mission, where the treadmill was used. In addition, although Skylab 3 and 4 crews showed approximately the same preflight levels of physical conditioning (as determined by oxygen consumption), a distinct improvement in VO_2 was noted during the last mission. Although the Skylab 4 Commander performed the least work on the bicycle ergometer, he did not exhibit losses in weight or os calcis mass postflight. Changes in his stressed heart level during maximum LBNP were also less pronounced than in the other two crewmembers. The main differences which account for this response might be walking and running on the treadmill and/or the in-

dividual physical fitness level which resulted in such a dramatic recovery postflight (Nicogossian et al., 1988).

Results of exercise on Soviet missions have shown similar patterns of reduced physiological deconditioning in response to more strenuous exercise programs (Gazenko, Genin, and Yegorov, 1981; Yegorov, 1980). These regimens have been successful: in flights of 6 months' duration on the Salyut-6 station some parameters, such as exercise capacity, did not change from preflight values. Body mass has tended to increase linearly during such missions—a result which can be attributed partly to exercise, particularly in view of the gradual restoration in leg volumes toward the end of the missions. In some instances, the response of heart rate and arterial pressure to lower body negative pressure tests in flight remained essentially unchanged from baseline values. Other cardiovascular parameters, such as cardiac ejection and filling times, output and pressure at rest and during stress, have continued to be affected by weightlessness; however, overall physical fitness has been adequately maintained.

Anti-Deconditioning Devices

A wide variety of onboard equipment has been developed for use in weightlessness. Most of these items are related to exercise, and all are designed for the maintenance of physical conditioning.

Ergometer

This device is a bicycle-like apparatus which can be pedaled with either the hands or the feet (Figure 18-1). A variety of cardiovascular and metabolic parameters can be monitored during work. Electrodes and a blood pressure cuff are attached to the user, and ventilation and aerobic capacity can be estimated (Sawin et al., 1975). Similar devices have been

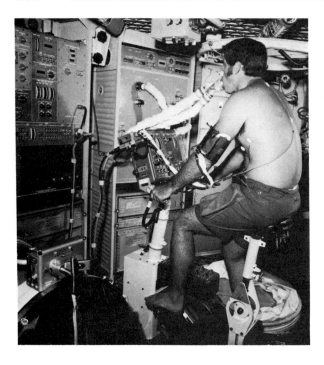

Figure 18-1. The ergometer device used on board Skylab. This apparatus permits both exercise and metabolic / cardiorespiratory analysis.

present on board Skylab and all Soviet space stations beginning with Salyut-4.

Treadmill

All Soviet space stations have featured treadmills (Figure 18-2) on which astronauts and cosmonauts could exercise the lower limbs more thoroughly than on the ergometer (Dodge, 1976; Hordinsky, 1977). The treadmill was used only on the final Skylab mission, Skylab 4, but is included onboard the Space Shuttle (Figure 18-3). In both the Soviet and American versions, elastic "bungee cord" straps are used to secure the individual to the treadmill and provide simulated gravitational force (1.1-g on Skylab; 0.62-g on Salyut).

"Penguin" Suit

Soviet cosmonauts use a special elasticized suit which provides passive stress on antigravity muscle groups of the legs and torso (Umanskiy, 1983). This constant-loading, or "Penguin" suit (Figure 18-4), is worn by cosmonauts not only through-

out exercise (the tie-down straps used with the treadmill can be attached), but also during the entire working day. It provides partial compensation for the absence of gravity by opposing movement, and places a constant gravitational load on

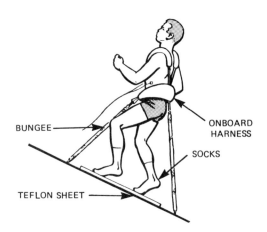

Figure 18-2. Representation of a passive treadmill used on board Skylab 4. Elastic bungee cords provide simulated gravitational loading. (From Thornton, 1981).

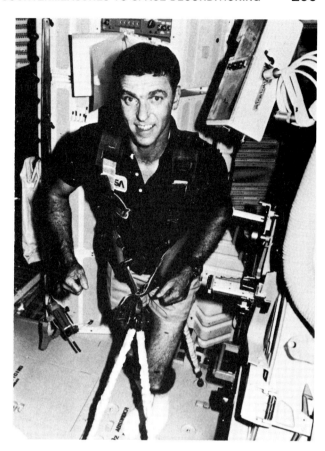

Figure 18-3. The STS-2 Commander using the Space Shuttle treadmill.

muscles of the legs and trunk (Yegorov, 1981).

Lower Body Negative Pressure Chamber

Lower body negative pressure, or LBNP, partially reverses headward fluid shifts, thus minimizing cardiovascular deconditioning. LBNP can also be used to assess levels of deconditioning during a mission, predicting the degree of postflight orthostatic intolerance. The LBNP chamber on Skylab (Figure 18-5) was used for this purpose (Johnson et al., 1977). The Soviets use LBNP for this purpose and as an inflight countermeasure to cardiovascular deconditioning. The "Chibis" vacuum suit (Figure 18-6) can be used while sitting or standing, freeing cosmonauts for other tasks. LBNP sessions in the Chibis are scheduled toward the end of long-term missions in order to subject the cardiovascular system to fluid shifts, helping to increase orthostatic tolerance upon return to Earth. Typically, LBNP is applied every 4 days for 20 minutes (5 minutes at each of four pressure levels), and for 50 minutes per day in the final 2 days of a mission (Gazenko et al., 1981). At the end of a mission, about 400 ml of water is consumed with 3 g of sodium chloride during application of LBNP, to restore fluid volume lost as a result of space flight.

Figure 18-7 shows an ambulatory LBNP suit for possible future use. It has not been evaluated in flight.

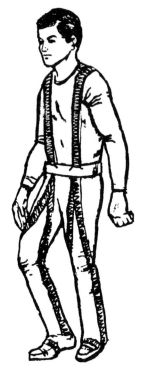

Figure 18-4. The "Penguin" constant-loading suit worn by cosmonauts.

lected muscles, a technique which relies partly on passive muscle conditioning. Various muscle groups are stimulated by an apparatus called the "Tonus," in an effort to reduce disuse atrophy of muscle tissue.

Other Devices

Numerous other exercise devices of lesser importance or more limited application have been employed in space. Most of these may be categorized as one of two standard types: the capstan-type "stretcher" or the elastic "chest expander." Representations of these are shown in Figure 18-8. Such devices are extremely lightweight, inexpensive, and easy to use; yet because of the nature of the forces they generate and the limited groups of muscles they exercise, they are not considered especially effective (Thornton, 1977). They are useful as accessory exercisers, however.

Antigravity Suit

Another countermeasure for minimizing postflight orthostatic intolerance used both by U.S. and U.S.S.R. crews is the antigravity suit (G-suit). This suit has somewhat the opposite function of the lower body negative pressure suit, as it increases pressure on the lower body, preventing blood from pooling in the extremities during reentry and postflight. The G-suit has been found to improve venous return and orthostatic stability postflight (Gazenko et al., 1981).

Electrostimulation

In the Soviet space program, a variety of procedures are experimented with and so far have not received wide acceptance by Western space medicine specialists. One of these is electrostimulation of se-

NUTRITION AND PHARMACOLOGICAL SUPPORT

Nutritional and pharmacological procedures have been investigated in a number of studies as possible countermeasures to space-induced physiological changes such as fluid shifts, cardiovascular deconditioning, muscle strength and mass losses, and bone mineral losses. Studies dealing with nutritional and pharmacological benefits are difficult to conduct and interpret. Drugs usually have broad effects across many body functions, and can produce potential iatrogenic side effects, especially when administered in conjunction with metabolic adaptive changes associated with space flight. Space pharmacology is in its infancy, since many of the mechanisms involved in the adaptation to weightlessness are poorly understood.

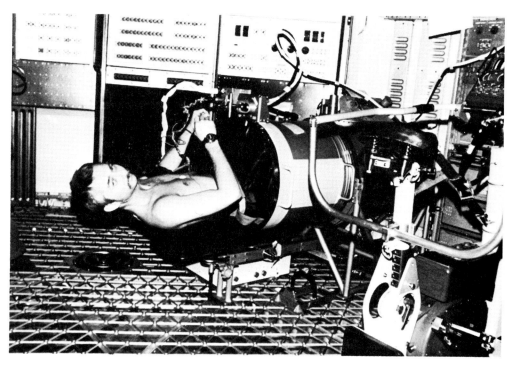

Figure 18-5. The LBNP apparatus in use on board Skylab.

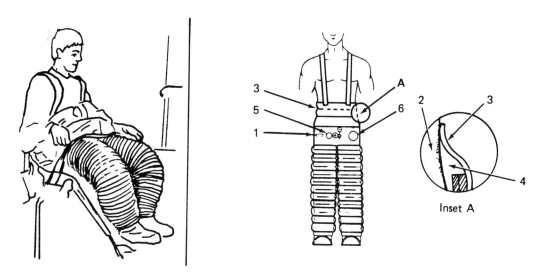

Figure 18-6. Subject wearing Chibis suit. At right is a general diagram of the garment. 1—Micropump, 2—body, 3—rubber shutter, 4—air space, 5—air intake valve, 6—manometer.

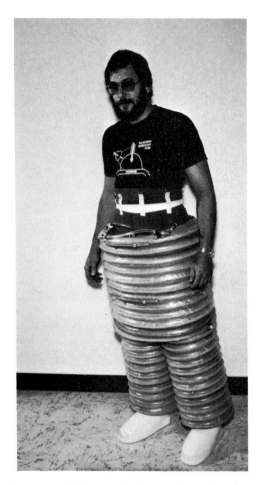

Figure 18-7. The NASA experimental ambulatory LBNP suit.

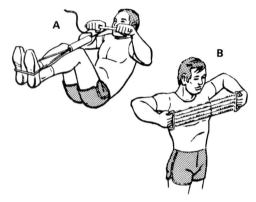

Figure 18-8. Two simple types of loading devices for arm exercise in weightlessness. On the left (A) is a rope/capstan device that allows development of high forces; on the right (B) is a simple elastic device.

Nutritional Considerations

The need for food, more precisely, the need for nutrient substances, is driven by the body's total energy expenditure as expressed in the activity of muscles, organs, systems, and mental/nervous processes. This need is regulated by thirst, appetite, digestion, and metabolism, and physical work output. Weightlessness results in a substantial loss of the fluids and electrolytes that govern many functions (Leach,

1981). The much-reduced physical work requirement results not only in altered energy output, but also in loss of protein nitrogen through muscle atrophy (Ushakov, 1980). The reduction in electromechanical stresses and other factors brings about a loss of calcium from bone. Some investigators have suggested that metabolic and digestive processes undergo substantial changes, partly as a result of the altered stress environments and physical confinement.

Much effort has been devoted in both the U.S. and Soviet space programs to determine the optimum diet for space missions. Considerations of storage time, size/weight restrictions, and practicality for consumption in weightlessness initially led to the use of freeze-dried food bars (Figure 18-9), and purees and juices packaged in squeeze tubes. The palatability of these early food items left much to be desired, which meant that the intended quantities were sometimes not consumed. In addition, early estimates of energy requirements on space missions were unrealistically low, and metabolic changes were not adequately taken into account. For these reasons, space diets have undergone considerable evolution.

Food Variety. The most significant changes in space diets over the years have been substantially increased diversity of foods, and improvements in packaging and presentation methods. For example, foods available to Skylab crews included 70 different items presented in the form of freeze-dried rehydratables, thermostabilized foods, dry and moist bite-sized foods, and a variety of beverages (Johnston, 1977). Hot and cold water were available for rehydration, as well as an oven for heating. Utensils could be used with solid foods covered by a plastic membrane (Figure 18-10). Spice packets added flavor and improved palatability. In the Space Shuttle, the Skylab innovations have been augmented by a food galley and pantry similar to those seen on airliners, and stocked according to crew preference (Sauer and Rapp, 1981). The Soviets have taken even larger steps to accommodate individual preferences, having customized menus on an individual basis since the early Soyuz flights (Dodge, 1976). In later Salyut missions, Progress cargo ships periodically supplied fresh fruits, vegetables, and condiments to supplement the diet. Crews were encouraged to "order out" for items they wanted. Overall, the tendency has been to establish meal patterns and food quality that approximate terrestrial standards while meeting energy and metabolic requirements.

Energy Content. On the basis of experience, and particularly with longer flights and extensive inflight exercise programs, total energy content of the diets in U.S./U.S.S.R. space programs has progressively

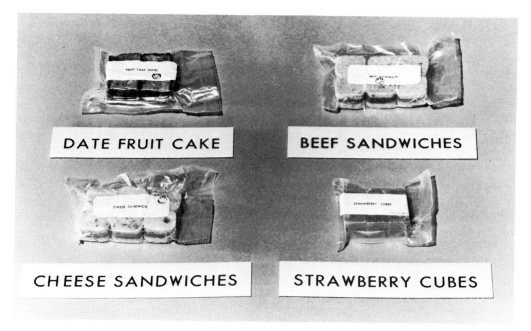

Figure 18-9. Typical space food developed for early Apollo missions.

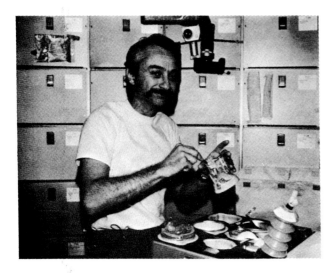

Figure 18-10. Astronaut reconstituting food during Skylab 3. Note use of normal utensils.

increased (Dodge, 1976; Johnston, 1977). In the first Soviet flights, for example, daily caloric intake was about 2,600 kcal, increasing to 2,800 kcal in the first phase of the Soyuz program. By the time of Salyut-1, this had been raised to 2,950 kcal. The Salyut-4 diet provided 3,000 kcal, and on Salyut-6, the caloric allowance was 3,150 kcal. Energy content of American space diets has been somewhat lower on average—about 2,500 kcal (except in the Apollo lunar landing missions, where it was 2,800-3,000 kcal). Table 18-2 shows the caloric and nutrient content of a typical Apollo meal. By the time of Skylab, the energy content of the space diet was equivalent to that of the normal preflight diet. The daily menu for the Space Shuttle provides 3,000 kcal per person, although individual intake is not necessarily this large. Table 18-3 shows estimated mean daily intake on board STS-1-4 flights.

Dietary Supplements. Attention has been paid to the potential impact of diets on higher cerebral function (via the neurotransmitters) and performance. This research is in the early stage of experimentation, and this approach of utilizing specially devised diet composition with respect to amino acids, needs to be further developed and validated (Fernstrom, 1981). Soviet scientists have indicated that intake of vitamins, amino acids, and minerals promotes the retention of fluids and electrolytes. These preparations are administered in larger doses just prior to reentry in order to facilitate the readaptation process (Yegorov, 1981). A lower level of potassium in the diet has been implicated in the cardiac arrhythmias and long postflight recovery period observed on Apollo 15; potassium supplements appeared to prevent these problems on subsequent missions (Berry, 1981).

Drugs

Pharmaceutical compounds are used in a variety of ways as countermeasures to the physiological effects of space flight, most significantly in preventing the symptoms of space motion sickness. (For a detailed treatment of this subject, see Chapter 8). Medical kits carried on board manned spacecraft include routine medications such as aspirin, antihistamines, stimulants, and sedatives, as well as a variety of emergency medications. These, however, are not intended for use as countermeasures, except in the case of motion sickness, to the problems discussed in this chapter. Although their research programs in this area are similar, American and Soviet biomedical specialists have adopted somewhat different approaches to the use of drugs as countermeasures in space flight. Inflight drug absorption studies such as acetaminophen and scopolamine seem to indicate that the pharmacokinetics of drugs in space flight is different from that observed on the ground (see Chapter 13).

Cardiovascular Deconditioning. More than their American counterparts, Soviet biomedical researchers favor the use of drugs as countermeasures to cardiovascular deconditioning. In conjunction with the Penguin, Chibis, and G-suits, and exercise regimens, cosmonauts have used drugs such as ephedrine, papazol, isoptin, ritmodan, novocainamid, cytochrome C, Aldactone, Nitrol, and mexitil to control cardiovascular disturbances resulting from weightlessness. Other drugs such as tropaphen, phenoxybenzamine, anapriline, octadine, cargocromene, and papaverine, separately or in combinations, have been used during missions to improve adrenergic regulation of blood circulation. Attempts have been made to normalize water-sodium metabolism by administra-

TABLE 18–2

TYPICAL COMPOSITION AND CALORIC CONTENT OF APOLLO DAILY MEAL

Food Composition of Daily Menu

Meal A	Meal B	Meal C
Fruit cocktail	Chicken salad	Beef stew
Bacon squares	Beef with vegetables	Potato salad
Strawberry cubes	Butterscotch pudding	Sweet pastry cubes
Cocoa	Fruitcake	Grapefruit drink
Orange drink	Pineapple-grapefruit drink	

Food Values

Constituents	Meal A	Meal B	Meal C	Total
Energy (kcal)	759	1123	911	2793
Protein (g)	28.5	45.2	28.7	102.4
Fat (g)	25.4	42.0	32.4	99.8
Carbohydrate	106.4	140.0	125.7	372.1
Ash (g)	7.0	6.8	7.3	21.1
Ca (mg)	176.0	505.0	486.0	1168.0
P (mg)	342.0	712.0	592.0	1646.0
Fe (mg)	3.3	4.8	4.9	13.0
Na (mg)	1659.0	1526.0	1916.0	5101.0
K (mg)	818.0	863.0	1047.0	2728.0
Mg (mg)	64.3	89.5	95.3	249.1
Cl as NaCl (g)	4.30	3.05	3.94	11.29

TABLE 18-3

ESTIMATED MEAN DAILY INFLIGHT NUTRIENT CONSUMPTION PER PERSON

Nutrient	STS Flights				Recommended Levels	
	No. 1 (2 days)	No. 2 (2 days)	No. 3 (8 days)	No. 4 (7 days)	(JSC)[a]	(RDA)[b]
RH$_2$O (g)[c]		1134	1393	1710.8		
NH$_2$O (g)[d]		88.4	353.0	325.5		
Kilocalories	2656	1100	1910	2446	3000	
Protein (g)	106.8	58.5	66.1	85.6	56	56
Fat (g)	83.1	28.0	49.6	73.5		
Carbohydrate (g)	358.6	152.0	280.2	319.2		
Calcium (mg)	1210	687	885	954	800	800
Phosphorus (mg)	1706	916	1210	1474	800	800
Sodium (mg)	4506	1782	3010	3506	3450	
Potassium (mg)	3238	1362	2244	2558	2737	
Iron (mg)	27.1	12.4	16.6	20.2	18	10
Magnesium (mg)	387	154	229	286	350	350
Manganese (mg)			1.6	2.2		
Copper (mg)			1.9	2.2		
Zinc (mg)	17.6	9.4	10.1	11.6		15
Chloride (mg)			4407	4784		

[a] JSC—Johnson Space Center
[b] RDA—Recommended Dietary Allowance
[c] RH$_2$O—rehydration water
[d] NH$_2$O—moisture in food
Sauer and Rapp, 1981, 1983.

tion of vasopressin, pitressin, desoxycorticosterone acetate, and nerobol (Shashkov and Yegorov, 1979). Antidiuretic hormone is sometimes administered to control fluid loss. In addition, isotonic solution loading prior to reentry is used to reduce postflight orthostatic intolerance.

Bone Mineral Loss. Considerable research has been directed at finding pharmaceutical means for halting the seemingly progressive loss of calcium. Soviet efforts in this area have so far been unsuccessful. However, American researchers have recently reported promising results with clodronate disodium, a diphosphonate compound which appears to prevent hypercalciuria during bed rest (Dietlein and Johnston, 1981).

Saline Ingestion Countermeasure. Bed rest studies have demonstrated and subsequent postflight studies have confirmed the usefulness of oral rehydration with saline solutions as a cardiovascular countermeasure to decrease the marked orthostatic intolerance which occurs during the first few hours after returning from microgravity or rising from bed rest. These saline solutions are isotonic sources of extracellular fluid (ECF) needed when the crewmember or bed rest subject first stands upright in gravity. At this time, the volume sensors of the cardiovascular system sense the sudden need for the additional circulating volume excreted during the early hours of bed rest or space flight. In addition to vasoconstriction, a profound thirst is felt and any available fluid in the gastrointestinal tract is absorbed to help replenish the deficit. As with most thirsts, water is needed, but unlike dehydration from heat, both salt and water are needed in proportion to that in the ECF. Hypertonic sugar beverages often used in athletic contests to replenish sweat and muscle glycogen may be used by the crewmember, but with less effect. During the first hour postflight, a crewmember may consume a liter or more of fluid in response to thirst sensations.

To aid the individual, both the U.S. and U.S.S.R. programs encourage crewmembers to ingest approximately 1 liter of drinking water made isotonic after ingestion, by simultaneously swallowing the appropriate number of coated salt tablets. For the Shuttle flights, each crewmember is furnished a 1-gram sodium chloride (salt) tablet for each 4 ounces (114 ml) of drinking water ingested, to a total of 8 tablets and 912 ml of water starting 2 hours before reentry. Postflight studies have indicated that this significantly decreases the degree of cardiovascular deconditioning as shown by the postflight blood pressure and heart rate response to a passive stand test (Bungo et al., 1985). However, preliminary assessments on short-duration missions of the Space Shuttle have shown that, starting with the fourth day in flight, there might be a tendency toward reduced efficiency of salt and water loading prior to reentry. Additional data will be required to confirm this finding (Bungo, personal communication). Postflight, additional fluids and electrolytes are given to returning crewmembers within the first 2 hours after landing, in order to further reduce the body fluid volume deficit.

The U.S.S.R. has used a similar regimen, but tends to start the rehydration program a week before reentry. Unlike U.S. crewmembers, cosmonauts use a flight LBNP device to enhance sequestration of the fluid in the interstitial space and thereby delay renal excretion of the fluid volume which is not needed in microgravity, but will be needed immediately on reentry.

SUMMARY

Undoubtedly, the reinterpretation of space flight data in light of new theories and accumulating evidence will have a profound impact on the development and utilization of countermeasures. Currently-proposed countermeasures to ameliorate undesirable effects of adaptation to weightlessness and/or prepare for return to Earth's gravitational field are shown in Tables 18-4 and 18-5. Their potential effect on specific target organs are also described. Obviously, their actions can also result in non-beneficial effects, i.e., sympatomimetic action of drugs in a hypovolemic situation.

It is clear from Tables 18-4 and 18-5 that a careful selection of several countermeasures alone or in combination could help maintain the capacity for rapid readaptation upon return to Earth or prevent inappropriate adaptive responses to space flight. The timing of these measures is also important. Use of the anti-motion sickness medications might affect the cardiovascular or central nervous systems such that unwanted side effects outweigh their benefits. Combining animal protein diets, high calcium and vitamin D supplements, and vigorous exercise, in light of negative water balance, might result in the appearance of nephrolithiasis in space (Sakhaee et al., 1987).

TABLE 18-4

POTENTIAL BODY SYSTEMS RESPONSES TO COUNTERMEASURES IN FLIGHT[a]

Countermeasure	Endocrine	Vestibular	Cardiovascular	Renal	Muscle	Bone
Drugs						
Anticholinergics	?	++	++	−	+	−
Antihistamines	+	+++	+++	−	−	−
Sympathomimetics	+	++	++	+	++	−
Exercise	+	?	+	+	++	+
Myoelectric stimulation	−	−	−	−	−	+
Salt/water supplements	+	−	+	+	−	−
Ca++ and vitamin D₃ supplements	+	−	−	++	−	++
Diphosphonates	−		−	−	?	++
LBNP[b]	++	?	++	++	?	−
Mineral corticosteroids	++	?	++	++	++	+

[a] Table key: ?—unknown; +—weak response; ++—strong response; −—no response.
[b] LBNP—lower body negative pressure device.
Adapted from Nicogossian et al., 1985.

TABLE 18-5

PROPOSED RESPONSES TO COUNTERMEASURES POSTFLIGHT[a]

Countermeasures	Cardiovascular	Vestibular	Muscle	Bone	Renal	Endocrine	Hematopoietic
Salt and water supplement	+ +	−	−	−	+ +	+ +	−
Ca⁺⁺ supplements	−	−	−	+ +	+ +	+ +	−
Vasoconstrictors	+ +	?	−	−	+ +	+ +	−
Physical rehabilitation	+ +	?	+ +	+ +	+ +	+ +	+ +
Vitamin supplements	−	−	−	−	−	−	+ +

[a] Table key: ?—unknown; +—weak response; + +—strong response; − —no response.
Adapted from Nicogossian et al., 1985.

Although empirically designed mainly from ground-based zero-g simulation experiments, countermeasures have provided some means of protection; their potential for unwanted side effects has not yet been fully clarified. It is obvious that current ground-based simulation techniques do not have a one-to-one relationship with adaptive changes occurring in space flight. Further approximation of results without adequate and reproducible space-documented data could further obfuscate the definition of the nature and time course of adaptation to space.

Answers to the above questions can be obtained only through well planned and integrated ground and flight studies, perhaps in combination with appropriate mathematical models of complex physiological systems. Dedicated life sciences missions are expected to provide scientific information which will contribute to the design of countermeasures by the mid 1990's.

REFERENCES

Berry, C.A. Physiological and psychological parameters of life in space stations. Spaceflight, 23(1):23–26, 1981.

Bungo, M.W., Charles, J.B., and Johnson, P.C. Cardiovascular deconditioning during spaceflight and the use of saline as a countermeasure to orthostatic intolerance. Aviation, Space, and Environmental Medicine, 56(10):985–990, 1985.

Dietlein, L.F., and Johnston, R. U.S. manned space flight: The first twenty years. Acta Astronautica, 8(9–10):893, 1981.

Dodge, C.H. The Soviet space life sciences. In: Soviet space programs, 1971–1975: Overview, facilities, and hardware, manned and unmanned flight programs, bioastronautics, civil and military applications, projections of future plans (Vol. 1). Library of Congress, Science Policy Research Division, Congressional Research Service, Washington, D.C., 1976.

Dodge, C.H. The space life sciences. In: United States civilian space programs, 1958–1978. Congressional Research Service, Science Policy Research Division, Washington, D.C., January 1981.

Fernstrom, J.D. Effects of the diet on brain function. Acta Astronautica, 8(9–10):1035–1041, 1981.

Gazenko, O.G., Genin, A.M., and Yegorov, A.D. Major medical results of the Salyut-6-Soyuz 185-day space flight. Preprints of the XXXII Congress of the International Astronautical Federation, Rome, Italy, 6–12 September 1981.

Graybiel, A. Observation on Human Subjects Living in an S.R.R. for Periods of 2 Days. AMA, Archives of Neurology, 3:55–73, 1960.

Henry, W.L., Epstein, S.E., Griffith, J.M., Goldstein, R.E., and Redwood, D.R. Effect of prolonged space flight on cardiac function and dimensions. In: Biomedical results from Skylab (NASA SP-377). Edited by R.S. Johnston and L.F. Dietlein, National Aeronautics and Space Administration, Washington, D.C., 1977.

Hooke, L., Radtke, M., Garshnek, V., Teeter, R., and Rowe, J. A physician on the flight crew (translation from Zemlya i Vselennaya, 5:49–57, 1985). U.S.S.R. Space Life Sciences Digest, NASA CR-3922 (05), 5:1–8, 1986.

Johnson, R.L., Hoffler, G.W., Nicogossian, A.E., Bergman, S.A., Jr., and Jackson, M.M. Lower body negative pressure: Third manned Skylab mission. Edited by R.S. Johnston and L.F. Dietlein, National Aeronautics and Space Administration, Washington, D.C., 1977.

Johnston, R.S. Skylab medical program overview. In: Biomedical results from Skylab (NASA SP-377). Edited by R.S. Johnston and L.F. Dietlein, National Aeronautics and Space Administration, Washington, D.C., 1977.

Lackner, J.R., Graybiel, A. The Effective Intensity of Coriolis Cross-Coupling Stimulation is Gravitoinertial Force Dependent. Aviation, Space, and Environmental Medicine, 57:229–235, 1986.

Leach, C.S. An overview of the endocrine and metabolic changes in manned space flight. Acta Astronautica, 8(9–10):977–988, 1981.

Nicogossian, A.E., Pool, S., Leach Huntoon, C.S., and Leonard, J.I. Development of Countermeasures for Use in Space Missions. Preprints 36th IAF Congress, Stockholm, Sweden, 1985.

Nicogossian, A., and McCormack, P. Artificial Gravity: A Countermeasure for Zero Gravity. Preprints 38th IAF Congress, Brighton, U.K., 1987.

Nicogossian, A., Sulzman, F., Radtke, and Bungo, M. Assessment of the efficacy of medical countermeasures in space flight. Acta Astronautica, Pergamon Press, 17(2):195–198, 1988.

Sakhaee, K., Nigam, S., Snell, P., Chue Hsu, M., and Pack, C.Y.C. Assessment of the pathogenetic role of physical exercise in renal stone formation. Journal of Clin. Endocrin. and Metab., 65(5):974–979, 1987.

Sauer, R.L., and Rapp, R.M. Food and nutrition. In: STS-1 medical report (NASA TM-58240). Edited by S.L. Pool, P.C. Johnson, Jr., and J.M. Mason, National Aeronautics and Space Administration, Washington, D.C., 1981.

Sauer, R.L., and Rapp, R.M. Food and nutrition. In: Shuttle OFT Medical Report: Summary of Medical Results from STS-1, STS-2, STS-3, and STS-4. NASA TM-58252. Edited by Pool, S.L., Johnson, P.C., Jr. and Mason, J.A., National Aeronautics and Space Administration, Houston, TX, p. 53–62, 1983.

Sawin, C.F., Rummel, J.A., and Michael, E.L. Instrumented personal exercise during long duration space flights. Aviation, Space, and Environmental Medicine, 46:394–400, 1975.

Shashkov, V.S., and Yegorov, B.B. Problems of pharmacology in space medicine. Farmakologiya i Toksikologiya, 42(4):325–339, 1979.

Thornton, W.E., and Rummel, J.A. Muscular deconditioning and its prevention in space flight. In: Biomedical results from Skylab (NASA SP-377). Edited by R.S. Johnston and L.F. Dietlein, National Aeronautics and Space Administration, Washington, D.C., 1977.

Toscano, W.B., and Cowings, P.S. Transference of learned autonomic control for symptom suppression across opposite directions of Coriolis acceleration. Preprints of the 1978 Annual Scientific Meeting of the Aerospace Medical Association, New Orleans, LA, 8–11 May, 1978.

Ushakov, A.S. Nutrition during long flight (NASA TM-76436). National Aeronautics and Space Administration, Washington, D.C., October 1980.

Vil'-Vil'yams, I.F. and Shul'zhenko, Ye.V. Functional condition of the cardiovascular system after 3 day immersion and prophylactic rotation on a short radius centrifuge (NASA TM-76299). Fiziologiya Cheloveka, 6(2):323–327, 1980.

Yegorov, A.D. Results of medical research during the 175-day flight of the third prime crew on the Salyut-6-Soyuz orbital complex (NASA TM-76450). National Aeronautics and Space Administration, Washington, D.C., 1981.

MEDICAL PROBLEMS OF SPACE FLIGHT

19 Toxic Hazards in Space Operations

MARTIN E. COLEMAN

Traditionally, submarine operations and certain industrial work environments have been the spheres of concern with respect to toxic gas contamination. The closed environment of spacecraft has presented a new focus for such concerns. As early as the Apollo Program, steps were taken to provide adequate protection for crews by eliminating, or at least minimizing, exposures to potentially harmful levels of trace contaminant gases and other hazardous substances in the spacecraft cabin (Rippstein, 1975). Accordingly, from the Apollo Program on, each NASA manned space flight program has incorporated a toxicology program as an element of biomedical support.

The NASA Johnson Space Center Toxicology Program has the following primary objectives: (1) establishment of atmospheric toxicity standards, (2) selection of materials with minimal atmospheric contamination potential, (3) atmospheric contaminant removal, (4) measurement of atmospheric contaminant levels, and (5) toxicological assessment of items that may affect spacecraft habitation (Rippstein and Coleman, 1983). This chapter summarizes several toxic hazard issues of concern to the Shuttle Toxicology Program, and presents some results of inflight atmospheric sampling and analysis from STS missions 1 to 41-C.

Many chemicals of concern to the NASA Toxicology Program have been assigned spacecraft maximum allowable concentration (SMAC) limits for habitable spacecraft atmospheres (Weeks, 1981). These limit values are expressed in milligrams per cubic meter (mg/m^3) or in parts per million (ppm). SMAC limits are generally only about one-tenth to one-half the industrial exposure limits established by OSHA, because crewmembers in space flight may be continuously exposed to atmospheric contaminants for 24 hours per day, and because the spacecraft atmosphere has always contained several other trace gas contaminants that may be additive to any given contaminant. Although this has not been proven experimentally, it is also likely that the general deconditioning, reduced body fluid volume, and other body changes experienced during space flight (Johnston and Dietlein, 1977) may reduce tolerance to the toxic effects of many chemical contaminants.

FLUIDS AND GASES ON THE SPACE SHUTTLE IN RELATIVELY LARGE QUANTITIES, OUTSIDE THE HABITABLE AREAS

The Space Shuttle's unique landing capability is toxicologically significant because the transition from reaction jet to aerodynamic control to landing depends on spacecraft systems that use fluids and gases with toxic potential. These materials, contained in storage tanks, could present problems in the event of leaks during normal operations or from containers ruptured during a crash and rescue episode (Rockwell International: Space Division, 1978). Figure 19-1 shows the location of these storage tanks on the orbiter. The amount of material in each tank at landing depends upon whether or not the full flight schedule was completed. Exposure to each of these substances presents specific toxicological problems. Those substances which present the most significant potential health hazards, along with the amounts contained in the Space Shuttle at launch, are described below.

- Ammonia (44.27 kg). Storage tanks are located in the aft fuselage, and are a part of the Shuttle environmental control and life support system (ECLSS). A colorless vapor with a pungent odor,

1. Ammonia
2. Breathing oxygen
3. Freon—21
4. Freon—1301
5. Fluorinert FC—40
6. Helium
7. Hydrazine
8. Hydraulic fluid
9. Liquid hydrogen
10. Liquid oxygen
11. Lube oil
12. Monomethyl hydrazine
13. Nitrogen
14. Nitrogen tetroxide

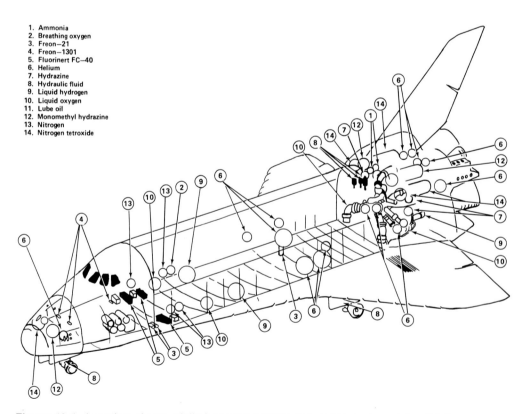

Figure 19-1. Location of potentially hazardous fluids and gases on board the Orbiter.

ammonia is a powerful irritant to the eyes and mucous membranes of the upper respiratory tract. Symptoms of exposure include irritation of the eyes, conjunctivitis, swelling of the eyelids, irritation of the nose and throat, coughing, dyspnea, vomiting, pulmonary congestion and pneumonitis. Systemic toxicity is low, since ammonia is rapidly converted into urea. Liquid anhydrous ammonia produces severe burns on contact (ACGIH*TLV** = 25 ppm, 18 mg/m³).

- Liquid and gaseous oxygen (3636 kg). The principal hazard associated with oxygen is fire. Materials in an oxygen-enriched atmosphere can be ignited by a spark. In the liquid state, oxygen can produce extensive "burns" on skin contact because of its low temperature. Oxygen tanks are located in the mid fuselage, and are part of the ECLSS. (The upper limit for the atmospheric concentration at one-atmosphere pressure is 100 percent for 6 hours; the lower limit is 19 percent.) Breathing 100 percent oxygen at ambient pressure for longer than 6 hours would cause oxygen toxicity; breathing less than 19 percent oxygen would cause hypoxia.

- Freon 21 (272.16 kg). Storage tanks for this colorless, odorless, nonflammable gas are located in the mid- and aft fuselage. Moderate concentrations in the atmosphere can produce lightheadedness, giddiness, shortness of breath, liver toxicity, and cardiac arrhythmia. In the event of light exposure, adrenaline, dextroamphetamine, or similar drugs should not be administered because of the possibility of initiating ir-

regular heartbeat (ACGIH TLV=10 ppm, 40 mg/m³).

- Flourinert FC-40 (35.34 kg). This fluorinated liquid is used as a dielectric coolant in the fuel cells of the Shuttle electrical power system. At normal ground temperatures and pressures it presents little or no health hazard, but exposures to temperatures of 600°F and above may produce toxic thermodegradation products.

- Helium (143.88 kg). Helium tanks are located throughout the orbiter. An inert, nonflammable, colorless, and odorless gas, helium acts as a simple asphyxiant in concentrations where the oxygen level is reduced to less than 15 percent.

- Hydrazine (476.28 kg) and monomethyl hydrazine (5578.35 kg). For fueling the auxiliary power unit, hydrazine and monomethyl hydrazine (MMH) tanks are located in the aft fuselage. At room temperature, the hydrazines are clear, oily liquids with an odor resembling ammonia. In liquid or vapor form, they are extremely toxic. Liquid hydrazines produce severe burns on contact with the skin or eyes, and can penetrate the skin to cause systemic effects similar to those produced when swallowed or inhaled. The vapor causes local irritation of the eye and respiratory tract, and systemic effects. Hydrazines produce effects on the central nervous system which can result in convulsions and even death. Rapid therapeutic treatment, using barbiturates or barbiturates in combination with other anticonvulsive drugs, suppresses the convulsive seizures and provides protection during the acute intoxication phase until the chemical can be metabolized (Azar et al., 1940). Repeated or prolonged exposure to hydrazines may cause toxic damage to the liver and kidneys. Pyridoxine (vitamin B₆) prevents fatty liver changes from hydrazine. The

---

*American Conference of Governmental Industrial Hygienists.

**Threshold limit value, the concentration of vapor at which workers, such as ground crews, may be repeatedly exposed day after day without significant irritation, injury, or impairment.

ACGIH TLV for hydrazine is 0.1 ppm, 0.1 mg/m³; the TLV for MMH is 0.2 ppm, 0.35 mg/m³. Table 19-1 presents the National Research Council's emergency exposure limits (EEL) for hydrazine and monomethyl hydrazine.

- Liquid hydrogen (309.35 kg). Part of the power generation system, liquid hydrogen tanks are located in the aft fuselage. In gaseous form, hydrogen acts as a simple asphyxiant. Liquid hydrogen produces serious "burns" on skin contact because of its low temperature.

- Nitrogen (103.42 kg). Tanks are located in the mid fuselage, and are part of the ECLSS. At room temperature, nitrogen is an inert, nontoxic, colorless, odorless, nonflammable gas. It acts as a simple asphyxiant when the oxygen level is reduced to less than 15 percent.

- Nitrogen tetroxide (9122.66 kg). This highly toxic chemical is used as an oxidant in the Reaction Control Subsystem and Orbital Maneuvering System. Brief skin contact with liquid nitrogen tetroxide results in a yellow stain. Severe chemical burns can result if contact is prolonged. The liquid can produce blindness. Inhalation of the gas results in irritation of the respiratory tract and may cause pulmonary edema (ACGIH TLV = 3 ppm, 6 mg/m³). When the three U.S. crewmembers of the Apollo-Soyuz Test Project inhaled gaseous nitrogen tetroxide upon reentry, resulting pulmonary edema forced cancellation of a number of postflight medical tests (Nicogossian et al., 1977).

TABLE 19-1

EMERGENCY EXPOSURE LIMITS OF HYDRAZINE AND MMH (Emergency Exposure Guidance Levels)

Exposure Limits	Hydrazine	MMH
1 hr	0.12 ppm	0.24 ppm
4 hr	0.03 ppm	0.06 ppm
8 hr	0.15 ppm	0.03 ppm
24 hr	0.005 ppm	0.01 ppm

From National Research Council, 1985.

from storage tanks, heat exchangers, fire extinguishers, reaction vessels, or payload experiments; (2) volatile metabolic wastes such as carbon dioxide, methane, and ammonia from crewmembers; (3) particulates such as lint or dust from fabrics or other materials; (4) thermodegradation products from electrical wire insulation or structural materials, or from fire extinguishants coming into contact with flames or hot surfaces; and (5) offgassing of nonmetallic materials such as electrical wire insulations, plastics, paints, adhesives, and lubricants. Heat produced by powering up equipment such as the furnaces in many types of payload experiments increases the rate of offgassing. Reduced atmospheric pressures may also increase offgassing. Trace gas contaminant levels were not remarkably increased, however, during reduction of the cabin atmospheric pressure from 14.7 to 10.2 psia in preparation for extravehicular activities during the STS 41-B and STS 41-C missions (Coleman, 1984).

SOURCES OF TOXINS IN SPACECRAFT ATMOSPHERES

Toxic substances in spacecraft atmospheres may arise from a number of different sources, including: (1) leaks or spills

SPACECRAFT CONTAMINANTS

In all missions, a wide variety of trace gas contaminants have been identified in habitable spacecraft atmospheres. Fortunately, the more toxic contaminants have generally remained at very low levels and no illnesses or injuries have resulted from exposures during the Shuttle era. Table 19-2 lists the general chemical classes of most trace gas contaminants found in spacecraft atmospheres, along with some specific examples and principal toxicological effects.

Table 19-3 lists specific chemicals that are most likely to pose health hazards to crewmembers during space flight, along with their potential sources, major toxic effects, and currently accepted means of treatment following exposure.

In most instances, the ECLSS has been remarkably effective in removing trace gas contaminants from spacecraft atmospheres. Shuttle decontaminant systems include the following:

- Lithium hydroxide / charcoal air filters. The lithium hydroxide in the canisters chemically reacts with carbon dioxide and acid gases. The charcoal absorbs a variety of chemical vapors on its porous surface. One or both of the two can-

isters are changed at 5–12 hour intervals, depending on the crew size.
- Dehumidifier unit. This unit condenses many water-soluble chemical vapors, along with water vapor.
- Ambient temperature catalytic oxidizer (ATCO) system. The platinum-coated charcoal in this system catalyzes the oxidation of carbon monoxide (Rippstein, 1983).

RESULTS OF SPACE MISSIONS

The Shuttle Toxicology Program provides for inflight air sampling and subsequent gas chromatographic / mass spectrometric (GC / MS) analyses during each STS mission. Table 19-4 lists the number of air samples taken and the maximum number of contaminants found in any one sample during a designated mission. Note that the maximum number of contaminants was usually found in air sampled from new or

TABLE 19-2

TRACE GAS CONTAMINANTS FREQUENTLY FOUND IN SHUTTLE CABIN ATMOSPHERE

Chemical Class	Common Examples	Prominent Toxicological Effects of Vapors
Aldehydes and ketones	Acetaldehyde, benzaldehyde, methylethyl ketone, acetone	Eye and respiratory tract irritation, central nervous (CNS) depression
Aliphatic hydrocarbons	Decane, butene, cyclohexane	CNS depression
Alcohols	Ethanol, isopropanol, n-butanol	CNS depression, slight eye and respiratory tract irritation
Aromatic hydrocarbons	Benzene, n-butylbenzene, toluene	CNS depression, dizziness, headache, blood dyscrasias, leukemia (benzine)
Chlorinated hydrocarbons	1,1-dichloroethane, trichloroethylene	CNS depression, sensitization of the heart to epinephrine, liver and kidney toxicity
Fluorinated hydrocarbons	Halon 1301 (bromotrifluoromethane, Freon 113 (1,1,2-trichloro-1,2,2-trifluoroethane)	CNS depression, sensitization of the heart to epinephrine

TABLE 19-3

POTENTIAL ATMOSPHERIC CONTAMINANTS IN SPACECRAFT

Contaminant	Description	Potential Source	NASA SMAC Limit mg/m^3 (ppm)	Acute Symptoms of Exposure	Treatment
Ammonia	Colorless gas, pungent odor	Heat exchanger	17.4 (25)	Eye, nose, and throat irritation; dyspnea, bronchospasm, chest pain, pulmonary edema, pink frothy sputum; skin and eye burns, vesiculation, rales, delayed respiratory infection, circulatory collapse. Liquid splashed on skin causes burns and vesiculation.*	If liquid is splashed on skin or eyes, flush with water. For high-level inhalation exposure, perform the following procedures if necessary: (1) Chest x-ray, (2) 60–80% O$_2$ by mask or cannula, (3) artificial respiration, (4) morphine for dyspnea, (5) epinephrine aerosol or I.V. aminophylline for bronchospasm, (6) 20–30% ethanol aerosol to remove frothy exudates, (7) barbiturates for sedation, (8) endotracheal intubation, (9) corticosteroids to reduce inflammation, (10) antibiotics for infection, (11) I.V. fluids to maintain blood pressure.**
Cadmium	Whitish metal	Heat vaporization of connectors in electrical equipment, explosion or venting of nickle cadmium batteries	0.02 (0.004)	Metallic taste, headache, liver or kidney damage, lower respiratory tract irritation causing pulmonary edema with accompanying shortness of breath, rales, chest pains	For liver or kidney damage, see dichloracetylene treatment For respiratory tract irritation, see ammonia treatment

Contaminant	Physical description	Source	mg/m³ (ppm)	Symptoms	Treatment
Carbon monoxide	Colorless, odorless gas	Crew metabolism, offgassing, thermodecomposition of structural materials	28.6 (25)	Headache, cyanosis, rapid breathing, weakness, dizziness, mental confusion, hallucinations, fainting, depression of S-T segment of EKG	Administer 100% oxygen (hyperbaric, if possible) For metabolic acidosis, treat with IV sodium bicarbonate For cerebral edema, treat with corticosteroids and diuretics
Dichloroacetylene	Colorless, odorless gas	Dehydrochlorination of trichloroethylene in ECLSS lithium hydroxide air filter	0.08 (0.026)	Difficulty in breathing, neurological injury causing sensory loss and paralysis of facial muscles, kidney injury, causing oliguria, hyperkalemia, manifest by muscle weakness, restlessness, paresthesis, cardiac arrhythmias and abnormal EKGs, liver injury resulting in anorexia, nausea, and vomiting, tender liver enlargement, jaundice and spontaneous nose bleeds	For respiratory tract irritation, see ammonia treatment For renal failure, if needed, treat by keeping blood potassium levels acceptably low with Kay; exalate or IV 10% glucose plus insulin; administer antibiotics for infection; or perform hemodialysis For liver toxicity, if needed, treat by bed rest and balanced diet For anorexia and vomiting, treat with IV nutrients and fluids For restlessness or nausea, treat with sedatives For spontaneous bleeding, treat with vitamin K
Freon 113 (1,1,2-trichloro,1,2,2,-trifluoroethane)	Colorless, odorless, low boiling liquid	Used preflight as a cleansing and degreasing agent in spacecraft	383 (50)	Dizziness, drowsiness, impaired mental performance, irregular heartbeat in conjunction with adrenalin release	Withdraw from source of exposure; it is rapidly excreted from lungs
Freon 502 (azetropic mixture of 48.8% Freon 22 and 51.2% Freon 115)	Colorless, odorless gas	Vapor phase refrigerators	456 (100)	Same as Freon 113 (above)	Same as Freon 113 treatment

TABLE 19-3 (Continued)

POTENTIAL ATMOSPHERIC CONTAMINANTS IN SPACECRAFT

Contaminant	Description	Potential Source	NASA SMAC Limit mg/m³ (ppm)	Acute Symptoms of Exposure	Treatment
Glutaraldehyde	A clear liquid with a pungent odor; the vapor pressure is slightly lower than water	Frequently used in space flight as a tissue fixative	0.4 (0.1)	The liquid is irritating to the skin and eyes. Vapors cause eye and respiratory tract irritation and CNS depression	Flush eyes or skin with water For respiratory tract irritation, see ammonia treatment
Halon 1301 (Bromotri-fluoromethane)	Colorless, odorless gas	Spacecraft fire extinguishers	608.8 (100)	Same as Freon 113 (above) plus slight eye and respiratory tract irritation and bronchoconstriction. May decompose into hydrogen fluoride and carbon monoxide plus other toxic chemicals upon contact with flames or hot surfaces[a]	Same as Freon 113 treatment For treatment of HF or CO toxicity, see these agents in this table
Hydrogen fluoride	Colorless, highly reactive gas	Thermodecomposition of Halon 1301 fire extinguishant and some plastic materials	0.5 (0.6)	Irritation of eyes and respiratory tract (see ammonia); systemic effects of fluoride include impaired blood clotting, impaired function of the heart, circulatory shock, and CNS depression	For eye and respiratory tract irritation, see ammonia treatment For impaired clotting or CNS depression, treat symptomatically

Isopropyl alcohol	A clear, volatile liquid, has a distinctive disagreeable odor	Cleansing and disinfection of skin prior to venipunctures, offgassed by many nonmetallic materials	98.3 (40)	Vapors cause intoxication with mental impairment, nausea, gastrointestinal upsets, and slight eye and upper respiratory tract irritation. Very high levels could cause breathing impairment, circulatory collapse and deep coma. Remains in the body much longer than ethanol	For breathing impairment, treat with oxygen and/or artificial respiration For circulatory collapse, treat with IV fluids and hemodialysis to assist removal from body
Mercury	Liquid, silvery metal, vapors have a metallic taste	Mercury vapor lamps, several payload experiments, mercury batteries	0.006 (0.001)	Vapors cause respiratory tract irritation, readily penetrate to lungs (see ammonia). CNS effects include mental disorientation, tremors, and emotional instability	For lower respiratory tract irritation, see ammonia treatment; remove from body with chelating agents such as penicillamine or EDTA to reduce systemic effects
Methyl ethyl ketone	Clear, volatile liquid, has a pungent odor	Used as a cleansing agent, offgassing from nonmetallic materials	59.0 (20)	Vapors cause irritation to eyes and respiratory tract (see ammonia), CNS depression with breathing impairment, sustained exposure may cause peripheral neuropathy	For eye and respiratory tract irritation, see ammonia treatment For respiratory depression accompanying CNS depression, treat with artificial respiration

* Wands, 1981
** Gosselin et al, 1976
[a] Pippen, 1983.

TABLE 19-4

NUMBER OF ATMOSPHERIC SAMPLES TAKEN AND TOTAL NUMBER OF CONTAMINANTS FOUND DURING STS MISSIONS THROUGH 41-C AND SKYLAB 4

STS Mission	Space Vehicle	Number of Atmospheric Samples Analyzed	Total Number of Contaminants Found
1	Columbia	4	61
2	Columbia	3	96
3	Columbia	4	50
4	Columbia	1	6
5	Columbia	1	17
6	Challenger	4	26
7	Challenger	3	16
8	Challenger	1	6
SL-1	Spacelab	8	24
41-B	Challenger	2	24
41-C	Challenger	4	14
Skylab 4	Skylab	3	81

refurbished Shuttle vehicles; the number usually decreased during subsequent missions, probably because the various nonmetallic structural materials are "seasoned out" over time. Most atmospheric contaminants were at levels below 0.1 mg/m^3 and below 0.05 ppm. A few were at levels exceeding 4 mg/m^3. These compounds, along with their SMAC limits, are listed in Table 19-5. Fortunately, most of the chemicals listed in Table 19-4 are of relatively low toxicity (see SMAC limits).

The number of different contaminants found in atmospheres sampled during the STS-1 and STS-2 missions was comparable to the number of atmospheric contaminants found during the 1974 Skylab 4 mission (see Table 19-4). Concentrations of most common atmospheric contaminants measured during STS-1 and STS-2 were much lower than the concentrations of the same or similar chemical contaminants found during Skylab 4, however. Specific chemicals and their concentrations are listed by Rippstein, 1981, 1982; Rippstein and Coleman, 1983; and Hartmut et al., 1975. The lower concentration of spacecraft atmospheric contaminants found

during the Shuttle era, as compared with the Skylab missions, was primarily due to the following factors:

1. Selection of nonmetallic materials with fewer offgassing characteristics.
2. Improved systems for removal of contaminants from spacecraft atmospheres (see above).
3. Maintenance of higher atmospheric pressures in spacecraft.

No trace gas contaminant was found to exceed its SMAC limit in any Shuttle air sample taken. Toluene, at 68.877 mg/m^3, was near its SMAC limit of 75.3 mg/m^3 in one sample taken during STS-2, and was rather high in other air samples taken during that mission. In this sample, the combined levels of toluene plus other chemicals classified as protoplasmic poisons were above acceptable levels for combined toxins of this type (Rippstein, 1982). Whether crewmembers suffered any illness or incapacitation because of this has not been reported.

As shown in Table 19-5, methane was frequently seen at levels above 4 mg/m^3, increasing progressively during most mis-

TABLE 19-5

ATMOSPHERIC CONTAMINANTS IN EXCESS OF 4 MG/M³ MAXIMUM CONTAMINANT CONCENTRATION IN AIR SAMPLES TAKEN DURING EACH MISSION

Chemical Compounds	STS Missions									SL-1	41-B	41-C	SMAC Limits
	1	2	3	4	5	6	7	8	9				
Bromotrifluoromethane (Halon 1301)			16.292 (2.674)							77.331 (12.778)		8.060 (1.323)	608.8 (100)
1,1,2-Trichloro-1,2,2-Trifluoromethane (Freon 113)	5.697 (0.749)	13.091 (1.707)		10.214 (2.332)		17.281 (2.254)			5.045 (0.658)				383 (50)
Methane	18.384 (28.10)		4.933 (7.54)	89.351 (135.54)	75.108 (114.774)		15.760 (24.089)	19.044 (29.108)	66.781 (102.074)	68.041 (104.280)	83.56 (102.2)	52.931 (89.904)	1771 (2700)
Ethanol		4.724 (2.626)							14.940 (7.943)	10.758 (5.719)			94 (50)
2-Propanol									8.784 (3.580)	34.580 (14.095)			98.3 (40)
Toluene		63.877 (16.980)											75.3 (20)

Note: Values not in parentheses are in mg/m³; those in parentheses are in ppm.

325

sions. This was largely due to the metabolic generation by crewmembers and the inability of any of the ECLSS decontaminant systems now in use to readily remove methane. Fortunately, methane is odorless and of very low toxicity (see SMAC limit). Halon 1301, a Freon gas of rather low toxicity, was seen at slightly elevated levels during the STS-3 and Spacelab 1 missions. It may have escaped from a fire extinguisher, but this could not be verified. Freon 113 levels were above 10 mg/m^3 on three occasions. This volatile liquid is commonly used preflight as a cleansing and degreasing agent. It probably permeates some materials during cleaning, vaporizing slowly during flight. It is also commonly detected during offgassing tests of various materials. Levels of 2-propanol (isopropyl alcohol) and ethanol were somewhat high during the STS-9/Spacelab 1 mission. Both are commonly detected during routine offgassing tests of space flight materials. Isopropyl alcohol swabs were also used during this mission for cleansing the skin of crewmembers prior to venipunctures.

During the STS-6 mission, crewmembers reported smelling smoke, which was later found to have been caused by overheating and fusion of Kapton-PTFE electrical wire insulations (Coleman, 1983). An atmospheric sample collected 91 minutes after this incident contained no detectable levels of thermodecomposition products. In a postflight pyrolysis test with the same Kapton-PTFE wiring, several highly toxic thermodecomposition products, including hydrogen cyanide and benzonitrile (benzyl cyanide), were found to evolve after heating to 650°C. These chemicals were not seen in any previous atmospheric sample, nor were they adsorbed by charcoal air filters from previous missions. The reduction in the concentration of the above pyrolysates to below detectable levels in the brief span of 91 minutes after the electric wire insulation fusion demonstrates the effectiveness of the Shuttle decontamination system in removing toxic substances.

TOXICOLOGICAL ASPECTS OF THE SPACE STATION

Toxicological support of the Space Station will be even more essential than in present-day spacecraft due to the long tenure envisioned for crews and the diversity of activities that could result in toxic chemical release (Coleman, 1984). Regenerable trace gas absorbents will be needed for atmospheric decontamination in order to minimize weight and bulk.

"Dumping" of many types of gases "overboard" after desorption from trace gas absorbents may not be permissible, because these gases would probably interfere with electronic and optical equipment. Therefore, other convenient means of disposal must be found. Adequate removal of methane and other contaminants that are not easily removed by present-day decontaminant systems must be ensured, since these materials could accumulate to dangerous levels over a period of months or years. New SMAC limits will have to be assigned to many potential chemical contaminants, especially the systemic toxins and suspected carcinogens, since crewmembers could be exposed continuously or intermittently for extended periods of time.

Considering the numerous potential sources of atmospheric contamination, the consequences of prolonged exposures, and the infrequency with which atmospheric samples could be returned to ground laboratories for analysis, some type of analytical capability will be needed on board the Space Station. This will probably be a GC/MS system that telemeters spectrographic tracings to Earth for analysis. Such a system would enable near-continuous monitoring of trace gas contaminant levels in the Space Station, provide early warning of chemical "spills," and assist in maintaining a clean, safe environment for crewmembers over long periods of time.

REFERENCES

Azar, A., Thomas, A.A. and Shillito, F.H. Pyridoxine and phenobarbital as treatment for aerozine-50 toxicity. Aerospace Medicine, 41:1, 1940.

Coleman, M.E. Postflight Report for STS-6 atmospheric analysis and analysis for Kapton-PTFE wire insulation pyrolysates. (Unpublished memo), June 3, 1983.

Coleman, M.E. Shuttle Toxicology: Cabin atmospheric verification with full cabin pressurization. DTO 623. May 1984 (unpublished).

Coleman, M.E. Atmospheric Contamination Control. In: Space Station Medical Sciences Concepts (NASA TM-58255). Edited by J.A. Mason and P.C. Johnson, Lyndon B. Johnson Space Center, Houston, TX, February 1984.

Gosselin, R.E., Hodge, H.C., Smith, R.P., and Gleason, M.N. Clinical Toxicology of Commercial Products: Acute Poisoning, Section IV: Therapeutics Index, Fourth Edition, Baltimore, Williams & Wilkins, 1976.

Hartmut, M.L., Bertsch, U., Zlatkis, A. and Schneider, H.J. Volatile organic components in the Skylab 4 spacecraft atmosphere. Aviation, Space, and Environmental Medicine, 1002–1007, 1975.

Biomedical results from Skylab (NASA SP-377). Edited by Johnston, R.S. and Dietlein, L.F. U.S. Government Printing Office, Washington, D.C., 1977.

National Research Council, Committee on Toxicology, Emergency and Continuous Exposure Guidance Levels for Selected Airborne Contaminants. Volume 5, page 3. National Academy Press, Washington, D.C., 1985.

Nicogossian, A.E., LaPinta, C.K., Burchard, E.C., Hoffler, G.W. and Bartelloni, P.J. Crew health. In: The Apollo-Soyuz Test Project Medical Report (NASA SP-411). Edited by A.E. Nicogossian. Springfield, VA, National Technical Information Service, 1977.

Pippen, D.L. Evaluation of toxic hazard to personnel from Halon 1301 fire extinguishant products. (WSTF unpublished memo) September, 1983.

Proctor, N.H. and Hughes, J.P. Chemical hazards in the workplace. Philadelphia, PA, J.B. Lippincott, 1978.

Rippstein, W.J. The role of toxicology in the Apollo space program. In: Biomedical Results of Apollo (NASA SP-368). Edited by R.S. Johnston, L.F. Dietlein, and C.A. Berry. National Aeronautics and Space Administration, Washington, D.C., 1975.

Rippstein, W.J. Shuttle toxicology. In: STS-1 medical report (NASA TM-58240). Edited by S.L. Pool, P.C. Johnson, Jr. and J.A. Mason. National Aeronautics and Space Administration, Washington, D.C., December 1981.

Rippstein, W.J. Shuttle toxicology. In: STS-2 medical report (NASA TM-58245). Edited by S.L. Pool, P.C. Johnson, Jr. and J.A. Mason. Lyndon B. Johnson Space Center, Houston, TX, May 1982.

Rippstein, W.J., Jr. Shuttle toxicology. In: Shuttle OFT medical report: summary of medical results from STS-1, STS-2, STS-3 and STS-4 (NASA TM-58252). Edited by S.L. Pool, P.C. Johnson and J.A. Mason. Lyndon B. Johnson Space Center, Houston, TX, July 1983.

Rippstein, W.J., Jr. and Coleman, M.E. Toxicological evaluation of the Columbia spacecraft. Aviation, Space and Environmental Medicine, Medical Supplement 1, 54(12):S60–S67, 1983.

Rockwell International: Space Division. Orbiter crash and rescue information, Space Shuttle Technical Manual U0000-9; SD74-SH-0336A, Revision A, 15 March, 1978.

Wands, R.C. Alkaline Materials. In: Industrial Hygiene and Toxicology (3rd ed.) G.D. Clayton and F.E. Clayton, editors. John Wiley and Sons, New York, 1981.

Weeks, L.M. Office of Space Transportation Systems: Flammability, odor and offgassing requirements and test procedures for materials in environments that support combustion (NASA NHB 8060.1B). Lyndon B. Johnson Space Center, Houston, TX, September 1981.

20 Radiation Exposure Issues

PERCIVAL D. McCORMACK

D. STUART NACHTWEY

Radiation has been described as "the primary source of hazard for orbital and interplanetary space flight" (Petrov et al., 1981). Data gathered over the past 25 years have characterized the radiation environment in Earth-orbital space (Chapter 2) as well as throughout much of the solar system. Results from numerous space probes present a picture of heightened radiation levels, changing character of radiation, and "radiation storms" occurring as solar activity waxes and wanes.

The success of U.S. and Soviet flight programs proves clearly that comparatively brief flights with carefully planned trajectories do not present a radiation hazard for space crews in the absence of solar flare activity. However, as the space programs of both nations expand and greater numbers of specialists spend more time in space, the problem of providing radiation protection grows in importance. Space medicine personnel must be knowledgeable concerning the extent of the danger, means of providing appropriate protection, and, most important, proper medical procedures for use in the event of a radiation emergency.

MEASUREMENT OF EXPOSURE

Measurement of radiation hazard and exposure risks for space crews requires an understanding of the units used for expressing radiation levels and their effects on biological systems. There are several interrelated units.

ABSORBED DOSE

The amount of radiation absorbed in any material is defined in terms of absorbed dose and has the dimensions of energy absorbed per unit mass. The S.I. unit of absorbed dose, the gray (Gy), is defined such that 1 gray is equal to 1 joule of energy absorbed in 1 kilogram of the material in question. Thus, the value of the absorbed dose depends on the material in which the energy is absorbed. Another unit of absorbed dose often used is the rad, originally defined as 100 ergs of energy absorbed per gram of material. One rad equals 0.01 Gy. The rad and the gray will be used here, and the material absorbing the energy will be assumed to be water, a material which can be used as an analog for human tissue.

DOSE EQUIVALENT

It is well established that different types of radiation produce different amounts of biological damage per unit of absorbed dose. In particular, charged particles with higher rates of energy loss per unit length of track, such as HZE particles and low-energy protons, are more effective in producing biological effects than particles with lower rates of energy loss, such as electrons and high-energy protons. The physical characteristic presently used to quantitate this difference is the rate of energy loss per unit length of track in the material; this quantity is called the linear energy transfer, or LET. In this chapter, we will refer to two related LET quantities: LET_{100} and LET_{∞}. The former indicates that only delta electrons with energies less than 100 electron volts are considered to deposit energy locally; the latter indicates that all delta electron energies are considered. The latter quantity will be designated simply as the LET.

In order to calculate the equivalent biological response from high-LET radiation, the standard procedure in radiation protection of introducing the quantity dose equivalent (DE) is adapted. For a given low dose of high-LET radiation (in the dose range relevant to radiation protection), this is the amount of low-LET radiation necessary to produce a biological effect equivalent to that produced by the high-LET radiation.

A factor called the quality factor (Q) that is related to the LET of a charged particle is used to convert an absorbed dose of a known high-LET radiation into a dose equivalent. It is necessary to determine average Q values for radiations in various environments in space. A measured or cal-culated LET spectrum is multiplied by the Q as a function of the LET and integrated over the entire spectrum. The ratio of this value to the integral without the Q weighting factor yields the average Q. In International Council for Radiation Protection (ICRP) Report 26 (ICRP, 1977), Q values were defined in terms of LET, and these values are used here. Recently, ICRP and the International Council for Radiation Units (ICRU) issued a report (ICRU, 1986) that resulted in the ICRP recommending a change in Q for fission neutrons from 10 to 20 (ICRP, 1985).

The Q value for proton irradiation from the South Atlantic Anomaly will be assumed to be 1.2. A single average Q value of 2.0 has been assumed as an upper limit for the composite of all galactic cosmic rays (Silberberg et al., 1985).

MEASURED RADIATION DOSES AND DOSE COMPONENTS ON MANNED MISSIONS

INTRODUCTION

On manned missions over the last 20 years, considerable effort has been dedicated to measuring overall absorbed dose at specific locations on astronauts' bodies and inside spacecraft. A more modest effort has focused on obtaining dose rates, LET spectra, and separate measurements of the neutron and HZE particle components. An adequate understanding has been complicated by many factors, including the diversity of radiation types, changes in radiation intensity due to the changing position of the spacecraft in orbit, complex and frequently changing shielding configuration, and severe limitations placed on the dosimetric effort by weight, power, and cost considerations.

In the U.S. program, radiation is monitored in flight with two types of dosimeter, passive and active (Barnes, 1981). Precise radiation information is obtained from passive dosimeters composed of thermoluminescent dosimeter (TLD) chips, plastic sheets, and metal foils, each affected by different kinds and energies of radiation. These dosimeters are contained in sealed units and must be processed in a laboratory following flight. Active dosimeters are used as a means of determining in real time the radiation danger being encountered, and may be read by a crewmember at any time. These are integrating dosimeters consisting of pen-sized ion chambers which measure three ranges of radiation exposure. The low-range pocket dosimeter (PDL) measures accurately in the range of 0 to 200 millirads. The high-range pocket dosimeter (PDH) measures accurately in the range of 0 to 100 rad. A contingency high rate dosimeter (HRD) is also provided for measurement of doses from 0 to 600 rad. This combination of passive and active dosimeters allows accurate monitoring and recording of radiation in space, including electron and proton radiation, and heavy cosmic rays.

Nuclear track detectors have been extensively used to measure the higher LET range produced by HZE particles. Preliminary attempts have also been made to assess the neutron component.

EARLY INFORMATION ON DOSES IN SPACE VEHICLES

Various types of manned spacecraft have been employed by the U.S. and the U.S.S.R. in their space programs. Obviously the size, mass, and therefore effective shielding within different spacecraft vary considerably. Frequently the shielding of detectors at the time of measurement is not precisely known, owing to such factors as distribution of components

within the spacecraft, changing amount of fluids such as propellants, water, etc., and even the movements of the astronauts.

Radiation doses measured on some early U.S. space flights are shown in Table 20-1. The Apollo and Skylab data were taken from Bailey's Summary (1977). A review of earlier data can be found in Curtis (1974). Dose rates for Earth-orbital flights vary from 11 mrad/day for Gemini 4 to nearly 90 mrad/day for the higher altitude and greater orbital inclination of the Skylab 4 mission. The exact shielding around the dosimeters, however, is not well known. Average dose rates inside the heavily shielded film vault drawers B (16–30 g/cm^2) and F (30–50 g/cm^2) of Skylabs 2 and 3 were 39.5 and 33.4 mrad/day, respectively, suggesting that even very heavy shielding is ineffective in reducing the dose rate from cosmic rays. Some of the results of joint U.S./U.S.S.R. dosimetry measurements conducted on Cosmos 936 and 1129 flights are shown in Table 20-2 (Benton et al., 1978; Benton et al., 1981a).

In addition to measuring absorbed dose with TLD detectors, dosimeters utilizing ^{6}Li, with and without Cd covers, and ^{23}OU, ^{232}Th, and ^{209}Bi were employed to measure the neutron components of space radiation. The neutron energy spectrum was divided into roughly three energy regions: thermal neutrons (< 0.2 eV), resonance neutrons (0.2 eV to 1.0 MeV), and high-energy neutrons (> 1.0 MeV). The recorded dose equivalents in the millirem involve the use of quality factors 2, 6, and 10, respectively for the three energy regions. The high-energy neutron data shown in Table 20-3 are uncertain, because the detector was operated at the limit of its sensitivity and separating the neutron from the high-energy proton events is difficult.

On the Cosmos 936 and 1129 flights, dose was measured as a function of shielding, where shielding was allowed to vary

TABLE 20-1

DOSIMETRY DATA FROM U.S. MANNED SPACE FLIGHTS

Flight	Duration (hr)	Inclination (deg)	Apogee-Perigee (km)	Average Dose Rate (mrad/day)[a]
Gemini 4	97.25	32.5	296–166	11
Gemini 6	25.25	28.9	311–283	23
Apollo 7[b]	260.1			15
Apollo 9[b]	241			20
Apollo 10[b]	192		lunar orbital flight	60
Apollo 11[b]	194		lunar orbital flight	22
Apollo 12[b]	244.5		lunar orbital flight	57
Apollo 14[b]	216		lunar orbital flight	127
Apollo 16[b]	265.8		lunar orbital flight	46
Apollo 17[b]	301.8		lunar orbital flight	44
Skylab 4[c]	90 days	50	alt = 435	86 ± 9
ASTP[d]	9 days	50	alt = 435	12

[a] One mrad = 1 Gy.
[b] Doses quoted for the Apollo flights are skin doses. The doses to the blood-forming organs are approximately 40% lower than the values measured at the body surface.
[c] Mean thermoluminescent dosimeter (TLD) dose rates from crew dosimeters.
[d] Apollo-Soyuz Test Project.
Adapted from Bailey: Dosimetry during space missions (1977).

down to extremely small values (Benton et al., 1978, 1981b). A power law relationship of dose rate vs. shielding thickness was observed, with dose rate varying from about 125 rad/day behind 0.02 g/cm^2 of Al, down to 0.5 rad/day behind 1 g/cm^2 of Al. Measurements were made utilizing TLD detectors, with thickness of 1.0 g/cm^2. The measured data generally support the prediction that, in low Earth-orbit, the dose encountered is strongly altitude-dependent with a weaker dependence on inclination (Watts and Wright, 1976). A recent compilation of dosimetric results for all STS flights through January 1, 1986, is presented in Table 20-3 (Benton, 1986). The two missions experiencing the highest dose rates (41-C and 51-J) orbited at the highest altitudes. The data show that the most important variable that determines the average dose rate is flight altitude.

HZE PARTICLE MEASUREMENTS

On Apollo, Skylab, ASTP, Cosmos, and STS flights, HZE particle exposure for individual astronauts has been measured by means of plastic nuclear track detectors. On Apollo, detectors were located in the passive dosimetry packs worn on the chest, thigh, and ankle of each astronaut (Benton et al., 1977a). On Skylab, each astronaut wore a single passive dosimeter on either the wrist or ankle (Benton et al., 1977b). On Apollo missions, each plastic packet consisted of two or three 190 μm-thick layers of type 8070-112 Lexan. Each detector had an area of about 8 cm^2.

The most heavily instrumented Apollo mission was Apollo 17. In addition to the passive personnel dosimeters, five other biologically related experiments utilized plastic nuclear track detectors. Experiments included the HZE dosimeters, the

TABLE 20-2

DOSIMETRY RESULTS OF JOINT U.S./U.S.S.R. COSMOS FLIGHTS

Cosmos Flight No.	1129	1887
Flight duration (days)	18.56	12.63
Inclination	62.8	62.8
Altitude (km, apogee/perigee)	394/226	406/224
TLD dose rate (mrad/day)[a]	18.0	24.8
Thermal neutrons (E < 0.3 eV)		
fluence	5.1×10^5 cm^{-2}	2.64×10^5 cm^{-2}
dose equivalent	0.52 mrem ± 20%	

[a] One mrad = 1 Gy.
[b] One mrem = 0.01 Sv.
Adapted from Benton (1981a).

Alfmed, the Biocore and two sets in the Biostack. Detailed results from the cellulose nitrate detectors are shown in Table 20-4.

The data clearly show the influence of shielding on HZE exposure, with the lightly shielded HZE dosimeter recording nearly four times the flux recorded with the Biocore detectors. At the same time, it is clear that even for a very heavily shielded detector such as the Biocore (30–40 g/cm^2 is a conservative estimate), there is still a significant number of HZE particle hits. Taking spacecraft weight limitations into account, it is clear that complete shielding from galactic cosmic rays is not practical.

On the second Skylab mission, a set of cellulose nitrate plastic detectors was used to measure the HZE component, with five dosimeters distributed throughout the Command Module during the 28-day mission. The measured Skylab HZE particle planar fluence and flux are listed in Table 20-5, in which the first column designates the dosimeter, the second the approximate shielding. The third and fourth columns contain the particle fluence data, with the planar fluence corrected for detector efficiency. The planar flux is shown in the fifth column and represents fluence divided by total mission time. The data

clearly show the effect of shielding on particle flux, with flux changing from a high of 3.33 to a low of 0.75 particles/cm^2-day. The average planar flux for the five dosimeters for particles with LET in tissue >105 keV/μm is 1.90 + 0.40 particles/cm^2-day.

RADIOBIOLOGICAL FEATURES OF THE SPACE RADIATION ENVIRONMENT

INTRODUCTION

The description of the biological effects of space radiation stems largely from experiments in fundamental radiation biophysics and radiation therapy research. The unique feature of the space radiation environments described above is the abundance of particulate radiations. Characteristic effects of electrons, protons, and heavy ions in those environments have been studied at various levels of biological organization. In the case of protons and heavy ions, the insufficient information about effects in humans makes it necessary to rely on experimental data. It is clear that molecular and cellular effects can help ex-

TABLE 20-3

SPACE SHUTTLE DOSIMETRY SUMMARY MEASUREMENTS FROM THE AREA PASSIVE DOSIMETERS: WHOLE BODY DOSE EQUIVALENTS (mrem)

Measurements	STS-2	STS-3	STS-4
Low-LET[a]	12.5 ± 1.8	52.5 ± 1.8	44.6 ± 1.1
Rate (/day)	5.2 ± 0.8	6.5 ± 0.2	6.3 ± 0.2
Neutron			
Thermal	<0.03	0.03	0.04
Total	<6	9.7	15.6
High-LET[b]	1.0 ± 0.4	6.3 ± 1.0	7.7 ± 2.9
Total Mission			
Dose Equivalent	<19	68.5	67.9
Mission Parameters			
Duration (hrs)	57.5	194.5	169.1
Inclination (deg)	38	40.3	28.5
Altitude (km)	240	280	297
	STS-6	STS-7	STS-8
Low-LET[a]	27.3 ± 0.9	34.8 ± 2.3	34.8 ± 1.3
Rate (/day)	5.5 ± 0.2	5.8 ± 0.4	5.8 ± 0.2
Neutron			
Thermal	0.03	0.02	0.02
Total	8.4	1.4[c]	2.6[c]
High-LET[b]	13.8 ± 1.8	11.7 ± 1.6	19.2 ± 3.5
Total Mission			
Dose Equivalent	49.5	47.9[c]	56.6 ± 3.7[c]
Mission Parameters			
Duration (hrs)	120	143	70 75
Inclination (deg)	28.5	28.5	28.5
Altitude (km)	284	297	297 222
STS-9	STS-41B	STS-41C	STS-41D
Low-LET[a]	43.6 ± 1.8	403 ± 12	42.0 ± 2.8
Rate (/day)	5.5 ± 0.2	57.6 ± 1.7	7.0 ± 0.5
Neutron			
Thermal	0.02	0.05	0.01
Total[c]	0.5	3.2	1.5
High-LET[b]	13.6 ± 1.5	98 ± 3	21 ± 1.3
Total Mission			
Dose Equivalent[c]	57.7 ± 2.3	504 ± 12	64.8 ± 3.1
Mission Parameters			
Duration (hrs)	191	168	145
Inclination (deg)	28.5	28.5	28.5
Altitude (km)	297	519	297

Adapted from Benton (1986).
[a] Photons and electrons of any energies. High LET at lower efficiency.
[b] HZE particles with LET > 20 keV/μm of water. All high-LET data is preliminary.
[c] Does not include high-energy neutron dose.

TABLE 20-4

HZE PARTICLE TRACK FLUENCES ON APOLLO 17[a]

Experiment	Absolute planar track fluence (tr / cm²)		Flux[d] (tr / cm²-day)
	LET_{tissue} > 225 keV / m[b]	LET_{tissue} > 105 keV / m[b]	LET_{tissue} > 105 keV / m[c]
HZE dosimeter (˜2 g / cm² shielding)	26.1 ± 3.9	153 ± 23	16.4
Biostack (˜10 g / cm² shielding)	16.2 ± 2.3	95 ± 14	10.2
	13.4 ± 1.8	78 ± 11	7.4
ALFMED (˜20 g / cm² shielding)	11.7 ± 1.5	69 ± 9	7.4

[a] All measurements are from cellulose nitrate processed for 10.0 hr at 40°C in 6.25N NaOH.
[b] Corresponds to an LET_{350}^{Lexan} > 150 keV / m in Lexan or LET_{350}^{CN} > 170 keV / m.
[c] Corresponds to an LET_{350}^{CN} > 8 0 keV / m.
[d] Flux is the planar flux in effective days in interplanetary space; mission duration is 301.5 hr or 9.33 effective days.
Adapted from NCRP (1989).

plain acute effects and interactions with other agents of high-LET particulate radiations. However, late effects can only be assessed in whole organisms, and in the two decades since the National Academy of Sciences Report (NAS/NRC, 1967) only some of the pertinent questions have been answered. This section considers, briefly, the salient features of the effects of electrons, protons, and neutrons, and in somewhat more detail, heavy ions. Neutrons are included because it is known that some level of neutron exposure occurs in spacecraft, although the contribution of neutrons to the total dose is currently considered to be very small.

BIOLOGICAL EFFECTS OF ELECTRONS

Electrons are small, negatively charged particles. Irradiation of matter with X- or gamma rays sets electrons in motion with adequate energy to ionize atoms. Thus, the biological effects of low-LET radiations, X- and gamma rays, and electrons are quantitatively similar. Much less is known about the biological effects of exposure to electron beams than about effects of photon irradiation (see Elkind and Whitmore, 1967; Alpen, 1979; Hall, 1982). Low-LET radiation causes a spectrum of DNA lesions, in particular, single-strand breaks and base damage. The ratio of induced single-strand to double-strand breaks is higher after exposure to low-LET than to high-LET radiations. The cellular capacity for repair of low-LET radiation-induced damage, such as single-strand breaks, is greater than for high-LET radiation-induced damage (see Elkind and Whitmore, 1967). This differential in repair accounts, in part, for the difference in relative biological effectiveness (RBE) among radiations. The importance of the repair of DNA lesions is reflected in increased cell survival, decreased mutation, decrease in chromosome aberrations, and decreases in *in vitro* malignant transformation and cancer induction when the dose is incurred at a low rate in small fractions (Meyn and Withers, 1980). Capacity for repair does not appear to be diminished by repeated

TABLE 20-5

HZE PARTICLE FLUENCE AND PLANAR FLUX IN THE SKYLAB (D-008-SL2) COMMAND MODULE[a]

Dosimeter (layer 11)	Approx. Shielding (g/cm² of Al)	Planar flux[b] (particles/cm²-day)
F1	⁻10	3.33 ± 0.38
F2	>20	1.01 ± 0.19
F3	>20	0.75 ± 0.19
F4	⁻10	3.08 ± 0.31
F5	⁻20	1.32 ± 0.19

[a] The data are averages arising from measurements performed with cellulose nitrate.
[b] Corresponds to particles with $LET_{350}^{CN} > 80$ keV/m which is equivalent to $LET_{tissue} > 105$ keV/m.
Adapted from NCRP (1989).

exposures (Joiner et al., 1986). However, repair and expression of damage are influenced by a number of postirradiation conditions. Dose rate and fractionation effects are important at doses above 10 rad (0.1 Gy).

Information about late effects of electron irradiation is scarce, but their carcinogenic effects have been studied in skin (see Burns and Albert, 1986). The results indicate that repair of potentially carcinogenic damage occurs in fractionation regimes and the dose-response curve for single exposures is curvilinear. It is assumed with confidence that late effects of electron irradiation in space can be predicted on the basis of knowledge of effects of photon irradiation and the energy spectrum of electron radiation.

BIOLOGICAL EFFECTS OF PROTONS

As they pass through tissues, protons lose energy principally by interacting with atomic electrons. Secondary particles are produced by nuclear interactions and contribute a small but important fraction of the total dose, except in the case of high energies (>1 GeV). These particles consist of secondary protons, neutrons, pions, heavy particles, and gamma rays. As the

particle slows, rate of energy loss increases. At low velocities, rate of energy loss decreases, in part because a slow positive ion can capture and lose electrons. The depth-dose distribution in tissue exposed to a beam of monoenergetic protons is characterized by a Bragg curve which reflects the relative ionization as a function of depth, the depth in tissue of the peak being dependent on the energy. The dose at the peak of the Bragg curve is, of course, greater than at the plateau region. After the peak, the dose decreases to almost zero as the particles stop. LET, which influences the degree of biological effect, increases with decreasing proton energy. The LET in the plateau region is low, approximately 0.5 keV/μm, but rises considerably over a very short range of the track as the particles decelerate and stop.

As noted earlier, a value for Q of 1.1 has been estimated from the energy spectra of protons encountered in low Earth-orbit (LEO) involving exposures in the inner radiation belt. While such a Q value is consistent with experimental data, there are no human data and no studies of late effects, in particular cancer, with low doses of protons.

In general, RBE values for protons are the same as for the 250 kV X-rays and, therefore, somewhat more effective than

^{60}Co gamma rays. An exception to the RBE of 1 were the estimates in mice of 30-day lethality of 2.4 and testicular atrophy of 4.9 (Storer et al., 1957). These RBE values were based on the effects of the 0.6 MeV proton obtained by subtraction of the gamma-ray effects in thermal column radiation, and therefore are not direct RBE estimates. Few estimates of RBE are relevant to the selection of a Q for proton radiation in LEO, but the RBE values of Urano et al. (1984) for jejunal crypt cells, skin, and lens range from 0.8–1.3.

In the case of proton-induced tumors, Clapp et al. (1974) found no RBEs greater than 1.0 for 60 MeV protons in their study of life shortening and tumor induction. Burns et al. (1975) exposed rats to 10 MeV protons and compared the induction of skin tumors with exposure to electrons. They estimated the RBE at about 3. The observed reduction of the tumorigenic effect with fractionation of the exposures to protons suggested repair, and the curvilinear response to single doses was typical of low-LET radiation.

Bettega et al. (1985) found that malignant transformation of cells *in vitro* was characterized by a curvilinear response and, although no RBE value was estimated, the response was similar to that induced by X- and gamma rays.

An important study of proton-irradiated monkeys has been underway for about two decades (Yochmowitz et al., 1985). The study involves exposures to 32, 55, 138, 400, and 2300 MeV protons. In females, a predominant finding was endometriosis that appears to be radiation-induced (Wood et al., 1986). There is no evidence that this lesion is related to radiation quality, or that humans will show comparable susceptibility. Eight of 41 monkeys that have died and were exposed to 55-MeV protons (400–800 rad, 4.0–8.0 Gy surface dose) had glioblastomas. It is not known whether or not this species, *Macacca mulatta,* is unusually susceptible to

this tumor. When data for different proton energies and all tumor types in both sexes are pooled, the dose response appears curvilinear and similar in general form to low-LET radiation responses for tumor induction.

Results obtained with a relatively broad range of proton energies suggest that risks for exposure to protons in space will not significantly exceed those for low-LET radiations such as electrons and gamma rays.

BIOPHYSICAL CHARACTERISTICS OF HEAVY IONS

Heavy ions are charged particles, but differ from electrons and positrons. In contrast to uncharged photons and neutrons, heavy ions lose energy almost continually by their electromagnetic interaction with atomic electrons as they penetrate matter. This mode of energy loss is described by Bethe's (1930) stopping-power formula, giving the mean linear rate of energy loss (dE/dx = LET), as a function of the ion's charge and velocity and the electronic density and mean excitation energy of the medium. At high energies, a complex ion (e.g., the nucleus of an atom other than H) can also undergo fragmentation when it strikes the nucleus of an atom. Fragmentation occurs when matter is radiated by a beam of heavy ions at high energies. Nuclear fragments of smaller mass appear to proceed from the collision site with little reduction in velocity. Some fragmentation products are radioactive and are deposited near the end of the primary beam's path. Tobias et al. (1971a) termed this phenomenon "autoactivity."

The precise details of track structures are matters of current study. For convenience in description, the concept of a core and a penumbra is useful. The heavy ion's energy is deposited along the core of the track, where the ionization events produced in glancing collisions are very dense. The core may be a few nanometers in width. Surrounding the core is the so-called penumbra of delta rays, where the density of ionization events is much lower than in the core, but extends a considerable distance. Because of these features and the length of the track of an energetic heavy ion, the traversal of a single heavy ion particle in tissue may affect a number of cells. It is the multiplicity of neighboring cells hit, and perhaps inactivated, by a single particle that presents features not encountered with other radiation qualities.

The core itself results from collisions between the heavy ions and electrons, and excitation is the common outcome of the transfer of energy to the electrons in a narrow central part of the core. Ionization is predominant in the more peripheral part of the core and in the penumbra (Magee and Chatterjee, 1980).

Cellular and subcellular effects of heavy ions have been reviewed recently (Ainsworth, 1986; Lett et al., 1986; and Raju, 1978). From the time of the early studies by Zirkle and Tobias (1953) there has been a slow but steady increase in knowledge about the comparative effects of high-LET radiations (Todd et al., 1973).

Studies of heavy ion effects on chemicals, macromolecules, cells, tissues, organs, and organ development indicate that the factors modifying low-LET radiation action do not modify significantly the action of very high-LET heavy ions (> 100 keV/ μm). Geard (1985) has shown the variations in sensitivity to induction of chromosomal aberrations through the cell cycle decrease with increasing LET. High-dose studies have shown that the effects of oxygen, radical scavengers, hydrogen donors, dose fractionation, and dose-rate changes have very little effect on cellular-level responses to heavy ions (Blakely et al., 1984). On the other hand, caffeine, an apparent inhibitor of post-irradiation poly (ADP)-ribose-dependent DNA repair, has a profound effect on the ability of eukaryotic cells to survive high-LET irradiation (Todd and Walker, 1984).

Effects of accelerated heavy ions, in some cases including argon and iron, in cells *in vivo* and in organs of experimental animals have been reviewed by Leith et al. (1983). As the LET of a single ion species is increased beyond the maximal effective LET, the action cross section (probability of effect per unit of fluence, in cm^2) decreases. There are several possible interpretations of this result, but, from the space radiation protection standpoint, it implies that action cross sections of very heavy ions do not exceed the area of the cell nucleus, and that every particle track has a maximally efficient segment (Blakely et al., 1984). When single-cell endpoints such as cell death are compared with multicellular effects, such as gut-colony suppression, a maximum RBE occurs around 200 keV/μm and RBE decreases at higher LET in tissue studies (Alpen et al., 1980, 1981; Todd and Walker, 1984).

There are very few studies on the carcinogenic effects of heavy ions; important questions remain concerning the relative carcinogenic effectiveness of HZE particles. A study on the induction of rat mammary cancer by Neon-20 suggests RBE in the 2–4 range, but since very low doses were not used, higher RBEs cannot be excluded. Burns and Albert (1981) studied the effect of Argon-40 on skin tumor induction. There is no single RBE (Argon/ electron), even at low doses, if the dose-response relationship for one or both radiations is a power function. Such a relationship would also result in a high value for RBE.

Using C_3H ^{10}T ½ cells, Yang et al. (1985) demonstrated an increase in RBE for neoblastic transformation up to about 10 with LET of the heavy ion beams increasing to about 100–200 keV/μm. At higher LET values, the RBE dropped to about 1 for 960 MeV/amu uranium-238. The authors suggest that transformation lesions in pro-liferating cells are probably not repaired.

Fry et al. (1985) reported RBEs of about 30 for induction of Harderian gland tumors by the heavy ions Argon-40 and Iron-56, and lower RBEs with beams of lower LET. The current results suggest that there may be no peak in the curve of RBE vs. LET in the vicinity of 100–200 keV/μm, but rather a plateau. Based on ratios of initial slopes of the dose response curves for ex-posure to an iron-56 beam and ^{60}Co, the RBE for carcinogenesis appears to be about 30. RBEs for Argon-40 and fission neu-trons in this system are of the same order.

HEALTH EFFECTS OF THE SPACE RADIATION ENVIRONMENT

INTRODUCTION

Biological and health effects of the dif-ferent radiations encountered in the space environment are considered in two general categories: 1) early or acute effects, and 2) late or delayed tissue effects. Early effects manifest within hours, days, or weeks fol-lowing high-dose whole-body exposure. Late or delayed effects usually occur after months or years following exposure and include tissue damage, impairment of fer-tility, lens opacification, cancer induction, heritable effects, and developmental ab-normalities in the newborn.

EARLY ORGAN EFFECTS

Early radiation health effects assume clin-ical significance only with whole-body doses of X- or gamma radiation greater than approximately 100 to 200 rads, and received in relatively brief time periods (minutes to hours). Equivalent exposure

levels are likely to be encountered in space only during major solar particle events, and almost exclusively in regions beyond the Earth's protective magnetosphere.

However, substantially lower doses pro-duce significant cell and organ injury. Doses of X- and gamma radiation at which subclinical and clinical effects can be ex-pected are shown in Table 20-6 (all for a single exposure delivered at high exposure rates). The principal sites of biological ac-tion of ionizing radiation are the prolif-erating cells of renewing tissues and body organs, particularly the bone marrow, lymphopoietic tissue, intestinal epithe-lium; the male gonadal tissues; and, to a lesser extent, the female gonadal tissues. Delay and inhibition of cell division, frac-tional cell population killing, cellular de-pletion of vital tissues and organs, organ malfunction, serious illness, and possibly death occur sequentially in the increas-ingly heavily-irradiated individual. Whole-body irradiation doses in the lethal range (200 to 400 rads) cause severe bone marrow depletion leading to symptoms re-lated primarily to a decrease of circulating neutrophils and platelets in the blood. The

TABLE 20-6

LOWEST EXPOSURE LEVELS AT WHICH HEALTH EFFECTS APPEAR IN THE HEALTHY ADULT (SINGLE, HIGH-DOSE RATE EXPOSURE)

Health Effect	Dose, X or gamma radiation (rads)[a]
Blood count changes in the population	15–25
Blood count changes in the individual	50
Vomiting, "effective threshold"	100
Mortality, "effective threshold"	150
LD$_{50}$, minimal supportive care	320–360
LD$_{50}$, supportive medical treatment	480–540

[a] 100 rad = 1 gray (Gy).
Adapted from NCRP (1989).

signs and symptoms of the resulting bone marrow syndrome are infection in a variety of body tissues due to neutropenia, severe bleeding in tissues and organs due to thrombocytopenia, and possibly death within 20 to 40 days after exposure.

Prodromal vomiting is of particular importance because it can have catastrophic consequences in space, especially to the helmeted individual. Although the occasional healthy, unmedicated adult may be nauseated and perhaps vomit at doses of whole-body irradiation below 100 rads, such signs and symptoms are likely to be mild and appear only after 10 hours or more (for a graph showing the time of appearance of signs and symptoms as a function of dose, see Baum, 1984). The ED50, or dose at which about one-half will vomit within 2 days, is in the range of 150–200 rads whole body. Modern antiemetics (e.g., metaclopromide) are quite effective in most patients. Oral medication should be given 1 hour prior to exposure: intravenous preparations can be given 15 minutes before, but by slow infusion.

The gastrointestinal (GI) and central nervous system (CNS) syndromes may be encountered above about 1,500 and 5,000 rads, respectively. There may be some mental performance decrement at these high dose levels, and treatment can only be symptomatic, and not curative.

Bone Marrow

Present evidence indicates that the poor regeneration capacity of the bone marrow may make damage to this organ one of the limiting factors for some space missions in which relatively large doses (10's of rads (cGys) or more) may be delivered even at a relatively slow rate.

Skin

Because the skin may receive the largest dose of any organ, particularly during EVA maneuvers, its absolute sensitivity, as well as its repair and regenerative capacities are discussed in more detail. Dose-response curves for absolute sensitivity of the skin in terms of erythema and moist desquamation, and the protraction dependence of these effects, can be found in the 1967 review of Langham. Although the data were obtained from humans exposed to X-rays in the 200–250 kVp range, the Compton electrons generated have the same effectiveness per rad (determined for the basal cell layer assumed to lie at 0.1 mm in depth) as primary electrons over a wide range of energies (epidermal thickness for various body surface regions is given by Whitton and Everall, 1973). Hence, the curves given by Langham et al. (1967) may be used in connection with exposure to electrons in space.

The median effective dose for erythema is of the order of 600 rads (60 Gy), while that for the much more serious moist desquamation is roughly three times this amount. Protraction of the dose for both endpoints increases the exposure required for a given degree of severity by a factor of approximately three. Thus, these types of injury would appear to be readily avoidable.

Fertility

Female. Sensitivity to radiation-induced sterility varies with age (Rubin and Casarett, 1968); women under 40 years require larger doses to induce menopause than do women over 40 years. Doses below 100 rads are likely to have no effect on fertility, but may produce transient sterility for a few months. Although a small percentage may be permanently sterilized by doses as low as 125 rads (1.25 Gy), doses of 200 (2 Gy) to 650 (6.5 Gy) rads are required to sterilize 5 percent of women for more than 5 years. Doses of 625 (6.25 Gy) to 2000 (20 Gy) rads or more are required to sterilize 50 percent of women (Lushbaugh and

Casarett, 1976). Protraction or fractiona-tion of dose reduces injury to the ovary, and fractionation of dose from therapeutic radiation up to total doses greater than 2000 rads (20 Gy) does not always produce sterility (Baker, 1971).

Male. The seminiferous epithelium is among the most radiosensitive tissues in the adult. A single acute dose of 15 rads (15 Gy) will cause a significant decrease in sperm count for about 40 percent of normal men within approximately 2 months (Langham, 1967; Poulsen, 1973). Doses up to 400 rads (4.0 Gy) cause tem-porary sterility and/or infertility lasting up to 30 months (Poulsen, 1973). With testes exposures up to 600 rads (6.0 Gy), sterility followed by infertility may last for a period of 5 years or more (Rowley et al., 1974), but recovery may occur without se-rious physiological alterations.

Human data also suggest that longer pe-riods of exposure to lower dose rates can also cause infertility. Men, receiving ra-diotherapy for Hodgkin's disease and un-avoidably receiving a daily dose of 10 (10 cGy) to 15 (15 cGy) rads to the testes (total of 150 (1.4 Gy) to 300 (3.0 Gy) rad), become sterile, with no evidence of recov-ery for up to 40 months (Speiser et al., 1973).

RADIATION QUALITY: EARLY EFFECTS

In the above discussion of early effects, amount of radiation was stated in terms of absorbed dose in rads; the quantity dose equivalent (units of rem) was not used, in order to avoid ambiguity. The relatively large quality factors for fast neutrons and other high-LET radiations used in radia-tion protection are supported principally by RBE values for carcinogenesis and mu-tagenesis. They do *not* apply to early effects or late non-cancer organ effects.

For most *early* effects, RBE values for neutron spectra with median energies in the range of about 1 to 7 MeV lie between unity and approximately 3. Values of 3 have been observed for several endpoints, including skin erythema (Field, 1969). However, for bone marrow using CFU de-pletion in mice (Carsten et al., 1976), the value is close to unity for neutron energies in the ranges given, and about 3 for "monoenergetic" neutrons in the 400 keV energy range (single values of RBE can be given because the dose-response curves for CFU depletion are essentially exponential over the region of interest).

Lethality from the bone marrow syn-drome can also be used as a criterion for evaluating the RBE of neutrons for bone marrow damage. Comparisons of LD50 values for mice (Carter et al., 1956) and dogs (Bond et al., 1956) indicate RBEs of about 2 and 1, respectively. The expla-nation for the RBE of 1 for large animals may lie in the observation from micro-dosimetry (Booz, 1978) that, even with uniform, large-dose whole-body irradia-tion in the conventional sense, some tens of percent of cells (1 micrometer diameter "sensitive sites" within the cell) may be completely unscathed. Thus, bone marrow regeneration would be expected to be markedly accelerated.

If protons are sufficiently penetrating to produce reasonably uniform whole-body radiation, RBE will not differ significantly from 1. Although less penetrating protons would be less effective, the magnitude of such a loss in effectiveness is so situation-specific as to preclude generalization. The protective effect of partial body exposure is discussed below.

PREVENTIVE AND THERAPEUTIC MEASURES

Preventive measures include the obvious increase in effective spacecraft hull thickness, installation of a "storm shelter" to reduce total body exposure, partial body shielding, and radioprotective chemicals (Conklin, 1986). The weight of increased hull mass or storm shelters may well be prohibitive. The effectiveness of partial body shielding in reducing mortality from large exposures can be assumed to be proportionate to the fraction of total bone marrow that is effectively shielded (Swift et al., 1956). However, in view of the poor regeneration capability of bone marrow, procedures involving sublethal exposures might be considered as well, in order to accelerate the return of the marrow to normal.

Partial-body shielding of a relatively small fraction of bone marrow is effective in reducing, by a factor of 3 or more, the severity of the bone marrow syndrome (Schick et al., 1981). This is because the intact cells are transported via the blood, to provide a continuous transfusion of progenitor and mature blood and bone marrow elements to the depleted regions.

A substantial amount of research has focused on development of radioprotective chemicals that would be effective and free of serious side effects. The Walter Reed Army Institute of Research has developed some 4500 such drugs, many of which are quite effective in increasing the lethal dose for low-LET radiation by a factor of 2 or more (much less for high-LET radiation). One such drug, WR2721, is currently under clinical trial. However, all such drugs to date must be administered in relatively large doses, usually parenterally, to be effective, and essentially all produce significant side effects with large doses. The most serious side effect is vomiting, and for this reason such protective agents are not recommended at present. Therapeutic measures include "replacement therapy" and use of bone marrow transfusions (Bond et al., 1960 and 1965; Wells et al., 1979; and Thomas et al., 1975, 1977).

Perhaps bone marrow or blood stem cell transfusions could be performed in space, but only with adequate preflight preparation. Serious immunologic side effects can be avoided by use of autologous marrow. Long-term marrow preservation by freezing (at least 10 years) is no longer unusual (Jin et al., 1985), so that marrow from the appropriate individuals could be removed prior to flight and stored. Amounts adequate for transfusion can be concentrated to volumes of 100 or even 50 ml.

However, because a minimum of 4 weeks may be required for the transfused marrow to supply significant amounts of blood elements, a period of severe hematopoietic depression, particularly of platelets, may have to be endured. This difficulty, coupled with the difficulties of marrow or blood cell replacement in space, makes it evident that prior shielding of part of the bone marrow would most likely provide a simpler, less traumatic, less costly, and more effective approach to restoring depleted elements to the marrow and blood.

SPACE RADIATION EXPOSURE LIMITS

CURRENT CONSIDERATION

Today, other non-radiation risks in the space program have been reduced, although not eliminated. As the program has matured, a number of astronauts have retired to assume civilian roles. The residuum of their experience in space, assuming recovery from any temporary physiological changes, is the still present risk of stochastic effects from the low, but not zero, doses of ionizing radiation they received. In the age group of astronauts in the past, the possibility of genetic effects being expressed has not been high. It may be increasingly necessary to consider genetic risk in the future. For the moment, however, the principal risk to be considered is that of induced cancer. There is an increasing tendency, while still recognizing the exceptional nature of space travel, to relate the risks from doses of ionizing radiation received in space to other occupational experiences on the ground.

It has been shown in occupational radiation circumstances on the ground that the average worker has a total risk of fatality, both from radiation and accident, no greater than those experienced in safe industries, with an annual risk (excluding travel) of up to 10^{-4}/year and a lifetime risk of about 0.5 percent. (Travel to and from work adds another 10^{-4}/year, or 0.5 percent/lifetime, to both circumstances.) Traditional industries such as agriculture and construction involve risks in the range $(2^{-6}) \times 10^{-4}$/year, with lifetime risks of up to about 3 percent. More hazardous occupations—steeplejacks, deep sea fishing, test pilots, etc.—involve much higher annual risks. Given the exceptional nature of the occupation, and the great difficulty of reducing exposures in space below a certain level, it seems unreasonable to confine space travelers to the average experience of radiation workers on the ground. It seems more reasonable to compare the space crewmember with a more highly exposed radiation worker on the ground, the limit for whom is 5 rem/year, or 250 rem/lifetime, corresponding to an approximate lifetime risk of 5 percent. Fortunately, no exposures of this magnitude actually occur. As noted in NCRP, 1986, steady radiation exposure at the present limit is discouraged and, indeed, NCRP believes that with the proper application of the radiation exposure ALARA (As Low As Reasonably Achievable) principle, few workers should ever exceed about age $\times$ 1 rem, or a lifetime limit of approximately 70 rem. A lifetime risk of 3 percent corresponds to about 150 rem, or about twice the level of the more highly exposed workers on the ground. Given all the circumstances, a career limit based on a lifetime risk of 3 percent for both sexes does not seem unreasonable.

A further method of comparison could be to compare lifetime risks of the various occupations noted above with those of space flight. Again, given the exceptional character of the latter, comparison with the safest occupations on the ground seems unreasonable. On the other hand, comparison of radiation risks with' the most hazardous occupations on the ground is also unreasonable, because crewmembers face other, additional risks. Consequently, comparison of radiation risks with the middle group of "less safe" occupations seems most reasonable, with lifetime risks of about 3 percent. As Table 20-7 shows, the risk of fatal cancer for a 25-year-old male is about 2 percent and for a 25-year-old female is about 3 percent after a chronic exposure of 100 rad of low-LET radiation. This suggests a career limit based on a lifetime risk of excess cancer of 3 percent for 25-year-olds of 100 rem (female) and 150 rem (male). It is also apparent from Table 20-9 that risk decreases with age, being almost a factor of 2 less at 35 than at 25, and a factor of about 3 less at 45–55 than at 25.

RECOMMENDED LIMITS

Given all the above considerations, the NCRP recommends that for all but exceptional exploratory circumstances in space (e.g., Mars mission or lunar base), a career radiation risk limit of 3 percent be adopted for regular space travelers or workers of all ages and both sexes. Career dose equivalents associated with this risk are given in Table 20-8. These career dose limits would permit a reasonable number of missions, e.g., a 25-year-old male could undertake about 12 Space Station missions

TABLE 20-7

PREDICTED LIFETIME RISK OF EXCESS CANCERS AMONG 1000 PERSONS WHO EXPERIENCE AN ACUTE EXPOSURE OF 100 RAD[a]

Sex	Age at Exposure	Lung	Breast	Colon
Male	25	17.30		7.51
	35	11.67		3.49
	45	8.45		1.95
	55	6.12		1.85
Female	25	13.72	31.23	8.87
	35	11.37	19.22	4.53
	45	10.31	3.44	2.68
	55	8.78	1.69	2.52

Sex	Age at Exposure	Pancreas	All Acute Leukemia	Chronic Granulocytic Leukemia	Total Cancers
Male	25	5.45	2.55	1.44	72.97
	35	2.51	2.82	1.49	40.05
	45	1.60	3.16	1.53	27.25
	55	1.64	3.17	1.51	22.71
Female	25	8.41	1.67	0.97	110.49
	35	3.62	1.94	1.02	67.68
	45	2.24	2.42	1.10	39.16
	55	2.23	2.71	1.16	32.77

[a] Type of exposure—acute.
 Type of risk—cancer incidence.
 Radiation dose—100 rad.
 Duration of exposure—within 20 days at a rate of more than 5 rad/day.
Adapted from NCRP (1989).

of 90 days over a 10-year period. Older persons could participate in more missions, females somewhat fewer missions than males.

The limits in Table 20-8 are based on a 10-year exposure duration. If a crewmember's career extends over a longer period (e.g., 20 years), career limit for the same

TABLE 20-8

RECOMMENDED DOSE EQUIVALENT LIMITS—ALL AGES

Period	BFO[a]	Eye	Skin
Career	[b]	400	600
Annual	50	200	300
30 days	25	100	150

[a] Blood-forming organs.
[b] 200 + 7.5 (Age−30) males.
 200 + 7.5 (Age−38) females.
Adapted from NCRP (1989).

lifetime risk could be higher (by about 20 percent). Correspondingly, for shorter intervals of exposure, the risk is higher per unit exposure. If exposure is on the order of a year or two, a 3 percent lifetime risk will correspond to a career limit of about 120 rem for a 25-year-old male (not 150 rem) and 210 rem (not 250 rem) for a 35-year-old male.

Careers starting at other than designated ages. Recommended career limits can be plotted as a function of age and simple rules derived from the near linear plots that result. The career dose equivalent is approximately equal to:

200 + 7.5 (age − 30) rem for males, up to 400 rem
200 + 7.5 (age − 38) rem for females, up to 300 rem

In addition to the career limit, it is necessary to establish other shorter-term limits in order to avoid nonstochastic effects in critical organs, such as the bone marrow, lens of the eye, and skin. Considering information on nonstochastic effects and past experience based on the former NAS guidelines, the limits shown in Table 20-8 are recommended. It is believed that if these limits are observed, no acute or nonstochastic late effects will be developed.

No specific limits are recommended for exploratory personnel in space, e.g., crewmembers on missions to Mars, certain exploratory EVA tours of duty, etc. Clearly these are circumstances which cannot be directly controlled and, thus, specific limits have little meaning. For planning purposes, however, it is recommended that in addition to the application of the principles of ALARA where possible, the career limits proposed in Table 20-9 be adhered to as guidelines, rather than as limits, wherever possible (e.g., during EVA, where length of exposure may be controllable).

The NCRP also recommends that under

TABLE 20-9

CAREER RISK LIMIT FOR SPACE TRAVELERS (BASED ON A 10-YEAR EXPOSURE DURATION)

Lifetime Excess Risk of Fatal Cancer (3×10^{-2})		
Age	Male	Female
25	150	100
35	250	175
45	325	250
55	400	300

Adapted from NCRP (1989).

no circumstances should a pregnant female fly in space. The special risks for the embryo-fetus are malformation and mental retardation, and the risk of cancer may be greater than that for adults.

PREDICTED DOSES AND SHIELDING FOR SPACE STATION CREWMEMBERS

The common module in the Space Station will be cylindrical in shape—43.7 feet long and 14.8 feet in diameter. Its wall consists of the inner pressure shell, outer bumper layer, plus spacers. For the purpose of initial dose calculation, a single-pressure layer of aluminum, .125 inches thick was assumed (.3175 cms. or .86 cm/cm^2). Doses were calculated for protons only, as the electron dose is negligible. Doses are expressed in millirem, with a quality factor of 1.2. The models used were AP8-Min, IGRF 1965 for epoch 1964, with a man target; and AP8-Max, Hurwitz (USC and GS) for epoch 1970 with a man target. There is a rapid rise in dose at altitudes over 450 Km. Doses to the skin and blood-forming organs in 90-day Space Station tours are shown in Table 20-10. Radiation

TABLE 20-10

ACCUMULATED DOSES—SPACE STATION[a]

Target	Dose Rate (mrem / day) (Skin)	(BFO)	90-day Dose (rem) (Skin)	(BFO)
Solar Min	390	180	35.1	16.2
Solar Max	195	110	17.6	9.9

[a] *Altitude* 500 Km
Adapted from McCormack (1986).

exposure limits for astronauts, as presently formulated by the NCRP, are shown in Table 20-11.

Table 20-9 shows career dose versus age for females and males. For a 40-year-old male, for example, the career limit would be 275 rem to the blood-forming organs. Even under Solar Min conditions, an astronaut could safely complete a 3-month tour every 2 years over a 20-year career. For a 1-year stay during Solar Min, the dose would be 65 rem, which exceeds the annual limit. One way to overcome this would be to double the module wall thickness to about .25 inches aluminum. This would reduce the dose by a factor of 1.2, and the annual dose to 54 rem—just under the annual limit.

Increasing radiation protection by increasing wall thickness is an expensive countermeasure: the module weight penalty would be about 3000 lb. For Space Station, a lower orbital altitude during Solar Min periods would be a more economical measure (constant drag strategy).

EVA workload on Space Station will be heavy, and it will not always be possible to program EVAs to avoid intersection with the South Atlantic Anomaly. Table 20-12 shows the shielding afforded by the present (Space Shuttle) space suit assembly. This shielding level is inadequate for Space Station EVA operations. In the more advanced space suits under development, shielding of over 1.5 g/cm^2 aluminum equivalent will be provided over the entire body and head of the crewmember.

Shielding crewmembers from ionizing radiation during long stay times on Space Station and deep space missions is a matter of great significance, both from the aspects of health and economy. Choice of materials and their arrangement are two critical factors.

TABLE 20-11

NCRP RADIATION EXPOSURE LIMITS (REM)

Period	BFO (5 cm)	Eye (.3 cm)	Skin (.001 cm)
30 days	25	100	150
Annual	50	200	300
Career	200 + 7.5 (age–38) females 200 + 7.5 (age–30) males	400	600

Adapted from McCormack (1986).

TABLE 20-12

SHUTTLE SPACE SUIT ASSEMBLY SHIELDING VALUES

MATERIAL COVERING ARMS AND LEGS

	Density (g/cm^2)	Thickness (inches)
Thermal Management Garment (TMG)	.091	.053
Restraint-Dacron/Bladder Fabric	.035	.020
Liquid Cooling Ventilation Garment (LCVG)	.039	.0295
Total	.165	.1025

Approx. Alum Equiv $\sim$ .2/cm^2

UPPER TORSO

TMG	.091	.053
Fiberglass Shell	.354	.075
LCVG	.039	.0275
Total	.484	.158

Approx. Alum. Equiv. $\sim$ .5 g/cm^2

EYE SHIELD

	Density (g/cm^2)	Thickness (inches)
Helmet Bubble	.182	.06
Protective Visor	.182	.06
Sun Visor	.190	.06
Center Eyeshades	.067	.07
Side Eyeshades	.238	.125
Total	.859	.375

Approx. Alum. Equiv. $\sim$ 0.9 g/cm^2

Adapted from McCormack (1986).

REFERENCES

Ainsworth, E.J. Early and late mammalian responses to heavy charged particles. Adv. Space Res., 1986.

Alpen, E.L., Powers-Risuis, P. and McDonald, M. Survival of intestinal crypt cells after exposure to high Z, high energy charged particles. Radiat. Res. 83, 677, 1980.

Alpen, E.L. and Powers-Risuis, P. The relative biological effect of high-Z, high-LET charged particles for spermatogonial killing. Radiat. Res. 88, 132, 1981.

Alper, T. Cellular Radiobiology (Cambridge University Press, London), 1979.

Bailey, I.V. Dosimetry during space missions. IEEE Trans on Nucl. Sciences, NS-23, No. 4, 1379, 1977.

Bailey, I.V., Hoffman, R.A. and English, R.A. Radiological Protection and Medical Dosimetry for the Skylab Crewmen. In: Biomedical Results from Skylab (NASA SP-377). Edited by R.S. Johnston and L.F. Dietlein, U.S. Government Printing Office, Washington, D.C., 1977.

Baker, T.G. Comparative Aspects of the Effects of Radiation during Oogenesis. Mutation Res. 11:9, 1971.

Barnes, L.M. Radiological Health. In STA-1 Medical Report (NASA TM-58240). Edited by S.L. Pool, Jr. and G.A. Mason, NASA Scientific and Technical Information Branch, Washington, D.C., 1981.

Baum, S.J., Anno, G.H., Young, R.W. and Withers, H.R. Nuclear Weapon Effect Research at PSR-1983, Vol. 10. Pacific-Sierra Research Corporation Report. Defense Nuclear Agency document DNA-TR-85-50, 1984.

Benton, E.V., Cassou, R.M., Frank, A.L., Henke, R.P. and Peterson, D.D. Space radiation dosimetry on board Cosmos 936: U.S. portion of experiment K-206. (University of San Francisco, Report TR-48), 1978.

Benton, E.V., Henke, R.P., Frank, A.L., Johnson, C.S., Cassou, R.M., Tran, M.T. and Etter, E. Experiment K309—Space radiation dosimetry aboard Cosmos 1129: U.S. portion of experiment. National Aeronautics and Space Administration, Tech. Memo. TM-81288, 1981b.

Benton, E.V., Henke, R.P., Frank, A.L., Johnson, C.S., Cassou, R.M., Tran, M.T. and Etter, E. Space radiation dosimetry on board Cosmos 1129. University of San Francisco, Report TR-53, 1981a.

Benton, E.V., Peterson, D.D., Bailey, J.V. and Parnell, T. High-LET particle exposure of Skylab astronauts. Health Physics 32:15, 1977b.

Benton, E.V., Peterson, D.D. and Henke, R.P. Summary of measurements of high-LET particle radiation in U.S. manned space missions. Space Research 15:119, 1977a.

Benton, E.V. Summary of Radiation Dosimetry Results on U.S. and Soviet Manned Spacecraft. Adv. Space Res. 6(11):315–328, 1986.

Bethe, H.A. Zur Theorie des Durchgungs schneller Korpuskulastrahlen durch Materie. Annalen der Physik 5:S.325, 1930.

Bettega, D., Calzolari, P., Pollara, P. and Tallone Lombardi, L. In vitro cell transformation induced by 31 MeV protons. Radiat. Res. 104:178, 1985.

Blakely, E.A., Ngo, F.Q.H., Curtis, S.B. and Tobias, C.A. Heavy-Ion Radiobiology: Cellular Studies. In: Adv. in Radiation Biology, Vol. 11, Edited by J.T. Lett, U.K. Ehmann, and A.B. Cox, 1984.

Bond, V.P., Carter, R.E., Robertson, J.S., Seymour, P.H., and Hechter, H.H. The Effects of Total-Body Fast Neutron Irradiation in Dogs. Rad. Res. 4:139, 1956.

Bond, V.P., Fliedner, T.M., and Cronkite, E.P. Evaluation and Management of the Heavily Irradiated Individual. Proc. 7th Ann. Meet., Soc. Nucl. Med., Colorado. J. Nucl. Med. 1:221, 1960.

Bond, V.P., Theodor, T.M. and Archambeau, J.O. Mammalian Radiation Lethality: A Disturbance in Cellular Kinetics. New York, Academic Press, 1965.

Booz, J. Mapping of fast neutron radiation quality. In: Proc. 3rd Symp. on Neu. Dos. in Biol. and Med. Commission of European Communities, report 5848DE/EN/FR, 1978.

Burns, F.J. and Albert, R.E. Dose Response for rat skin tumors induced by single and split doses of argon ions. In: Biological and Medical Research with Accelerated Heavy Ions at the Bevelac, 1977–1980. Edited by M.C. Pirucciello, and C.A. Tobias. Report LBL-11220, Lawrence Berkeley Laboratory, Berkeley, CA, 1981.

Burns, F.J. and Albert, R.E. Radiation carcinogenesis in rat skin. In: Radiation Carcinogenesis. Edited by A.C. Upton, R.E. Albert, F.J. Burns, and R.E. Shore. New York, Elsevier, 1986.

Burns, F.J., Albert, R.E., Vanderlaan, M., Strickland, P. The dose response curve for tumor induction with single and split doses of 10 MeV protons. Radiat. Res. 62:598, 1975.

Carsten, A.L., Bond, V.P. and Thompson, K. The RBE of Different Neutrons as Measured by the Hematopoietic Spleen Colony Technique. Int. J. Rad. Biol. 29:65, 1976.

Carter, R.E., Bond, V.P. and Seymour, P.H. The Relative Biological Effectiveness of Fast Neutrons in Mice. Radiat. Res. 4:413, 1956.

Clapp, N.K., Darden, E., Jr. and Jernigan, M.C. Relative effects of whole-body sublethal doses of 60 MeV protons and 300 kVp X rays on disease incidences in RF mice. Radiat. Res. 57:158, 1974.

Conklin, J.J. Research issues for radiation protection for man in prolonged space flight. Advances in Radiation Biology, Vol. 13, New York, Academic Press, 1986.

Curtis, S.B. Radiation physics and evaluation of current hazards. In: Space Radiation Biology and Related Topics. Edited by C.A. Tobias and P. Todd. New York, Academic Press, 1974.

Elkind, M.M. and Whitmore, G.F. The radiobiology of cultured mammalian cells. New York, Gordon and Breach, 1967.

Field, S.B. The relative biological effectiveness of fast neutrons for mammalian cells. Radiology 93:915, 1969.

Fry, R.J.M., Powers-Risuis, P., Alpen, E.L. and Ainsworth, E.J. High-LET radiation carcinogenesis. Radiat. Res. 104:S188, 1985.

Geard, C.R. Charged particle cytogenetics: Effects of LET, fluence, and particle separation on chromosome aberrations. Radiat. Res. 104:S112, 1985.

Hall, E.J. Radiobiology for the Radiologist, 2nd Edition, New York, Harper and Row, 1982.

ICRP Publication 26. Recommendations of the International Commission on Radiological Protection. Annals of the ICRP 1, #3, New York, Pergamon Press, 1977a.

ICRP Publication 27. Problems Involved in Developing an Index of Harm. Annals of the ICRP, Vol. 1, No. 3, New York, Pergamon Press, 1977b.

ICRP Publication 32. Limits for Inhalation of Radon Daughters by Workers. Annals of the ICRP 6, #1, 1–24, 1981.

ICRP Publication 39. Principles for Limiting Exposure of the Public to Natural Sources of Radiation. Annals of the ICRP 14, #1, 1–8, 1984.

ICRP Statement from the 1985 Paris Meeting of the International Commission on Radiological Protection, Paris, March 20–22, 1985. Annals of the ICRP, Vol. 15, No. 3, New York, Pergamon Press, 1985a.

ICRP Publication 45. Quantitative Bases for Developing a Unified Index of Harm, Annals of the ICRP, Vol. 15, No. 3, New York, Pergamon Press, 1985b.

ICRU Report 39. Determination of Dose Equivalent Resulting from External Radiation Sources. International Commission on Radiation Units and Measurements, Bethesda, MD, 1984.

ICRU Report 40. The Quality Factor in Radiation Protection, Report of a Joint Task Group of the ICRP and the ICRU to the ICRP and the ICRU, International Commission on Radiation Units and Measurements, Bethesda, MD, 1986.

Jin, N.R., Hall, R.S., Petersen, F.P., Buckner, C.D., Stewart, P.S., Amos, D., Appelbaum, F.R., Clift, R.A., Bousinger, W.I., Sanders, J.E. and Thomas, E.D. Marrow harvesting for autologous marrow transfusion. Expt. Hematol. 13:879, 1985.

Joiner, M.C., Denekamp, J., and Maughan, R.L. The use of 'top-up' experiments to investigate the effect of very small doses per fraction in mouse skin. Int. J. Radiat. Biol. 49:565, 1986.

Langham, W.H., ed. Radiobiological factors in manned space flight. NAS-NRC Publication 1487, 1967.

Leith, J.T., Ainsworth, E.J. and Alpen, E.L. Heavy-Ion Radiobiology: Normal Tissue Studies. In: Adv. in Radiation Biol, Vol. 10. Edited by J.T. Lett, U.K. Ehmann, and A.B. Cox, 1983.

Lett, J.T., Cox, A.B. and Bergtold, D.S. Cellular and tissue responses to heavy ions: basic considerations. Radiat. Environ. Biophys. 25:1, 1986.

Lushbaugh, C.C. and Casarett, G.W. Effects of gonadal irradiation in clinical radiation therapy: a review. Cancer 37:2, 1111–1120, 1976.

Magee, J.L. and Chatterjee, A. Radiation chemistry of heavy-particle tracks. General considerations. J. Phys. Chem. 84:3529, 1980.

McCormack, P.D. Radiation dose predictions for the Space Station. Paper presented at the 37th IAF Congress, Innsbruck, Austria. Acta Astronautica (in press), October, 1986.

Meyn, R.E. and Withers, H.D., Eds. Radiation Biology in Cancer Research New York, Raven Press, 1980.

NCRP. National Council on Radiation Protection and Measurements. NCRP Report—High-LET Radiation. Washington, D.C., 1989.

NAS/NRC. National Research Council. Radiobiological factors in manned space flight, report of space radiation study panel of the life sciences committee. Edited by W.H. Langham, Space Science Board, National Academy of Sciences, Washington, D.C., 1967.

Petrov, V.M., Kovalev, E.E. and Sakovich, V.A. Radiation: risk and protection in manned space flight. Acta Astronautica, 8(8–10):1091–1098, 1981.

Poulsen, C.A. The Study of Irradiation Effects on the Human Testes: Including Histologic, Chromosomal and Hormonal Aspects. Terminal Report, AEC Contract AT(45-1)-2225, 1973.

Raju, M.R., Bain, E., Carpenter, S.G., Cox, R.A. and Robertson, J.B. A comparative study of heavy particles in radiation therapy. II. Cell survival as a function of depth of penetration. Brit. J. Radiol. 51:704, 1978.

Rowley, J.J., Leach, D.R., Warner, G.A., and Heller, C.G. Effects of graded doses of ionizing radiation on the human testes. Radiat. Res. 59(3):665, 1974.

Rubin, P. and Casarett, G.W. Chemical Radiation Pathology, vol. I, Chapt. VIII. Philadelphia, PA, Saunders, 1968.

Schick, P., Messerschmidt, O. and Sailer, J. Proceedings of the 1981 Workshop of the Research Study Group on the Assessment of Ionizing Radiation Injury in Nuclear Warfare. NATO, H1-7, Paris, 1981.

Speiser, B., Rubin, P. and Casarett, G. Aspermia following lower truncal irradiation for Hodgkin's disease. Cancer 32:692, 1973.

Storer, J.B., Harris, P.S., Furchner, J.E. and Langham, W.H. The relative biological effectiveness of various ionizing radiations in mammalian systems. Radiat. Res. 6:188, 1957.

Swift, M.N., Taketa, S.T. and Bond, V.P. Efficacy of hematopoietic protective procedures in rats X-irradiated with intestine shielded. Radiat. Res. 4:186, 1956.

Thomas, E.D. and Buckner, C.D. et al. One hundred patients with acute leukemia treated by chemotherapy, total body irradiation and allogenic marrow transplantation. Blood 49:511, 1977.

Thomas, E.D. and Storb, R., et al. Bone marrow transplantation. N. Engl. J. Med. 292:832, 1975.

Tobias, C.A., Chatterjee, A. and Smith, A.R. Radioactive fragmentation of N+7 ion beam observed in a beryllium target. Phys. Lett. 37A:119, 1971a.

Todd, P. and Walker, J.T. The microlesion concept in HZE particle dosimetry. Adv. Space Res. 4:187, 1984.

Todd, P., Schroy, C.B., Schimmerling, W., and Vosburgh, K.G. Cellular Effects of Heavy Charged Particles. Life Science and Space Research, 11:261, 1973.

Urano, M., Verhey, L.J., Goitein, M., Tepper, J.E., Suit, H.D., Phil, D., Mendiondo, O., Gragoudas, E. and Koehler, A. Relative biological effectiveness of modulated proton beams in various murine tissues. Int. J. Radiat. Oncol. Biol. Phys. 10:509, 1984.

Watts, J.W., Jr. and Wright, J.J. Charged particle radiation environment for the Spacelab and other missions in low Earth orbit—Revision A. NASA Tech. Memo. TMX-753358, 1976.

Whitton, J.T., and Everall, J.D. The Thickness of the Epidermis. Brit. J. Dermatol. 89:467, 1973.

Wood, D.H., Yochmowitz, M.G., Hardy, K.A. and Salmon, Y.L. Animal studies of life shortening and cancer risk for space radiation. Adv. Space Res. (in press).

Yang, T.C., Craise, L.M., Mei, M.T. and Tobias, C.A. Neoplastic cell transformation by heavy charged particles. Radiat. Res. 104:5, 1985.

Yochmowitz, M.G., Wood, D.M., and Salmon, Y.L. Seventeen-year mortality experience of proton radiation in Macaca mulatta. Radiat. Res. 102:14, 1985.

Zirkle, R.E. and Tobias, C.A. Effects of ploidy on LET on radiobiological survival curves. Arch. of Biochem. and Biophys. 47:282, 1975.

NCRP Report No. 98 (1989). Guidance on Radiation Received in Space Activities.

21 Medical Care and Health Maintenance In Flight

ARNAULD E. NICOGOSSIAN

SAM L. POOL

The demands and potential hazards of space flight require that crewmembers maintain health and peak proficiency at all times. The preventive medicine program used in preparation for a mission is designed to ensure that astronauts are in excellent health at the moment of launch. The extensive preflight precautions, however, do not guarantee that medical episodes will not occur during a mission; indeed, the history of space flight indicates that isolated episodes are inevitable. These are for the most part minor, but with occasional events of real medical consequence. While the principal effort of space medicine is preventive, planning and preparation for inflight problems must be sufficient to address and resolve these relatively rare events at the time of their occurrence.

Procedures for handling medical problems that arise during a mission include:

1. Ground-Based Monitoring. Space missions are monitored continuously by a flight control team, which includes medical personnel. The medical team receives health-related information via spacecraft telemetry. This is supplemented by private medical conferences, as necessary, with crews. Information obtained during monitoring concerns direct medical problems and evaluation of circumstances which appear to be leading toward such problems. This data includes status of environmental control systems, radiation exposure, food supply, water condition, and personal hygiene. Any malfunction of a spacecraft life-support system having a potential effect on crew health can be examined.

Additional health monitoring can be carried out using data from onboard biomedical experiments and instrumented physical exercise. In the Skylab era, flight motion sickness studies, cardiovascular studies, and metabolic load experiments provided invaluable information to medical teams via biotelemetry. Instrumented physical exercise sessions on Skylab and more recent Shuttle flights were useful adjuncts in the implementation of an inflight health monitoring and maintenance program. Environmental data, such as partial pressures of oxygen and carbon dioxide, as well as cabin temperature, can be obtained as required. In addition, noise and radiation exposure surveys are conducted at selected points of a mission to evaluate long-term effects of potential environmental hazards. Finally, during critical inflight operations, such as extravehicular activities, biomedical monitoring can proceed through voice communications supported by one-lead electrocardiography and information on metabolic expenditure during work.

2. Medical Training. Each astronaut is trained for both prevention and management of inflight medical problems. This training, described at greater length in the chapter on biomedical training, includes general medical training, augmented by special courses for handling onboard medical systems and biomedical experiments. As part of mission preparation, additional briefings are designed to review pre- and postflight medical procedures, discuss crew preventive medicine measures, instruct the crew in the contents and use of the onboard medical kit, demonstrate the configuration and operation of the biomedical harness, and familiarize the crew with toxicological considerations (Vanderploeg, 1981). Finally, if a physician-astronaut is included in the crew complement, he or she can direct the management of an inflight emergency.

3. Onboard Medical Kit. An onboard medical kit is provided for treatment and stabilization in life-threatening emergencies, and diagnosis and treatment of all minor injuries and illness events.

INFLIGHT DISEASE AND INJURY

Space crews are given detailed medical examinations during the month prior to launch, and a final physical examination is administered on the day of launch. Combined with the use of a Health Stabilization Program to minimize disease contact prior to flight, these examinations ensure, to the extent possible, the health of space crews at the time of launch.

Extensive preflight preventive programs have held inflight medical problems to a minimum. Table 21-1 lists the illnesses and injuries experienced by U.S. space crews to date, including inflight episodes which required management by the flight crew. Instances of trauma and toxic pneumonia encountered during landing were dealt with by members of the medical recovery team. Incidents of space motion sickness are discussed in a previous chapter.

Some caution should be observed when using the results in Table 21-1 to define medical care requirements for future space missions. The data in this table are based on findings from the Gemini Program through the Apollo-Soyuz Test Project. Each new program introduces a new spacecraft environment and different crewmember work demands. In Space Shuttle missions, for example, astronauts work for the first time in a sea-level atmosphere. They also perform a variety of unique work activities related to the various payloads that can be carried. These features

TABLE 21-1

ILLNESS / INJURY OCCURRENCE IN U.S. SPACE CREWS

Illness / Injuries	Number
Inflight	
Dysbarism	2
Eye-skin irritation (fiberglass)	3
Skin infection	2
Contact dermatitis	2
Urinary tract infection	2
Arrhythmias	2
Serious otitis	1
Eye and finger injury	1
Sty	1
Boil	1
Rash	
Recovery and Landing	
Trauma (scalp laceration from detached camera)	1
Toxic pneumonia (inadvertent atmosphere contamination by N_2O_4)	3
Postflight	
Back strain (due to lifting of heavy object)	1

From data of Furukawa et al., 1982.

may well alter the potential for injury from that found, for example, in the Skylab Program.

ONBOARD MEDICAL EQUIPMENT

All U.S. spacecraft have included an onboard medical kit. In the Mercury Program, this kit was rudimentary, containing only an anodyne, an anti-motion sickness drug, a stimulant, and a vasoconstrictor for treatment of shock (Link, 1965). As Project Mercury evolved into Project Gemini, additional medications were included in the medical kit. The contents for the 14-day Gemini 7 kit are listed in Table 21-2. Similar drugs have been included in the medical kits for the subsequent Apollo, Skylab, and Space Shuttle Programs. Onboard medical supplies for Skylab were more elaborate, including surgical instru-

ments and diagnostic equipment, in view of the longer durations of these flights.

The Space Shuttle Orbiter carries a specially designed medical system that allows crewmembers to deal with medical emergencies in flight. This package, known as the Shuttle Orbiter Medical System (SOMS), has three configurations—SOMS A, SOMS B, and SOMS C. The smallest unit, SOMS A, is designed for use on flights of 21 man-days or less. SOMS B is designed for flights of up to 44 man-days. The largest unit, SOMS C, is designed for flights extending beyond this period. Since the nominal Space Shuttle mission in the immediate future will be on the order of 7 days, only the smallest system, SOMS A, is described here.

The SOMS includes two medical kits, a Medications and Bandage Kit (MBK) plus an Emergency Medical Kit (EMK), and a medical checklist for crewmember use. Other Orbiter systems such as the Portable Oxygen System (Vanderploeg, 1981) are used on occasion. Each kit contains three

TABLE 21-2

GEMINI 7 INFLIGHT MEDICAL AND ACCESSORY KITS

Medication	Dose and Form	Label	Quantity
Cyclizine HCl	50-mg tablets	Motion sickness	8
d-Amphetamine sulfate	5-mg tablets	Stimulant	8
APC (aspirin, phenacetin, and caffeine)	Tablets	APC	16
Meperidine HCl	100-mg tablets	Pain	4
Triprolidine HCl	2.5-mg tablets	Decongestant	16
Pseudoephedrine HCl	60-mg tablets	Decongestant	16
Diphenoxylane HCl	2.5-mg tablets	Diarrhea	16
Tetracycline HCl	250-mg film-coated tablets	Antibiotic	16
Methyl cellulose solution	15 cc in squeeze-dropper bottle	Eye drops	1
Parenteral cyclizine	45 mg (0.9 cc in injector)	Motion sickness	2
Parenteral meperidine HCl	90 mg (0.9 cc in injector)	Pain	2

From Berry, 1975.

pallets with items stowed on both sides of each pallet. The general contents and purpose of each pallet are shown in Table 21-3.

The SOMS medical kits contain an array of drugs for use as dictated by illness and injury conditions. As part of the preparation for a mission, each astronaut is evaluated for sensitivity to the drugs in the kit. This drug sensitivity evaluation involves two steps (Vanderploeg, 1981). First, each crewmember's health record is reviewed and a listing is made of all medications received. Any reported reactions or side effects are noted. In the second step,

each crewmember is tested for sensitivity to those medications felt to have a high likelihood for inflight use. Any reactions are noted in a listing maintained at the Mission Operations Control Room as reference information for use by mission medical personnel.

Figure 21-1 shows the two medical kits included in SOMS A. The three pallets can be seen stored within each of these kits. Figures 21-2 and 21-3 show the contents of one pallet from the Emergency Medical Kit and one from the Medications and Bandage Kit, respectively.

The medicine and supplies contained in

TABLE 21-3

SOMS MEDICAL KIT

Pallets	Pallet Contents	General Purpose of Equipment in Pallet
A	Injectables	Medications to be administered by injection
B	Emergency items	Minor surgery equipment
		Diagnostic/therapeutic items
		Instruments for measuring and inspecting the body
D	Oral medications	Pills, capsules, and suppositories
E	Bandage items	Material for covering or immobilizing body parts
F	Non-injectables	Medications to be administered by topical application

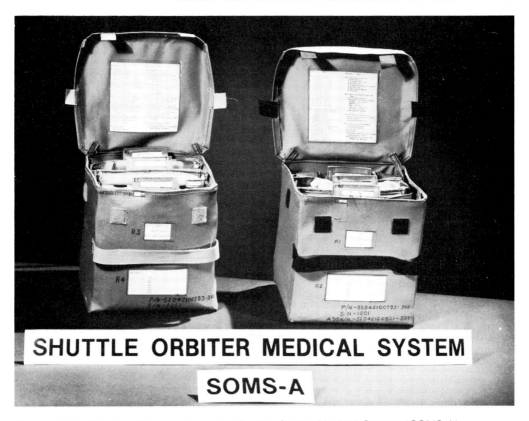

SHUTTLE ORBITER MEDICAL SYSTEM

SOMS-A

Figure 21-1. The two kits comprising the Shuttle Orbiter Medical System (SOMS-A).

each of the six pallets of the two medical kits are listed in Tables 21-4 through 21-9. Periodically, the items in these pallets are reviewed against growing flight experience and contents are revised as appropriate. In addition, medications are periodically refurbished according to consideration of the manufacturer's specification for shelf life and possible effects of the space environment on pharmacological activity of the drugs.

In the event of a serious mishap, such as a cervical spine injury or an illness requiring immobilization of a crewmember in the weightless environment, special procedures utilizing available Orbiter equipment have been devised. Figures 21-4 and 21-5 show these procedures as developed by the medical support team.

The medical system carried on the Space Shuttle Orbiter includes a limited capability for inflight laboratory tests, such as microbial analyses. The possibility of an infectious disease undetected during preflight examinations could require inflight diagnosis. Equipment is carried to facilitate inflight microbiological sampling and analyses of samples from the throat, urine, and wounds or obvious areas of infection. A hematology kit is being designed for future flights. This kit will allow drawing of blood and limited clinical analyses of hematocrit, hemoglobin, and, with a microscope, white-cell counts.

In the event of a minor illness in space, a crewmember, in consultation with the crew physician, may use the medical kit to administer aid. If the condition is serious

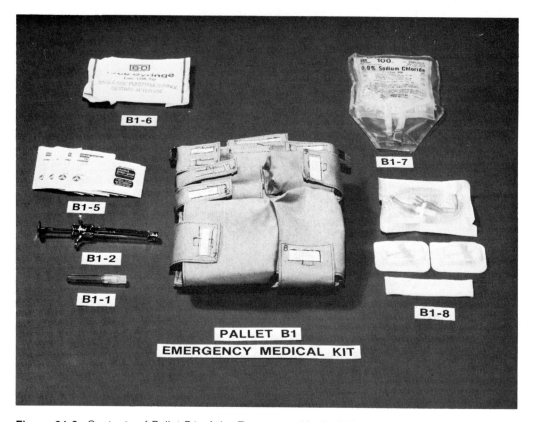

Figure 21-2. Contents of Pallet B1 of the Emergency Medical Kit.

TABLE 21-4

CONTENTS OF PALLET A (SOMS)

Aramine 10 mg/cc	Lidocaine HCl 20 mg/cc
Epinephrine 1:1000	Lidocaine 20 mg/cc
Atropine 0.4 mg/cc	Valium 5 mg/cc
Phenergan 25 mg/cc (IV)	Xylocaine 2% with epinephrine
Compazine 5 mg/cc	Xylocaine 2% without epinephrine
Pronestyl 500 mg/cc	Demerol 25 mg/cc
Morphine sulfate 10 mg/cc	Benadryl 50 mg/cc
Decadron 4 mg/cc	Vistaril 50 mg/cc

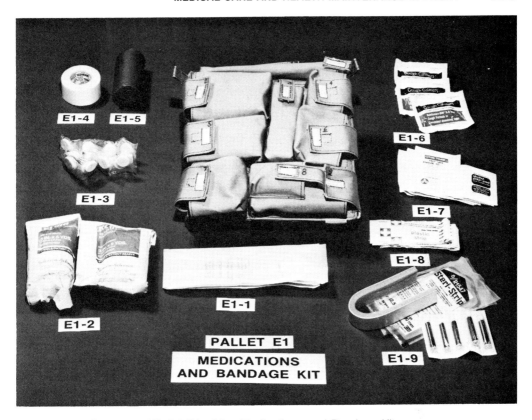

Figure 21-3. Contents of Pallet E1 of the Medications and Bandage Kit.

enough to require definitive treatment so that it does not become life-threatening, the mission can be aborted and an emergency rescue made at a landing facility. An orbital rescue with a second vehicle is also possible, although more complicated. In this event, astronauts trained in EVA procedures would transfer using the space suit and, if needed, the manned maneuvering units (MMU). Other crewmembers or passengers who are not trained for EVA would use the personal rescue system shown in Figure 21-6. This is an inflatable sphere with a diameter of 86 centimeters which allows transfer of personnel to another spacecraft. The system includes the

TABLE 21-5

CONTENTS OF PALLET B (SOMS)	
Needles, 22 g, 1.5 inch	Suture 4-0 Dexon with needle
Tubex injector	Bili-lab Stix and chart
Syringes, 10 cc	Forceps, small point
Needle, 21 q, butterfly (IV)	Needle holder and small hemostat
Normal saline, 100 cc	Tweezers, fine point
Tubing, IV, without chamber	Scalpel No. 13, Scalpel No. 11, and curved scissors

TABLE 21-6

CONTENTS OF PALLET C (SOMS)

BP cuff and stethoscope	Foley catheter, No. 11 Fr., with 30 cc balloon
Tourniquet and cotton balls	Penlight
Oral airway and cricothyrotomy set	Ophthalmoscope head
Disposable thermometers	Fluorescein strips
Tongue depressors	Binocular loupe
Otoscope specula	Sterile drape
Otoscope	Sterile gloves
Cobalt light	

personal rescue enclosure, constructed of a gas-tight restraint and thermal protection garment; a rescue support umbilical line to provide life support functions and communications capability during the pre- and post-rescue modes; and a portable oxygen system. The oxygen system provides pressurized gas for the rescue system sufficient for a 1-hour rescue period. Suited astronauts would transfer their crewmates to the rescue ship by rigging a pulley-and-clothesline device between the two vehicles, using the Canadian Remote Manipulator System, or physically towing the enclosures through space with the power of the MMUs.

After the Challenger accident, new means for escape during the powered phases of the Space Shuttle flights were considered. Specifically, three modes of crew extraction from the Orbiter were evaluated. The three modes consist of total ejection and parachute recovery of the pressurized cabin; individual escape system consisting of tractor rockets for each crewmember's extraction from the cabin and parachute landing; and use of a guide pole to clear the vehicle, with subsequent parachute landing. The last mode of rescue has been adopted for the early Space Shuttle flights. Additional or modified capabilities for rescue will be installed in the mid-1990's on subsequent missions.

Currently, studies are underway to de-

TABLE 21-7

CONTENTS OF PALLET D (SOMS)

Actifed tablets	Nitroglycerin tablets, 0.4 mg
Dexedrine tablets, 5 mg	Periactin tablets, 4 mg
Donnatal tablets	Sudafed tablets, 30 mg
Lomotil tablets	Pen VK tablets, 250 mg
Dalmane capsules, 15 mg	Phenergan/Dexedrine, 25/5 mg
Ampicillin capsules, 250 mg	Compazine suppositories, 25 mg
Erythromycin tablets, 250 mg	Keflex capsules, 250 mg
Tetracycline capsules, 250 mg	Aminophyllin suppositories, 500 mg
Throat lozenges, Cepacol	Digoxin, 0.25 mg
Scop/Dex capsules, 0.4/5 mg	Phenergan suppositories
Pyridium capsules, 200 mg	Dulcolax tablets
Valium tablets, 5 mg	Parafon Forte
Tylenol tablets, No. 3	Aspirin
Benadryl capsules, 25 mg	

TABLE 21-8

CONTENTS OF PALLET E (SOMS)	
Q-tips	Steri-strips
3-in Kling	Finger splint
Mylanta tablets	Benzoin wipes
Dermicel tape, 1 in	2 x 2 sponges
Gauze	Eye patch
Robitussin Cough Calmers	Adaptic dressing
Wipes, alcohol	Toothache kit
Wipes, Betadine	Ace bandage
Bandaids	

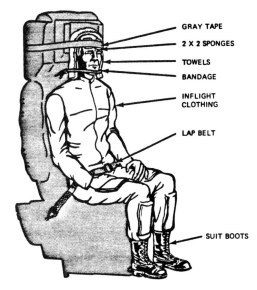

Figure 21-4. Procedure for immobilizing a Space Shuttle crewmember in the event of serious neck injury.

velop a small reusable space vehicle which can double as a space ambulance in case of inflight injuries, to be used in conjunction with the Space Station complex.

HEALTH PRACTICES

Medical personnel are primarily responsible for direct medical issues arising during manned space flight. However, they share with spacecraft designers and engineers the responsibility to ensure that spacecraft procedures and living conditions are conducive to good health and performance. Health maintenance is a broad area which includes more than simply prevention of disease. For example, in order for crewmembers to be at peak mental and physical condition during a launch period, circadian rhythms are adjusted as needed. In the event of an early morning or late night launch, circadian rhythms may be adjusted by altering the work schedule for the days immediately prior to launch. During missions, the general rule is that crew schedules are correlated with Houston or Cape Canaveral time. Schedules may also be adjusted or modified before landing, but care is taken to ensure

TABLE 21-9

CONTENTS OF PALLET F (SOMS)	
Afrin Nose Spray	Neocortef
Methylcellulose eyedrops	Halotex
Kerlix dressing	Neosporin
Povidone-Iodine Ointment, tube	Pontocaine, 15 ml bottle
Anusol-HC cream	Blistex
Kenalog cream, 0.1%	Cortisporin otic solution
Mycolog cream	Triangular bandage
Sulfacetamide	Surgical masks

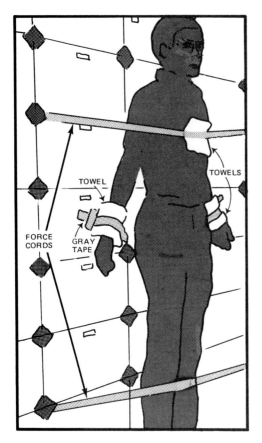

Figure 21-5. Procedure for restraining a Space Shuttle crewmember at the first aid station in the event of spinal injury or illness requiring immobilization.

that adjustments do not interfere with biomedical experiments.

In Space Shuttle operations, every attempt has been made to provide food service in a relatively normal manner. Special care is taken to ensure palatability, quality, nutritional value, and ease of preparation. Prior to flight, available foodstuffs are discussed with individual crewmembers and daily menus are established based on their preferences. Since unforeseen events could extend a mission beyond the planned time lines, contingency rations are included in the pantry of the Orbiter. These foods re-

quire special containers and utensils for use in weightlessness. Figure 21-7 shows a Space Shuttle astronaut preparing beverages in weightlessness.

Housekeeping on orbit and provisions for hygiene are considered important from the dual perspective of preventive medicine and morale. Considerable effort has been devoted to designing efficient and acceptable waste management systems. These systems are much improved over earlier bag collection devices and, in the Space Shuttle (see Chapter 4), resemble small bathrooms which accommodate male and female crewmembers. Provisions are made in the Space Shuttle for personal hygiene activities such as shaving (Figure 21-8). In longer missions such as Skylab, equipment was provided for hair grooming (Figure 21-9) using specially designed vacuum sources to prevent contamination of the cabin environment. Space showers also have been incorporated into the design of space vehicles. Figure 21-10 shows the shower system used on Skylab.

Considerations of human comfort and hygiene will grow in importance as plans for future space stations evolve. These stations will support a much larger work force over longer periods than do current programs. Important as they are now, issues of food service, personal hygiene, waste management, and scheduling of leisure time will be of even greater consequence for health maintenance.

THE FUTURE OF MEDICAL CARE AND HEALTH MAINTENANCE IN FLIGHT

The space programs of the next few decades will bring important advances in the utilization of the near-Earth orbital environment. It is envisioned that space stations will be permanently manned, with

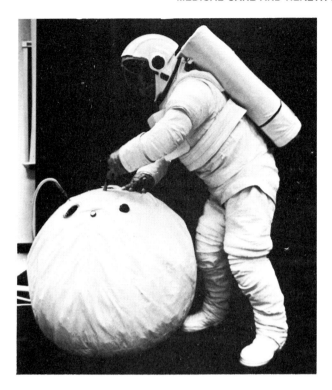

Figure 21-6. The personal rescue system used for transferring personnel to a rescue vehicle.

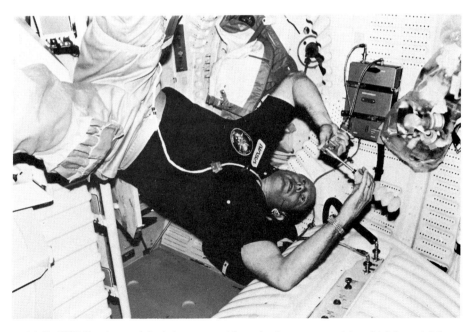

Figure 21-7. STS-3 astronaut Jack Lousma adds water to prepare a juice drink in weightlessness.

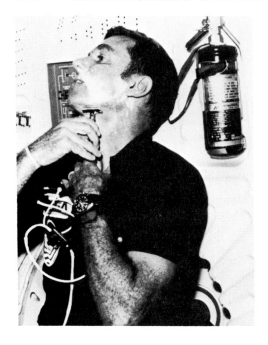

Figure 21-8. STS-2 astronaut Joe Engle shaving in the mid-deck area of the Space Shuttle.

rotating crews. The health and medical needs of these crews will place substantial demands on the growing field of space medicine. For space medicine to fulfill its charter as a specialty within preventive medicine, additional knowledge must be obtained concerning both short- and long-term adaptation to weightlessness. To what extent do problems of space motion sickness, cardiovascular deconditioning, and loss of bone mineral constrain future space missions? What are the critical psychological and habitability needs for crews working routinely in space?

Medical support for space station operations will require new philosophies and new technologies. The epicenter of medical care will shift from ground-based mission control centers to a space-based medical unit. For situations requiring the return of an ill crewmember to Earth, appropriate medical criteria must be established for allowing a patient to reenter the

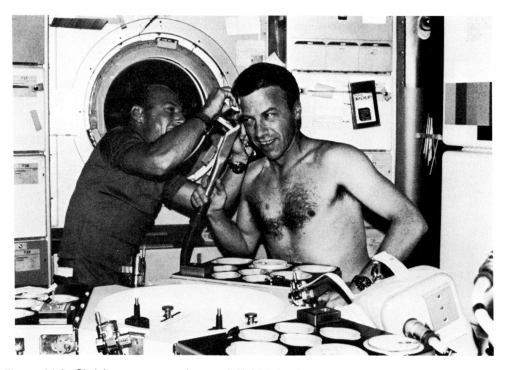

Figure 21-9. Skylab crewman receives an inflight haircut.

one-gravity environment, following weightlessness, without endangering his or her condition. These considerations demand that a space station contain personnel, facilities, and technologies qualified to provide adequate medical care and health maintenance services in zero gravity.

The Health Maintenance Facility envisioned for the Space Station (Figure 21-11) is intended to provide inflight preventive, diagnostic, and therapeutic capabilities, within limitations, to: 1) ensure the health and safety of Space Station crews, 2) eliminate unnecessary rescue operations, and 3) increase the probability of success when rescue is necessary. Through careful and thorough analysis of the requirements and limitations of the Space Station, and upon recommendations of a committee of recognized medical consultants, the most appropriate capabilities have been selected for integration into the Health Maintenance Facility. Capabilities

for handing all possible medical contingencies are, of course, not practical. However, it is possible to furnish medical knowledge, advice, and assistance equivalent to that available on Earth, through state-of-the-art diagnostic monitoring systems downlinked to a consultant network. This will allow highly specialized consultants to review data and images, observe procedures, provide instructions, prescribe treatment, and assist Space Station personnel in reaching well informed decisions consistent with existing capabilities and circumstances.

Within the Health Maintenance Facility 11 major subsystems fit into the categories of diagnostics, therapeutics, monitoring, countermeasures, and information management. These subsystems are summarized as follows:

Health Maintenance Computer—integrates the independent instruments of the HMF, maintains complete medical records on

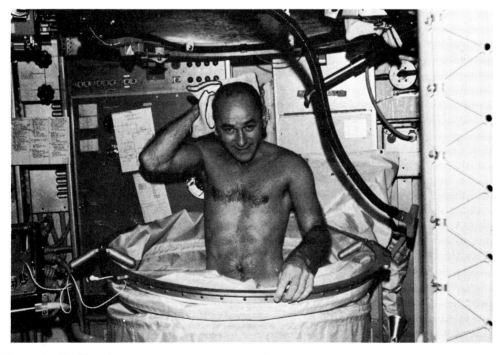

Figure 21-10. The shower system in use aboard Skylab.

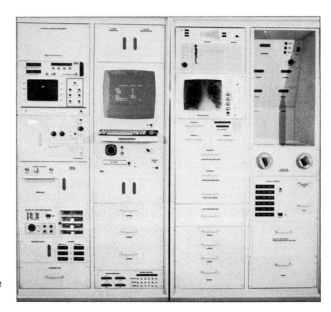

Figure 12-11. Health Maintenance Facility.

crewmembers, and provides protocols for prevention, diagnosis, and treatment.

IV Fluid and Nutritional Support—short-term IV fluid therapy and long-term parenteral nutrition.

Medical Life Support—bedside patient monitoring and conventional "crash cart" capability, in tandem with ventilation therapy.

Imaging—Radiographic imaging supports diagnostics and therapeutic procedures. Micro- and macroscopic imaging will include transmission and receiving of images by ground facilities.

Clinical Laboratory—clinical chemistries, hematology, dissolved gas analysis, microbiology analysis, and other tests and analyses as required.

Ventilation—provides ventilatory support to critically ill patients.

Pharmacy, Safe Haven, and Central Supply—includes inventory management and security, provides for crew support up to 28 days.

Surgery, Dentistry, and Anesthesiology—capability to perform minor surgery, dental procedures and administer anesthesia.

Physician's Instruments—provide wide variety of instruments to meet medical officers' needs, including noninvasive diagnostic capabilities.

Hyperbarics—treatment tables, protocols, and instrumentation to meet hyperbaric treatment requirements. Does not include chamber.

Exercise Countermeasures—provide appropriate exercise capability to preclude deleterious effects of microgravity on bone and muscle tissue.

In the future, as humans move beyond the Space Station toward advanced missions of longer duration, capabilities must be perfected for maintaining human health and well-being. The challenges for space medicine will undoubtedly match those presented by missions of the future.

REFERENCES

Berry, C.A. Medical care of spacecrews (medical care, equipment, and prophylaxis). In: Foundations of space biology and medicine (Vol. III) (NASA SP- 374). Edited by M. Calvin and O.G. Gazenko. U.S. Government Printing Office, Washington, D.C., 1975.

Furukawa, S., Nicogossian, A., Buchanan, P., and Pool, S. Medical support and technology for long-duration space missions. Paper presented at the 33rd International Congress of the International Astronautical Federation, Paris, France, 27 September–2 October, 1982.

Link, M.M. Space medicine in Project Mercury (NASA SP-4003). U.S. Government Printing Office, Washington, D.C., 1965.

National Aeronautics and Space Administration. MED EQ 2102 medical equipment workbook (CG3-027). Crew Training and Procedures Division, Training Integration Branch, Lyndon B. Johnson Space Center, Houston, TX, 1979.

Vanderploeg, J.M. Shuttle orbital medical system. In: STS-1 medical report (NASA TM-58240). Edited by S.L. Pool, P.C. Johnson, Jr., and J.A. Mason. National Aeronautics and Space Administration, Scientific and Technical Information Branch, Washington, D.C., December 1981.

22 Human Capabilities in Space Exploration and Utilization

VICTORIA GARSHNEK

JERI W. BROWN

Manned space flight can be viewed as an interaction of three general elements: the crewmember (selection, protection, training); spacecraft systems (function, design, performance); and the environment (external, internal, and combined) (Figure 22-1). To ensure the greatest possible mission productivity and success, these elements must be properly integrated, compatible, and mutually supportive. Within such a systems perspective, the three elements become highly interdependent: typically, variations in one component have repercussions in one or more of the others (Nicogossian, 1988).

The human operator is a crucial element in this system. His capacity for fine sensory and perceptual discriminations of the environment both inside and outside the vehicle, and the swiftness and accuracy of his responses to specific stimuli, have often proved critical to mission success. These abilities, however, may be compromised by certain physiological, psychological, environmental, and spacecraft systems factors which can negatively influence behavior and performance (Christensen and Talbot, 1985). Table 22-1 lists some of these space flight factors, along with certain appropriate measures that can be implemented to achieve maximum mission productivity.

The purpose of human factors research is to optimize the interface between operators and machines, so that the resulting systems operations meet specified performance and mission requirements. There are four important interfaces to be considered:

- Hardware elements, such as controls, displays, and workstations
- Computer software
- The operational environment, including temperature, vibration, acceleration, radiation, and ambient pressure

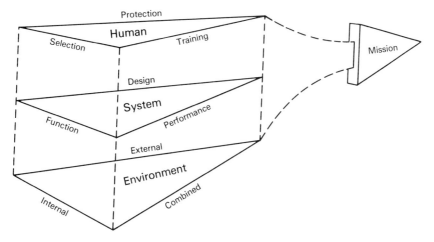

Figure 22-1. Elements of mission design (Nicogossian, 1988).

- Social interaction with other individuals (Sheridan and Young, 1985).

Human factors research examines human abilities and limitations in the operational environment of space flight, and the interfaces between the crewmember and automated spacecraft systems. For it is only by considering the human in the context of mission operations, vehicle design, and crew provisions that his or her abilities can be most effectively utilized. Investigations in this area, therefore, serve to bridge the gap between theoretical research and "real-world" engineering and planning, where practical constraints and limitations may determine the final configuration.

GENERAL FUNCTIONS OF THE HUMAN OPERATOR

In space flight, the general functions of the human operator can be divided into sensory, control, processing/memory, and motor. On the machine side of the interface are displays that convert electrical and mechanical signals into data recognizable to the human senses. Control devices, such as push-buttons, toggle switches, pedals, or joysticks, in turn transduce the operator's voluntary motor responses to electrical and mechanical signals capable of controlling the system. With increasing automation and reliance on computers, however, the human operator has been relieved of such tasks as closing a feedback loop or driving the vehicle: the computer serves as a direct controller, while the human operator's role has evolved to that of supervisor of an otherwise automatic control loop (Sheridan and Young, 1985).

Man's inherent ability to discern patterns, make decisions, and plan ahead is generally superior to inbuilt capabilities of existing hardware of comparable cost, weight, and size. On the other hand, the human senses are inferior in the time required to detect and process incoming signals, discriminate small variations in these signals, select a course of action, and execute a response (Wargo et al., 1967). The flexibility of human response is also limited. A poor match between the displays/controls and the human operator's capabilities (mental and physical) further complicates man's ability to perform rapidly and efficiently. Operator delays are a key area of concern in the use of man in complex systems: receptor-effector, cognitive, and perceptual delays are inherent and cannot be modified to any significant degree.

Man is fundamentally a single-channel sequential recorder with a reasonably wide base and low sensitivity input-output capacity in relation to his cost and size (Hartman, 1971). He has an advantage over machines in his capacity to select (or ignore), interpret, and store many units of information. Much of this input-output capacity is compromised, however, under conditions of stress and fatigue. Under these circumstances, man has a marked predilection for reverting to a more primitive mode, in which he deals with signals and responses singly and sequentially; competing signals must wait for his attention and action.

TABLE 22-1

SOME FACTORS THAT INFLUENCE BEHAVIOR AND PERFORMANCE OF SPACE CREWS AND OTHER OPERATIONAL PERSONNEL[a]

Psychological, Social and Physiological Factors	Environmental Factors	System Design and Operation	Protective Measures for the Human Operator
Psychological	Spacecraft habitability	Mission duration and complexity	Training
Limits of performance	Confinement	Organization for command and control	Preflight environmental adaptation training
Cognitive abilities	Weightlessness	Crew performance requirements	Social sensitivity training
Decision-making	Lack of privacy	Division of work: man/machine	Training for team effort
Motivation	Artificial life support	Information load	Cross training
Attitudes	Noise	Task load/speed	Inflight maintenance of proficiency
Emotions/moods	Work-rest cycles	Crew composition	Self-control training
Psychological stability	Shift changes	Space crew autonomy	
Personality variables	Desynchronization	Physical comfort/quality of life	Selection
Human reliability (error rate)	Simultaneous and/or sequential multiple stresses	Communications (intra-crew and space-ground)	Selection criteria
Productivity	Hazards	Competency requirements	
Adaptability	Boredom	Time compression	Protection/support
Time compression	Physical isolation		Inflight psychosocial support
	Social isolation		Work-rest/avoiding excess workloads
Social			Ground contacts
Leadership			Job rotation
Crew composition			Job enrichment
Social skills			Recreation
			Exercise
Physiological			Recognition, awards, benefits
Space adaptation syndrome			
Spatial illusions			
Fatigue (physical and mental)			

[a] Adapted from Christensen and Talbot, 1985.

MAJOR ROLES OF THE HUMAN IN SPACE

In the initial years of space flight, man's role was limited to a few tasks. His capabilities had yet to be demonstrated, although he could act in a reserve capacity should the automated system fail. Astronaut performance, however, particularly during unscheduled and emergency events, removed many doubts concerning human adaptability to and effectiveness in the space environment.

Man's role in spacecraft operations has evolved from operator (in U.S. Mercury and U.S.S.R. Vostok) to mission manager (in U.S. Space Shuttle and U.S.S.R. Soyuz-TM/Mir), supervising highly automated spacecraft systems and manually executing critical operations. According to Yeremin, Bogdashevskiy, and Baburin (1975), the duties of a space flight crew have traditionally involved the following tasks:

- Controlling and monitoring onboard systems
- Controlling and performing dynamic spacecraft operations
- Performing extravehicular activities; assembling and disassembling individual spacecraft units; operating special gear
- Conducting visual observations and scientific investigations.

On future manned missions, the human crewmember will undoubtedly assume increasing responsibilities as the overall system manager and decision maker. Complexity of tasks such as maintenance, repair, construction, and scientific observation will be increased. As supervisor of automated spacecraft systems, the human crewmember will be free to pursue tasks of a more creative and less repetitive nature, while retaining the capability to manually execute critical operations when the need arises.

SYSTEM MANAGEMENT AND DECISION MAKING

Increasingly, the role of the astronaut is becoming that of information manager and processor (Loftus, 1982). The magnitude of information management in space operations is indicated in Table 22-2, which shows the rate at which information sources within a spacecraft have increased

TABLE 22-2

CREW DISPLAYS AND CONTROLS

Program	Panels	Work Stations	Control Display Elements	Computers Number/ Modes
Mercury	3	1	143	0
Gemini	7	2	354	1
Apollo	40	7	1374	4/50
Skylab	189	20	2980	4
Shuttle	97	9	2300	5/140
Space Station[a]	200	40	3000	8/200

[a] Assumes real-time control on board, database management from the ground.

Loftus, 1982.

as American manned spacecraft have increased in complexity. Table 22-3 shows the corresponding growth, over the same time period, in the number of information items displayed, both to crewmembers and ground controllers.

Man determines priorities, goals, and risks, recognizes targets and opportunities, and improvises under unforeseen and unscheduled circumstances (Bejczy, 1982). While man is capable of assessing alternatives and determining a course of action, his decision will not necessarily be optimal in all cases. Studies have shown that decisions are a function of several types of cognitive information (Marques and Howell, 1979): 1) prior knowledge of the data source, 2) memories of past and similar occurrences, 3) simplification rules of heuristics employed by the operator, and 4) the operator's inherent biases. Some of these variables can be modified through training; others, however, are remarkably resistant.

Although major decisions in past space flight activities have largely been the responsibility of ground support personnel, it is expected that increased automation and more sophisticated systems will result in greater crew autonomy in future missions such as the U.S. Space Station and, particularly, piloted missions to Mars and a manned base on the moon. Onboard capabilities will allow the human crewmember to modify planned mission activities in real time, accurately determine resupply needs, and assess the spacecraft's functional status.

VEHICLE / SYSTEM CONTROL

As shown in the following paragraphs, systems management and timely manual spacecraft control are among the most useful skills exhibited by astronauts.

In 1966, Neil Armstrong and David Scott successfully completed the first docking of two spacecraft when they docked the Gemini 6 capsule with the Agena target satellite. Armstrong and Scott also expe-

TABLE 22-3

SPACE SYSTEM INFORMATION

Program	Total Measurements		Displayed to Crew		Displayed to Mission Control	
Mercury	100		53		85	
Gemini	225		75		202	
Apollo						
Command Module	475	} 948	280	} 494	336	} 615
Lunar Module	473		214		279	
Skylab						
Command Module	521	} 2241	289	} 615	365	} 2034
Airlock Module	1720		326		1669	
Shuttle	7831		2170		3826	
Space Station[a]	10,000		4000		4000	

[a] Assumes real-time control on board, database management from the ground.

Loftus, 1982

rienced the first emergency in space during this operation. After docking with the Agena, the vehicle began to spin out of control. The crewmembers were able to correct this unstable situation by firing the retro-rockets, returning to Earth 2 days early. Manual docking of spacecraft has subsequently become an important phase of many American and Soviet missions.

During the Apollo 11 mission, manual spacecraft control was tried for the first time under lunar conditions, and was accomplished flawlessly. In this case, the Commander was able to respond rapidly to an emergency during lunar touchdown. The Lunar Module was about to land in a crater surrounded by large boulders. To prevent a possible disaster, the Commander manually redirected the craft to a more suitable landing site. Another near-miss was experienced during Apollo 16, when the crew averted the spacecraft from a crater.

Such piloting skills have been crucial to the success of the Space Shuttle Program. To accomplish its scientific objectives, the Spacelab-1 mission required a number of different orientations during orbital flight. The preflight maneuvering schedule called for 182 attitude changes, with 90 additional changes requested to maximize scientific return. The piloting skills of the two astronauts proved invaluable in this dynamic maneuvering profile (Nicogossian, 1984).

The Space Shuttle Program expanded the scope of vehicle control with the Remote Manipulator System (RMS). With the operator remotely located on the orbiter's flight deck, the RMS has been used to control payload movements and assist crewmembers in EVA.

Crew control has also been successfully demonstrated with the Manned Maneuvering Unit (MMU) in EVA (Figure 22-2), where untethered astronauts have moved in free flight to a distance of over 300 feet from the Shuttle (Nicogossian,

1984). With the MMU, astronauts can leave the orbiter to inspect for suspected damage, repair satellites, and conduct rescue missions, should they be necessary. The ability of astronauts to move freely and independently outside the spacecraft was made possible through new protocols for prebreathing and nitrogen washout, and the establishment of optimum cabin/EVA suit pressure profiles. In the future, space workers will be able to perform useful labors on the Space Station's exterior surfaces and participate in the construction of other space structures.

MAINTENANCE, REPAIR, AND CONSTRUCTION

Space systems are complex and costly; therefore, reliability is a prime objective in their design and operation. The space crew, as individuals and as a team, makes valuable contributions by monitoring systems, inspecting for possible damage and malfunction, and making necessary repairs. To the extent that man can recognize and diagnose problems, the need for redundancies in the many components is reduced, with corresponding reductions in weight, complexity, and cost.

Khachatur'yants (1981) cites studies showing that the human crewmember greatly enhances the reliability of space flight systems, especially when he or she is capable of making in-flight repairs. He concludes that the capability for human intervention in flight may prove optimal to mission success. The following paragraphs detail instances from both the American and Soviet programs when space crewmembers have successfully performed emergency repairs.

Without direct intervention by astronauts, the Skylab vehicle would have been rendered uninhabitable because of the overheating caused by the loss of the micrometeoroid shield and the failure of the

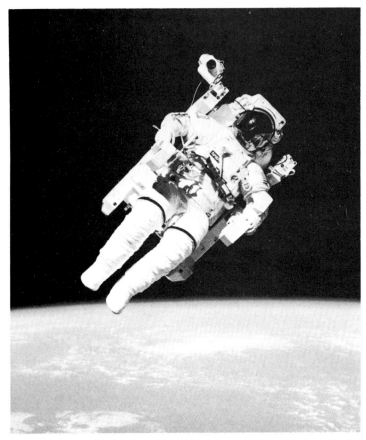

Figure 22-2. Astronaut Bruce McCandless during operation of the MMU in February, 1984, on STS mission 41-B.

solar array wing to deploy properly. In a difficult orbital repair job, the Skylab Commander and Scientist Pilot spent nearly 4 hours in EVA working to release the solar panel and restore vehicle operation. Their actions were instrumental in salvaging the $2.5 billion Skylab Program (Nicogossian, 1984).

Repair of the Solar Max satellite during Shuttle mission 41-C demonstrated important capabilities, including: 1) rendezvous and inspection of a satellite by free-flying, untethered crewmembers; 2) demonstration that docking is feasible with a moving satellite; 3) successful rotating grapple with the RMS; 4) repair of multiple components of the Solar Max satellite; and 5) repair of the satellite in the payload bay, and subsequent redeployment.

The orbital refueling system experiment conducted on Shuttle mission 41-G demonstrated human-tended capabilities to refuel orbiting satellites. Mission specialists performed an EVA to the aft end of the payload bay, where they connected a hydrazine servicing tool to a fuel supply tank. After pressure-checking the hook-up, the crewmembers returned to the cabin, where actual transfer of hydrazine is controlled.

Future satellite servicing procedures will be performed in a "shirtsleeve" environment, eliminating most of the limitations associated with EVA.

Construction procedures have been tested on orbit to determine the relative effectiveness of assembly techniques (Figure 22-3). It was discovered that hands-on EVA is five to ten times more efficient than use of manipulators or teleoperators. Similar assembly procedures will be utilized for on-orbit construction of the U.S. Space Station Freedom.

Soviet space crews have demonstrated invaluable capabilities for scheduled and unscheduled orbital maintenance and repair. The Salyut 6 space station had a pro-

jected design life of 18 months (Office of Technology Assessment, 1983). Largely as a result of the cosmonauts' efforts as on-orbit repairmen, the Salyut continued its mission for almost 5 years.

Unplanned repairs were also instrumental in saving the Soviet Salyut-7 program. A solar array malfunction reduced electrical power and seriously compromised the vehicle's environmental control system (Aviation Week and Space Technology, 1983). Without repair, the Salyut 7 would have been unusable for later missions due to internal damage resulting from excessive moisture. A repair crew was unable to reach the space station because of a fire during the launch sequence which caused

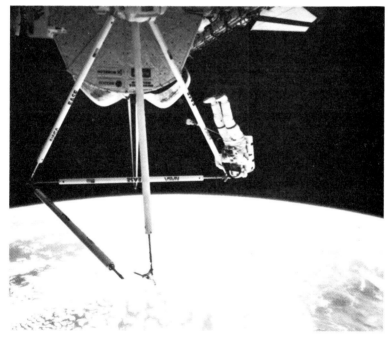

Figure 22-3. EASE is the Experimental Assembly of Structures in Extravehicular Activity. This experiment required the crewmember to float freely in space and move himself and the assembly elements by conservation of momentum. On-orbit assembly times were equivalent to water immersion simulation at the end of training.

the mission to be aborted. As a result, the next Salyut crew, who had not been specifically trained for repair operations of this kind, successfully repaired the station by following detailed instructions from ground controllers.

The first dedicated laboratory module for the Soviet space station Mir, the "Kvant" astrophysics module, failed in two docking attempts. Docking was successful on the third attempt, after the two cosmonauts inhabiting the Mir performed a 3-hour, 40-minute EVA to remove a foreign object from the docking apparatus. Thus, this costly module was "rescued," along with the many international experimental instruments which it contained (Soviet Aerospace, 1987).

FACTORS AFFECTING HUMAN PERFORMANCE IN SPACE

To date, crewmembers have shown remarkable versatility in space operations. However, some problems and areas for further study have been identified.

WEIGHTLESSNESS

The first manned flights dispelled many concerns about the ability of astronauts to carry out routine perceptual-motor activities in weightlessness. Although movement was restricted in the small Mercury capsule, motor difficulties did not prevent effective spacecraft management (Nicogossian and Parker, 1982). However, the repair, construction, and maintenance operations associated with more complex vehicles and missions are highly dependent on the accuracy of human motor and visual systems. Therefore, particular interest has centered on the extent to which weight-lessness disrupts the precise movements required in these activities.

Gerathewohl (1957) conducted a perceptual-motor performance study in which human subjects participated in an eye-hand coordination test. The subjects were required to aim for and strike the center of a test chart during vertical dives in a jet aircraft. Initially, subjects showed moderate disturbances from the decreased gravity. However, compensation was rapid and performance improved over the six trials, until it was comparable to performance under normal conditions.

During the Skylab Program, astronaut task performance in one gravity was compared to performance in zero gravity. Routine intravehicular activities such as donning and doffing EVA suits were evaluated through fine and gross motor coordination tests which required visual, tactile, or auditory feedback. Results showed that performance time for the majority of tasks increased after initial entry into weightlessness. However, after several days in flight, proficiency increased as crewmembers developed techniques to adjust their movements to the weightless condition. By the end of the second week in flight, more than 50 percent of the experimental tasks were performed as efficiently in space as on the ground. There was no evidence of performance deterioration with further time in space (Kubis et al., 1977).

CIRCADIAN RHYTHMS / SLEEP-WAKE-WORK CYCLES

Many functions of the body are regulated on a near 24-hour basis (Conroy and Mills, 1970; Colquhoun, 1971). Unusual environments or displaced or disrupted sleep or work schedules disrupt the body's normal circadian rhythms. This disruptive state is known as desynchronosis. Desynchronosis can produce physical symptoms such as insomnia, anorexia, malaise, and nervous stress (Hauty and Adams, 1966a, 1966b, 1966c).

In space, desynchronosis has been associated with disrupted sleep or work schedules. In all space missions up to and including Apollo 9, crewmembers' sleep schedules were staggered. This resulted in shifts of 6 to 10 hours from the Earth-based time during which sleep normally occurred. Even during later flights, when crewmembers slept simultaneously, hectic schedules required displacement of the sleep period by several hours, leading to fatigue and sleep disturbances (Connors et al., 1985). Disturbed sleep patterns noted in early flights were not improved until the 14-day Gemini flight, in which the work/rest schedule allowed crewmembers to sleep during the hours corresponding to night at Cape Canaveral (Gemini Midprogram Conference, 1966). The importance of synchronizing crew schedules with ground control is also well recognized by the Soviets. One of many improvements initiated in the Salyut Space Station Program was the establishment of a sleep-wake-work cycle keyed to normal Moscow time (Gurovskiy et al., 1981).

Variables that regulate the 24-hour clock are referred to as zeitgebers. Zeitgebers consist of a wide range of physical, temporal, and social "cues" that serve to entrain sleep and wakefulness to a particular rhythm. When zeitgebers are not present, certain rhythms become "free running" and may vary from a 24-hour schedule. A significant diurnal cue is the day/night cycle. In space, this familiar cue is lacking. For example, the orbital path of the Space Shuttle exposes crews to multiple sunrises and sunsets in a single Earth day. Given that circadian rhythms have a range of implications for performance in space, methods of entraining rhythms to the most advantageous sleep-wake cycles are important. Regulation of artificial lighting serves as a strong cue to perio-dicity. Social cues revolving around meals, work-rest schedules, and leisure activities can be even more important for regulating work performance (Aschoff, 1978).

PSYCHOLOGICAL FACTORS

Overall, psychological adjustment to space flight conditions has been good in both the American and Soviet programs. However, crew irritability and fatigue have been noted in relation to minor inflight illness. Irritability produced by fatigue has also been observed when schedules become too demanding (Cooper, 1976).

The Soviets have made detailed studies of psychological stresses. Of particular interest are those stresses associated with long-term missions. Performance has been evaluated against reported psychological state, and five general phases of task performance have been identified (Space Biology and Medicine Guide, 1983):

- Familiarization Phase (5–7 days): Individuals are adapting to the unusual conditions of space. Characterized by fluctuations in productivity and development of individually effective work rhythms. Errors (requiring intervention by ground control) committed on occasion. Emotional tension accompanies performance of critical tasks.
- Optimal Phase (10–15 days): Stable and efficient performance, with appropriate psychological responses. Major physiological functions are adequately adapted to weightlessness.
- Full Compensatory Period: Symptoms of fatigue are compensated by high motivation. Productivity and quality of work are not affected, and transitory fatigue disappears after sufficient sleep. High tension levels are associated with high workload.
- Unstable Compensatory Period: In-

creasing periods of fatigue, with decreased work capacity. Evidence of emotional instability with periodic sleep disturbance. Changes in perception levels, including visual, auditory, attention span, memory, and other sensory functions. Changes are highly individual, and work capacity is affected only slightly, manifested by decrease in motor reaction times, usually toward the end of the work day.

- Final Phase (2–3 days prior to return): High emotional and work efficiency levels.

Soviet scientists have noted that the above phases have no distinct demarcations, and are dependent on environmental habitability, and personal variables such as training, experience, general physical health, personal motivation, and willpower.

Cosmonauts showed signs of psychological stress during the final days of the Salyut and Mir long-term flights. As a result, to boost morale during the last stages of the 211-day Salyut 7 mission, the cosmonaut work day was reduced from 16 to 13 hours (Office of Technology Assessment, 1983). During the 326-day Mir mission, the work day was reduced from $8\frac{1}{2}$ hours to $6\frac{1}{2}$ hours, then further reduced to $4\frac{1}{2}$ hours near the end of the mission (FBIS, 1987). In addition, work that could not be accomplished during designated working hours was rescheduled. The Soviets have also implemented a comprehensive psychological support program, including the transport of letters, news, and favorite foods to space station crews. Frequent two-way video communication with families, entertainers, and research colleagues on the ground also helps to counter the stresses associated with long-term isolation, confinement, and busy work schedules (Office of Technology Assessment, 1983).

WORKLOAD

Work regimes of space crewmembers are structured to avoid fatigue and maintain an optimal workload. Fatigue may become a problem when the astronaut's reserve capacity is depleted, either from overloading or underloading. Gartner and Murphy (1976) suggest four broad categories of behavioral deterioration associated with over- or underloading: 1) decrements in skill or proficiency, 2) psychological stress, 3) decrements in motivation, and 4) decrements in performance. In addition, fatigue can result in slowed, irregular, or disordered performance (Welford, 1968).

After the first four Space Shuttle flights it was found that there was a significant task overload during the reentry phase of the mission. A third crewmember was added to the team of Commander and Pilot, and workload has been redistributed to accommodate different workloads during different activity phases. This has resulted in significantly improved performance and a marked reduction in work overloading.

In the Soviet program, the daily schedules of the Salyut 6 missions provide an example of overloading. In the course of the four main Salyut 6 flights, there was a total of 27 dockings of spacecraft with the space station, 4 redockings from one part of the station to another, 15 landings of Soyuz and Soyuz-T crew delivery vehicles, as well as 12 dockings of the Progress unmanned supply craft. One Salyut 6 crew performed 55 materials processing experiments and about 50 biomedical experiments (Myasnikov, 1983). The workload was exhausting; it was necessary to reduce the work day by 25 percent during the course of the mission (Office of Technology Assessment, 1983).

Proper sequencing of tasks is also important. Simple tasks can be performed effectively at much higher levels of fatigue than more complex ones (Welford, 1968).

In designing daily schedules, the assignment of complex tasks at the beginning of the workday or after rest periods might be the best approach. Simple tasks could then be assigned to follow complex tasks, or could be completed at the end of the day, when fatigue is probably greatest.

The delicate problem of balancing workload was demonstrated on Skylab, where mission programmers may have planned too busy a schedule in an attempt to prevent underloading (Cooper, 1976). A need exists to explore how mission activities might be juxtaposed and integrated to minimize fatigue, both with respect to the amount of work required and the sequencing of tasks.

HABITABILITY

Spacecraft habitability concerns not only the sustenance of human life in space, but assurance of the highest possible quality of life in that remote setting. Issues include environmental safety, sanitation, nutrition, and subtler factors such as environmental richness, temperature, humidity, and crew compatibility.

Designed with consideration both for ground training and flight operations, Spacelab and Skylab are excellent examples of a well-engineered habitat and workplace in terms of stowage and crew access to material, and layout of equipment and workstations. However, modules such as Spacelab can support only a limited number of crewmembers without crowding. Larger crews will require a new layout of workstations and additional habitable area.

With the launch of Salyut 6 in 1977, Soviet space station designers greatly increased their emphasis on "liveability" and a more "home-like" interior (Bluth and Helppie, 1986). Improved food service and hygiene systems, as well as entertainment items, helped reduce problems noted in earlier Salyut missions (irritability, boredom). Improvements continued with Salyut 7 (launched in 1982) and Mir (launched in 1986), incorporating suggestions from cosmonauts who had previously lived on board the space stations.

ANTHROPOMETRY AND BIOMECHANICS

Human factors engineering employs statistical information in the specification of equipment panels, workstations, seating, and the placement of displays and controls within the operator's reach envelope and field of vision. Design criteria must be established and evaluated according to characteristics averaged from the entire population of expected users.

Anthropometrics and biomechanics are focal points for investigations that seek to quantify human capabilities and physical limitations of spacecraft configurations. An anthropometric database provides systems equipment designers pertinent information about future flight personnel. As personnel of both sexes, various nationalities, and diverse age groups participate in space missions, the data collected help to better accommodate the broader anthropometric range of future crewmembers.

Major changes to human anthropometry and biomechanics under zero-g space flight conditions have been documented. These include adoption of a "fetal" resting posture as the limbs settle toward equilibrium in the weightless condition (Thornton et al., 1977). This postural change can adversely affect the ability to reach and position the arm and hand accurately. Prior to adaptation, there is a tendency to overshoot a target to be grasped. Therefore, space system designers should ensure that switches are easy to manipulate and do not require unnecessarily delicate tuning (Connors et al., 1985).

Measures of human strength and motion

also constitute an important research area. "Shirtsleeved" personnel can be accurately measured for individual joint (e.g., elbow range of motion) and torque generation for typical motions (e.g., push, pull). Pertinent variables include space suit design, crew restraints, and the measurement environment (e.g., one gravity, neutral buoyancy, and parabolic flight providing brief periods of zero gravity).

Although the requirements for crew restraints for on-orbit operations are closely examined preflight, inefficiencies have been observed during inflight activities, and crewmembers have reported fatigue. By collecting human strength and motion data in ground-based simulations and during space flight, tasks, crew procedures, vehicle subsystems, and crew equipment can be better paired with human performance capabilities.

Tests under parabolic flight conditions indicate that the space suit can augment as well as limit effective crew strength (Figure 22-4). Hand grip performance and EVA assembly testing provide insight into the driving parameters for designing the interfaces of the human hand, space suit glove, and various tools (Figure 22-5). Such scientifically rigorous testing also provides objective measures for comparing suit components, operating environments, and support required (e.g., restraints) during inflight use.

More efficient methods are also being sought to incorporate the vast amounts of information gathered in human factors research into spacecraft design. As an example, a reach envelope is a three-dimensional area (possibly four-dimensional if one considers the time course of motion). The envelope is described as a set

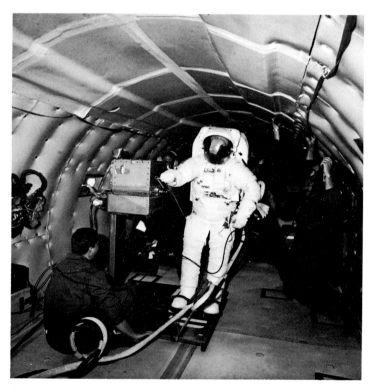

Figure 22-4. Astronaut strength measurement during simulated zero-g flights.

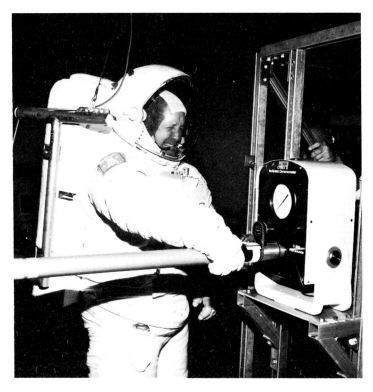

Figure 22-5. Crewmember applies maximum load during Space Station truss / connection testing.

of digitized points on the object's surface. Measurements of reach at varying cross-sections are useful in assessing workstation design, and the computer provides rapid access to the points along the cross section. The envelope can be manually traced or computer-generated, but differences in the final traces are evident and must be researched if accurate reach envelopes are to be defined.

Related to anthropometry / biomechanics research are computer man-modeling techniques (Figure 22-6), through which zero-g and reduced-g biodynamic models of the human are developed. These models extend the capabilities for design and planning and help to ascertain the efficiency of alternative approaches with relative speed, economy, and accuracy.

Computers can provide realistic graphics for assessment of crew activities, visual access, lighting, general habitability, and man/systems/equipment interfaces. Biodynamic models also allow the designer to place any crewmember at the workstation, assess reach and strength, check for fit, ease of access, and, in general, evaluate the man-machine interface during the design and development phases (Figure 22-7).

SUMMARY

Human factors engineering is essential to successful manned space flight. Although

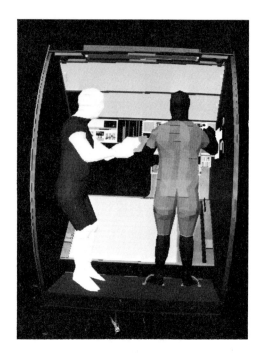

Figure 22-6. Computer man-model at work-station.

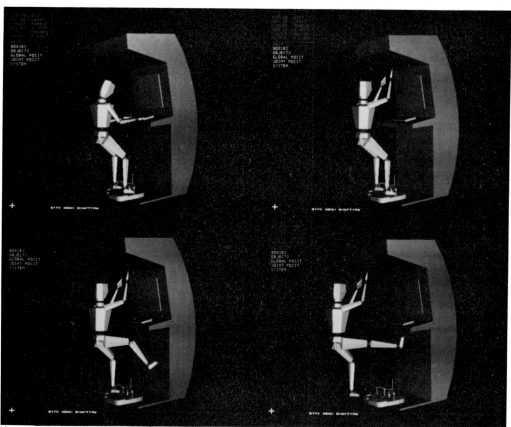

Figure 22-7. Example of workstation design activities.

research continues, and results are applied as soon as possible to space flight programs, major challenges remain: to quantify the capabilities and limitations of the human operator in progressively complex technological systems; to further understand symbiotic man-machine relationships; and to develop predictive models for designing safe and productive manned space flight systems and operations.

REFERENCES

Aschoff, J. Features of circadian rhythms relevant for the design of shift schedules. Ergonomics, 21:739–754, 1976.

Bejczy, A.K. Distribution of man-machine controls in space teleoperations. Proceedings of the Behavioral Objectives in Aviation Automated Systems Symposium, p. 114. Society of Automotive Engineers, Warrendale, PA, 1982.

Bluth, B.J., and Helppie, M. Soviet Space Stations as Analogs, 2nd ed. NASA Headquarters, Washington, D.C., August 1986.

Christensen, J.M., and Talbot, J.M. Research Opportunities in Human Behavior and Performance. NASA CR-3886, National Aeronautics and Space Administration, Scientific and Technical Information Branch, 1985.

Colquhoun, W.P. Circadian variations in mental efficiency. In: Biological Rhythms and Human Performance. Edited by W.P. Colquhoun, Academic Press, pp. 39–107, 1971.

Connors, M.M., Harrison, A.A., and Faren, R.A. Living Aloft: Human Requirements for Extended Space Flight, NASA SP-483, Washington, D.C., 1985.

Conroy, R.T., and Mills, J.N. Human Circadian Rhythms. J. and A. Churchill, London, 1970.

Cooper, H.S.F., Jr. A House in Space. Bantam Books, 1976.

Cosmonauts recover Kvant—Enter module to begin work. Soviet Aerospace, Vol. 49, no. 14, Phillips Publishing, Inc., Washington, D.C., April 13, 1987.

Faulty solar array caused Salyut 7 crew discomfort. Aviation Week and Space Technology, 119(24):24, 1983.

Frost, J.D., Shumate, W.H., Salamy, J.G., and Booher, C.R. Experiment M133-Sleep monitoring on Skylab. In: Biomedical Results from Skylab. Edited by R.S. Johnston and L.F. Dietlein. NASA SP 377, U.S. Government Printing Office, Washington, D.C., 1977.

Gartner, W.B., and Murphy, M.R. Pilot Workload and Fatigue: A Critical Survey of Concepts and Assessment Techniques. NASA TM D-8365, 1976.

Gemini Midprogram Conference. Manned Spacecraft Center, Houston, Texas, February 23–25, 1966, National Aeronautics and Space Administration, Washington, D.C., 1966.

Gerathewohl, S.J., Strughold, H., and Stalling, H.D. Sensorimotor performance during weightlessness. In: The Journal of Aviation Medicine (Vol. 28). Edited by R.J. Benford. The Bruce Publishing Co., St. Paul, MN, 1957.

Gurovskiy, N.N., Kosmolinskiy, F.P., and Melnikov, L.N. Designing the Living and Working Conditions of Cosmonauts (translation of "Proyektirovaniye Usloviy Zhizni i Raboty Kosmonavtov." Moscow, Mashinostroyeniye, 1980, pp. 1–168). NASA TM-76497, National Aeronautics and Space Administration, Washington, D.C., 1981.

Hartman, B.O. Psychologic Aspects of Aerospace Medicine. In: Aerospace Medicine, 2nd Ed. Edited by H.W. Randel. The Williams and Wilkins Co., Baltimore, MD, 1971.

Hauty, G.T., and Adams, T. Phase shifts of the human circadian system and performance deficit during the periods of transition: I. East-west flight. Aerospace Medicine, 37(7):668–674, 1966a.

Hauty, G.T., and Adams, T. Phase shifts of the human circadian system and performance deficit during the periods of transition: II. West-East flight. Aerospace Medicine, 37(10):1027–1033, 1966b.

Hauty, G.T., and Adams, T. Phase shifts of the human circadian system and performance deficit during the periods of transition: III. North-south flight. Aerospace Medicine, 37(12):1257–1262, 1966c.

Khachatur'yants, L.S. Present problems of psychophysiology of space work. In: Cosmonaut Activity in Flight and Means to Increase its Effectiveness. Edited by G.T. Beregovoy, and L.S. Khachatur'yants. Mashinostroyeniye Press, Moscow, 1981.

Kubis, J.F., McLaughlin, E.J., Jackson, J.M., Rusnak, R., McBride, G., and Saxon, S. Task and work performance on Skylab missions. Experiment M151. In: Biomedical Results from Skylab. Edited by R.S. Johnston and L.F. Dietlein. NASA SP-377, U.S. Government Printing Office, Washington, D.C., 1977.

Loftus, J.P., Jr. Evolution of the Astronaut's Role. In:

Workshop Proceedings—Space Human Factors (Vol. 1). Edited by M.D. Montemerlo and A.C. Cron. National Aeronautics and Space Administration, Washington, D.C., 1982.

Marques, T.E., and Howell, W.C. Intuitive Frequency Judgments as a Function of Prior Expectations, Observed Evidence, and Individual Processing Strategies (Tech. Rep. #79-06). Rice University, December, 1979.

Mir Cosmonauts' Fatigue Building Up. FBIS-SOV-87-243, LD180406, Moscow in English to North America, 2300 GMT, December 17, 1987.

Myasnikov, V.I. Mental status and work capacity of Salyut-6 station crewmembers. Kosmicheskaya Biologiya i Aviakosmicheskaya Meditsina, 17(6):22–25, 1983.

Nicogossian, A.E. Human capabilities in space. NASA TM-87360, National Aeronautics and Space Administration, Washington, D.C., 1984.

Nicogossian, A.E. Human Factors for Mars Missions. In: The NASA Mars Conference. Edited by D.B. Reiber. Vol. 71, Science and Technology Series, American Astronautical Society, San Diego, 1988.

Nicogossian, A.E., and Parker, J.F. Space Physiology and Medicine. NASA SP-447, U.S. Government Printing Office, Washington, D.C., October, 1984.

Office of Technology Assessment. Salyut—Soviet steps toward permanent human presence in space (OTA-TM-STI-14). U.S. Government Printing Office, Washington, D.C., 1983.

Sheridan, T.B., and Young, L.R. Human Factors in Aerospace Medicine. In: Fundamentals of Aerospace Medicine. Edited by R.L. DeHart. Lea and Febiger, Philadelphia, PA, 1985.

Space Biology and Medicine Guide. Moscow: Nauka, 1983.

Thornton, W.E., Hoffler, G.W., and Rummel, J.A. Anthropometric changes and fluid shifts. In: Biomedical Results from Skylab. Edited by R.S. Johnston and L.F. Dietlein. NASA SP-377, National Aeronautics and Space Administration, Washington, D.C., 1977.

Wargo, M.J., Kelly, C.R., Mitchell, M.B., and Prosin, D.J. Human Operator Response Speed, Frequency, and Flexibility, NASA CR-874, National Aeronautics and Space Administration, Washington, D.C., September, 1987.

Welford, A.T. Fundamentals of Skill. Methuen and Co., London, 1968.

Yeremin, A.V., Bogdashevskiy, R.M., and Baburin, Ye.F. Preservation of Human Performance Capacity Under Prolonged Space Flight Conditions. Weightlessness: Medical and Biological Research. NASA TTF-16105, pp. 365–383, 1975.

Author Index

Index

Page numbers in italics indicate figures; numbers followed by t indicate tables.